Early-Onset Neonatal Sepsis

Guest Editors

KAREN D. FAIRCHILD, MD
RICHARD A. POLIN, MD

CLINICS IN
PERINATOLOGY

www.perinatology.theclinics.com

June 2010 • Volume 37 • Number 2

SAUNDERS an imprint of ELSEVIER, Inc.

W.B. SAUNDERS COMPANY
A Division of Elsevier Inc.

Elsevier, Inc. • 1600 John F. Kennedy Blvd. • Suite 1800 • Philadelphia, PA 19103-2899

http://www.theclinics.com

CLINICS IN PERINATOLOGY Volume 37, Number 2
June 2010 ISSN 0095-5108, ISBN-13: 978-1-4377-1855-3

Editor: Carla Holloway
Developmental Editor: Theresa Collier

Clinics in Perinatology (ISSN 0095-5108) is published quarterly by Elsevier Inc., 360 Park Avenue South, New York, NY 10010-1710. Months of issue are March, June, September, and December. Business and Editorial Offices: 1600 John F. Kennedy Blvd., Ste. 1800, Philadelphia, PA 19103-2899. Customer Service Office: 3251 Riverport Lane, Maryland Heights, MO 63043. Periodicals postage paid at New York, NY and additional mailing offices. Subscription prices are $239.00 per year (US individuals), $347.00 per year (US institutions), $281.00 per year (Canadian individuals), $441.00 per year (Canadian institutions), $345.00 per year (foreign individuals), $441.00 per year (foreign institutions) $116.00 per year (US students), and $168.00 per year (Canadian and foreign students). Foreign air speed delivery is included in all Clinics subscription prices. All prices are subject to change without notice. **POSTMASTER:** Send address changes to *Clinics in Perinatology*, Elsevier Health Sciences Division, Subscription Customer Service, 3251 Riverport Lane, Maryland Heights, MO 63043. **Customer Service: Telephone: 1-800-654-2452** (U.S. and Canada); **1-314-447-8871** (outside U.S. and Canada). **Fax: 1-314-447-8029. E-mail: journalscustomerservice-usa@elsevier.com** (for print support); **journalsonlinesupport-usa@elsevier.com** (for online support).

Reprints. For copies of 100 or more, of articles in this publication, please contact the Commercial Reprints Department, Elsevier Inc., 360 Park Avenue South, New York, NY 10010-1710. Tel. (212) 633-3812; Fax: (212) 482-1935; email: reprints@elsevier.com.

Clinics in Perinatology is also publilshed in Spanish by McGraw-Hill Interamericana Editores S.A., P.O. Box 5-237, 06500 Mexico D.F., Mexico.

Clinics in Perinatology is covered in *MEDLINE/PubMed (Index Medicus) Current Contents, Excepta Medica, BIOSIS and ISI/BIOMED.*

Printed in the United States of America.

Contributors

GUEST EDITORS

KAREN D. FAIRCHILD, MD
Associate Professor of Pediatrics, Division of Neonatology, University of Virginia Hospital, Charlottesville, Virginia

RICHARD A. POLIN, MD
Professor of Pediatrics; Vice Chairman for Clinical and Academic Affairs, Department of Pediatrics; Director, Division of Neonatology, College of Physicians and Surgeons, Columbia University; Morgan Stanley Children's Hospital of New York, New York, New York

AUTHORS

WILLIAM W. ANDREWS, PhD, MD
Charles E. Flowers Professor and Chairman, Division of Maternal-Fetal Medicine, Department of Obstetrics and Gynecology, School of Medicine, University of Alabama at Birmingham, Birmingham, Alabama

WILLIAM E. BENITZ, MD
Professor of Pediatrics, Division of Neonatal and Developmental Medicine, Stanford University School of Medicine, Stanford, California; Chief of Neonatology, Packard Children's Hospital, Palo Alto, California

IRINA A. BUHIMSCHI, MD
Associate Professor, Department of Obstetrics, Gynecology and Reproductive Sciences, Yale University School of Medicine, New Haven, Connecticut

CATALIN S. BUHIMSCHI, MD
Director, Perinatal Research, Division of Maternal-Fetal Medicine, Department of Obstetrics, Gynecology and Reproductive Sciences, Yale University School of Medicine, New Haven, Connecticut

SOURABH DUTTA, MD, PhD
Additional Professor, Newborn Unit, Department of Pediatrics, Postgraduate Institute of Medical Education and Research, Chandigarh, India

HAMMAD A. GANATRA, MBBS
Research Associate, Department of Pediatrics and Child Health, Aga Khan University, Karachi, Pakistan

DAVID ISAACS, MBChB, MD, FRCP, FRACP
Clinical Professor, Department of Immunology and Infectious Diseases, University of Sydney, Children's Hospital at Westmead, New South Wales, Australia

JEANNE A. JORDAN, PhD
Professor, Department of Epidemiology and Biostatistics, School of Public Health and Health Services; Director, GWU-APHL International Institute for Public Health Laboratory Management, Washington, DC

OFER LEVY, MD, PhD
Staff Physician, Division of Infectious Diseases, Department of Pediatrics, Children's Hospital Boston; Assistant Professor, Department of Pediatrics, Harvard Medical School, Boston, Massachusetts

STEPHANIE J. SCHRAG, DPhil
Respiratory Diseases Branch, Division of Bacterial Diseases, National Center for Immunization and Respiratory Diseases, Centers for Disease Control and Prevention, Atlanta, Georgia

BARBARA J. STOLL, MD
Professor and Chair, Department of Pediatrics, Emory University School of Medicine; Children's Healthcare of Atlanta, Atlanta, Georgia

WILLIAM TARNOW-MORDI, MBChB, MRCP(UK), DCH, FRCPCH
Professor of Neonatal Medicine, Westmead International Network for Neonatal Education and Research (WINNER) Institute, Centre for Newborn Care, Westmead Hospital, University of Sydney, New South Wales, Australia

ALAN T.N. TITA, MD, PhD
Assistant Professor, Division of Maternal-Fetal Medicine, Department of Obstetrics and Gynecology, School of Medicine, University of Alabama at Birmingham, Birmingham, Alabama

JENNIFER R. VERANI, MD, MPH
Respiratory Diseases Branch, Division of Bacterial Diseases, National Center for Immunization and Respiratory Diseases, Centers for Disease Control and Prevention, Atlanta, Georgia

ROSE M. VISCARDI, MD
Professor, Department of Pediatrics, University of Maryland School of Medicine, Baltimore, Maryland

JAMES L. WYNN, MD
Medical Instructor, Division of Neonatology-Perinatal Medicine, Department of Pediatrics, Duke University, Durham, North Carolina

HECTOR R. WONG, MD
Professor and Director, Division of Critical Care Medicine, Cincinnati Children's Hospital Medical Center, Cincinnati, Ohio

ANITA K.M. ZAIDI, MBBS, SM
Professor of Pediatrics and Child Health, Department of Pediatrics and Child Health, Aga Khan University, Karachi, Pakistan

Contents

Neonatal sepsis continues to take a devastating toll globally. Although adequate to protect against invasive infection in most newborns, the distinct function of neonatal innate host defense coupled with impairments in adaptive immune responses increases the likelihood of acquiring infection early in life, with subsequent rapid dissemination and death. Unique differences exist between neonates and older populations with respect to the capacity, quantity, and quality of innate host responses to pathogens. Recent characterization of the age-dependent maturation of neonatal innate immune function has identified novel translational approaches that may lead to improved diagnostic, prophylactic, and therapeutic modalities.

Chorioamnionitis is a common complication of pregnancy associated with significant maternal, perinatal, and long-term adverse outcomes. Adverse maternal outcomes include postpartum infections and sepsis whereas adverse infant outcomes include stillbirth, premature birth, neonatal sepsis, chronic lung disease, and brain injury leading to cerebral palsy and other neurodevelopmental disabilities. Research in the past 2 decades has expanded understanding of the mechanistic links between intra-amniotic infection and preterm delivery as well as morbidities of preterm and term infants. Recent and ongoing clinical research into better methods for diagnosing, treating, and preventing chorioamnionitis is likely to have a substantial impact on short and long-term outcomes in the neonate.

Intrauterine infection is a unique pathologic process that raises the risk for early-onset neonatal sepsis (EONS). By acting synergistically with prematurity, EONS increases the risk for adverse neonatal outcomes, including intraventricular hemorrhage and cerebral palsy. Although several pathways for the pathogenesis of fetal damage have been proposed, the basic molecular mechanisms that modulate these events remain incompletely understood. Discovery of clinically and biologically relevant biomarkers able to reveal key pathogenic pathways and predict pregnancies at risk for antenatal fetal damage is a priority. Proteomics provides a unique opportunity to fill this gap.

The burden of early-onset disease caused by group B *Streptococcus* (GBS) has decreased dramatically in the United States over the past 20 years. Universal culture-based screening at 35 to 37 weeks gestational age and use of intrapartum antibiotic prophylaxis are the cornerstones of prevention measures that have led to this decline. GBS, however, remains the leading cause of early-onset neonatal sepsis in the United States. Revised guidelines for prevention of perinatal GBS are planned for issuance in 2010. This article discusses implementation challenges for clinicians caring for pregnant women and newborns and presents an updated algorithm for neonatal management.

There is accumulating epidemiologic and experimental evidence that intra-uterine or postnatal infection with *Ureaplasma* species is a significant risk factor for adverse pregnancy outcomes and complications of extreme preterm birth such as bronchopulmonary dysplasia and intraventricular hemorrhage. In a cohort of very low birth weight infants, *Ureaplasma* spp were detected by culture or polymerase chain reaction in respiratory secretions, blood, or cerebrospinal fluid of almost half of the subjects, suggesting that this organism is the most common pathogen affecting this population. This review summarizes the evidence supporting the hypothesis that *Ureaplasma*-mediated inflammation in different compartments (intrauterine, lung, blood, or brain) during a common developmental window of vulnerability contributes to preterm labor and lung and brain injury. Appropriate methods for detecting these fastidious organisms and potential strategies to prevent or ameliorate the effects of *Ureaplasma* infection are discussed.

Several molecular testing options are now or will soon be available for diagnosing bloodstream infections in the neonate. The advantages include the speed at which results would be available and the ability to use those results to tailor empirical therapy and reduce the amount of unnecessary or ineffective antibiotics an infant receives. However, there are still difficult challenges before this potential can be realized. A variety of technological advances are needed, including (1) improved recovery of microorganisms in whole blood extractions, (2) increased assay sensitivity, (3) simpler testing platforms that could be run 24/7, and (4) more assays to detect antibiotic resistance genes to reduce reliance on culture-based protocols for antimicrobial susceptibility testing. Although considerable hurdles remain, this challenge is now a priority for investigators in academia and industry.

Early-onset sepsis remains a major diagnostic problem in neonatal medicine. Definitive diagnosis depends on cultures of blood or other normally sterile body fluids. Abnormal hematological counts, acute-phase reactants, and inflammatory cytokines are neither sensitive nor specific, especially at the onset of illness. Combinations of measurements improve diagnostic test performance, but the optimal selection of analytes has not been determined. The best-established use of these laboratory tests is for retrospective determination that an infant was not infected, based on failure to mount an acute-phase response over the following 24 to 48 hours.

Neonatal septic shock is a devastating condition associated with high morbidity and mortality. Definitions for the sepsis continuum and treatment algorithms specific for premature neonates are needed to improve studies of septic shock and assess benefit from clinical interventions. Unique features of the immature immune system and pathophysiologic responses to sepsis, particularly those of extremely preterm infants, necessitate that clinical trials consider them as a separate group. Keen clinical suspicion and knowledge of risk factors will help to identify those neonates at greatest risk for development of septic shock. Genomic and proteomic approaches, particularly those that use very small sample volumes, will increase our understanding of the pathophysiology and direct the development of novel agents for prevention and treatment of severe sepsis and shock in the neonate. Although at present antimicrobial therapy and supportive care remain the foundation of treatment, in the future immunomodulatory agents are likely to improve outcomes for this vulnerable population.

Because of inadequate sample sizes of randomized controlled trials, few immunologic interventions to treat or prevent neonatal sepsis have been reliably evaluated. International collaboration is essential in achieving timely, adequate samples to assess effects on mortality or disability-free survival reliably. Promising or possible therapeutic interventions in severe or gram-negative sepsis include exchange transfusions, pentoxifylline, and IgM-enriched intravenous immunoglobulin. Promising or possible prophylactic interventions include lactoferrin, with or without a probiotic; selenium; early curtailment of antibiotics after sterile cultures; breast milk; and earlier initiation of colostrum in high risk preterm infants. Prophylactic oral probiotics are safe and effective ($P<.00001$) in reducing all-cause mortality and necrotizing enterocolitis in preterm infants by over half, but do not reduce sepsis.

Hammad A. Ganatra, Barbara J. Stoll, and Anita K.M. Zaidi

> Infections are a major cause of neonatal death in developing countries. High-quality information on the burden of early-onset neonatal sepsis and sepsis-related deaths is limited in most of these settings. Simple preventive and treatment strategies have the potential to save many newborns from sepsis-related death. Implementation of public health programs targeting newborn health will assist attainment of Millennium Development Goals of reduction in child mortality.

GOAL STATEMENT

The goal of *Clinics in Perinatology* is to keep practicing neonatologists and maternal-fetal medicine specialists up to date with current clinical practice in perinatology by providing timely articles reviewing the state of the art in patient care.

ACCREDITATION

The *Clinics in Perinatology* is planned and implemented in accordance with the Essential Areas and Policies of the Accreditation Council for Continuing Medical Education (ACCME) through the joint sponsorship of the University of Virginia School of Medicine and Elsevier. The University of Virginia School of Medicine is accredited by the ACCME to provide continuing medical education for physicians.

The University of Virginia School of Medicine designates this educational activity for a maximum of 15 *AMA PRA Category 1 Credits*™ for each issue, 60 credits per year. Physicians should only claim credit commensurate with the extent of their participation in the activity.

The American Medical Association has determined that physicians not licensed in the US who participate in this CME activity are eligible for a maximum of 15 *AMA PRA Category 1 Credits*™ for each issue, 60 credits per year.

Credit can be earned by reading the text material, taking the CME examination online at http://www.theclinics.com/home/cme, and completing the evaluation. After taking the test, you will be required to review any and all incorrect answers. Following completion of the test and evaluation, your credit will be awarded and you may print your certificate.

FACULTY DISCLOSURE/CONFLICT OF INTEREST

The University of Virginia School of Medicine, as an ACCME accredited provider, endorses and strives to comply with the Accreditation Council for Continuing Medical Education (ACCME) Standards of Commercial Support, Commonwealth of Virginia statutes, University of Virginia policies and procedures, and associated federal and private regulations and guidelines on the need for disclosure and monitoring of proprietary and financial interests that may affect the scientific integrity and balance of content delivered in continuing medical education activities under our auspices.

The University of Virginia School of Medicine requires that all CME activities accredited through this institution be developed independently and be scientifically rigorous, balanced and objective in the presentation/discussion of its content, theories and practices.

All authors/editors participating in an accredited CME activity are expected to disclose to the readers relevant financial relationships with commercial entities occurring within the past 12 months (such as grants or research support, employee, consultant, stock holder, member of speakers bureau, etc.). The University of Virginia School of Medicine will employ appropriate mechanisms to resolve potential conflicts of interest to maintain the standards of fair and balanced education to the reader. Questions about specific strategies can be directed to the Office of Continuing Medical Education, University of Virginia School of Medicine, Charlottesville, Virginia.

The faculty and staff of the University of Virginia Office of Continuing Medical Education have no financial affiliations to disclose.

The authors/editors listed below have identified no professional or financial affiliations for themselves or their spouse/partner:
William W. Andrews, PhD, MD; William E. Benitz, MD; Robert Boyle, MD (Test Author); Irina A. Buhimschi, MD; Catalin S. Buhimschi, MD; Sourabh Dutta, MBBS (AIIMS), MD, PhD; Karen D. Fairchild, MD (Guest Editor); Hammad A. Ganatra, MBBS; Carla Holloway (Acquisitions Editor); David Isaacs, MBChB, MD, FRCP, FRACP; Stephanie Schrag, D Phil; Barbara J. Stoll, MD; William Tarnow-Mordi, MBChB, MRCP(UK), DCH, FRCPCH; Alan T.N. Tita, MD, PhD; Jennifer R. Verani, MD, MPH; Rose M. Viscardi, MD; Hector R. Wong, MD; James L. Wynn, MD; and Anita K.M. Zaidi, MBBS, SM.

The authors/editors listed below identified the following professional or financial affiliations for themselves or their spouse/partner:
Jeanne A. Jordan, PhD is an industry funded research/investigator for Roche, is a patent holder with the Patent Office, and is a consultant for Arcxis.
Ofer Levy, MD, PhD is an industry funded research/investigator for Idera Pharmaceuticals and VentiRx.
Richard A. Polin, MD (Guest Editor) serves on the Advisory Committee for Discovery Laboratory.

Disclosure of Discussion of Non-FDA Approved Uses for Pharmaceutical Products and/or Medical Devices.
The University of Virginia School of Medicine, as an ACCME provider, requires that all faculty presenters identify and disclose any off-label uses for pharmaceutical and medical device products. The University of Virginia School of Medicine recommends that each physician fully review all the available data on new products or procedures prior to clinical use.

TO ENROLL

To enroll in the Clinics in Perinatology Continuing Medical Education program, call customer service at 1-800-654-2452 or visit us online at www.theclinics.com/home/cme. The CME program is available to subscribers for an additional fee of $196.00

THE CLINICS ARE NOW AVAILABLE ONLINE!

Access your subscription at:
www.theclinics.com

Preface

Early-Onset Neonatal Sepsis—Recent Advances in Diagnosis and Prevention

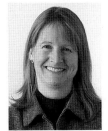 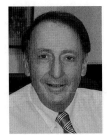

Karen D. Fairchild, MD   Richard A. Polin, MD
Guest Editors

Perinatal and neonatal practitioners know much about infection, encountering it nearly every working day. Our goal in this issue of the *Clinics in Perinatology* is to present a state-of-the-art review of the causes, prevention, pathophysiology, diagnosis, and treatment of chorioamnionitis and early-onset neonatal infection.

The fetal immune system is adapted to survive the normally sterile uterine environment, but when pathogens are encountered near the time of birth, the immature first-line host defenses prove to be maladaptive. Drs Wynn and Levy provide up-to-date information on innate host defenses in the fetus and neonate. A better understanding of the mechanisms of immature host-pathogen recognition and clearance allows for the design of more effective adjunct immunological therapies. Drs Tita and Andrews, and Buhimschi and Buhimschi focus on infection in the antepartum period. They review chorioamnionitis and the fetal inflammatory response, and the use of state-of-the art proteomic technology for detection of a hostile (infected or inflamed) intra-uterine environment. Increasing evidence linking neonatal morbidities such as chronic lung disease and periventricular white matter damage to chorioamnionitis justifies intense efforts to prevent, detect, and treat (through medication or through delivery) fetal infection.

Other articles review new information related to two pathogens, which are, arguably, the best-known and least known pathogens in early-onset neonatal infection: group B *Streptococcus* (GBS) and *Ureaplasma* species, respectively. In the current era of widespread screening and intrapartum antibiotic prophylaxis, GBS has dropped

Clin Perinatol 37 (2010) xi–xii
doi:10.1016/j.clp.2010.03.005
0095-5108/10/$ – see front matter © 2010 Elsevier Inc. All rights reserved.

from being the number one cause of early-onset sepsis in preterm infants, but remains a significant threat at all gestational ages. The Centers for Disease Control is developing new guidelines for the management of colonized women and infants at risk for GBS sepsis. Drs Verani and Schrag summarize the data supporting a change in the guidelines and present a new neonatal algorithm for the management of infants at risk. *Ureaplasma* species, the smallest free-living microorganisms, are a proven cause of chorioamnionitis and are associated stillbirth, preterm birth, and bronchopulmonary dysplasia. Dr Viscardi reviews the evidence supporting the role of *Ureaplasma* in the cause of chronic lung disease.

Two articles review laboratory tests beyond the traditional complete blood cell count and blood culture, which may facilitate decisions about antibiotic therapy. Using molecular diagnostics for rapid detection of pathogen DNA in the bloodstream is an exciting prospect for the future, and Dr Jordan highlights the challenges to implementation. Dr Benitz provides a framework for the rational use of antibiotics in infants with suspected sepsis. Drs Wynn and Wong, and Drs Tarnow-Mordi, Isaacs, and Dutta discuss therapies beyond antibiotics to support the hemodynamically compromised patient and boost the immune response.

Finally, in this issue we go beyond the technologically advanced medical centers in which most of us practice to resource-poor areas of the world. Drs Ganatra, Stoll, and Zaidi give us a sobering reminder that millions of newborns still die of sepsis each year for lack of hygiene and basic medical care, including vaccines and antibiotics.

We are indebted to the authors for their superb contributions. We also wish to thank Ms Carla Holloway from Elsevier for her expert guidance and editorial assistance on this and the next issue of the *Clinics in Perinatology*, which will cover healthcare-associated infections in the neonatal intensive care unit. Finally, we thank our families for their continued patience and support.

Karen D. Fairchild, MD
Department of Pediatrics
Division of Neonatology
University of Virginia Hospital
Box 800386
Charlottesville, VA 22908, USA

Richard A. Polin, MD
Department of Pediatrics
Division of Neonatology
College of Physicians and Surgeons
Columbia University, New York, NY, USA

Morgan Stanley Children's Hospital of New York
3959 Broadway, CHC 115
New York, NY 10032, USA

E-mail addresses:
KDF2N@hscmail.mcc.virginia.edu (K.D. Fairchild)
rap32@columbia.edu (R.A. Polin)

Role of Innate Host Defenses in Susceptibility to Early-Onset Neonatal Sepsis

James L. Wynn, MD[a],*, Ofer Levy, MD, PhD[b,c]

KEYWORDS

- Neonate • Early-onset sepsis • Innate immunity
- Acute phase reactant • Neutrophil
- Pathogen recognition receptor

Infection claims the lives of approximately 3000 neonates worldwide every day.[1] Preterm newborns are the most affected because they exhibit the highest sepsis-related morbidity and mortality among pediatric patients.[2] The distinct neonatal immune system, although adequate to protect against infection in most neonates, contributes to a newborn's enhanced susceptibility to infection.[3–6] The innate immune system represents the first line of prevention against microbial invasion and of defense once infection has occurred. Initial immunomodulatory efforts directed at improving neonatal sepsis survival through enhancement of innate immune function (see the article by Tarnow-Mordi and colleagues elsewhere in this issue for further exploration of this topic), including intravenous immunoglobulin (IVIG), granulocyte-macrophage colony-stimulating factor (GM-CSF), and granulocyte colony-stimulating factor (G-CSF), have thus far not yielded major benefit.[3] Dramatic progress in molecular characterization of innate immunity has been made over the past decade, paving the way for new prophylactic and therapeutic approaches. Although the roles of innate immunity in adult sepsis have been examined in great detail,[7–12] the distinct neonatal innate immune response remains incompletely characterized. In the context of

OL's laboratory is funded by NIH RO1 AI067353 and by the Bill & Melinda Gates Foundation.
[a] Division of Neonatal-Perinatal Medicine, Department of Pediatrics, Duke University, 2424 Hock Plaza, Suite 504, DUMC Box 2739, Durham, NC 27710, USA
[b] Department of Pediatrics, Division of Infectious Diseases, Children's Hospital Boston, Boston 300 Longwood Avenue, MA 02115, USA
[c] Harvard Medical School, 25 Shattuck Street, Boston, MA 02115, USA
* Corresponding author. Division of Neonatal-Perinatal Medicine, Department of Pediatrics, Duke University, 2424 Hock Plaza, Suite 504, DUMC Box 2739, Durham, NC 27710.
E-mail address: james.wynn@duke.edu

Clin Perinatol 37 (2010) 307–337
doi:10.1016/j.clp.2010.04.001
0095-5108/10/$ – see front matter © 2010 Elsevier Inc. All rights reserved.
perinatology.theclinics.com

increasing incidence of prematurity and the potential for neurodevelopmental impact in sepsis survivors,[13] there is an unmet medical need for novel approaches to prevention and therapy.

EARLY-ONSET SEPSIS

Early-onset neonatal sepsis (EONS) typically occurs during the first 24 hours of life, and is a fulminant multisystem infection acquired by vertical transmission from the mother.[14] Maternal factors that increase the risk of EONS include preterm labor and delivery, colonization with group B streptococcus (GBS), prolonged rupture of membranes, chorioamnionitis, and intrapartum fever.[15] A neonate can present with signs of respiratory distress, including apnea, temperature instability, hypotension, bradycardia, tachycardia, lethargy or irritability, and abdominal distension or feeding intolerance, requiring prompt evaluation and appropriate treatment from a physician. Once overtly symptomatic, mortality is unacceptably high.[16]

The incidence of EONS in term neonates is 1 to 2 per 1000 live births with a mortality of approximately 3%.[17,18] Responsible pathogens are dominated by 2 individual bacteria, GBS (41%) and *Escherichia coli* (17%).[17] GBS emerged as the leading pathogen of EONS in the 1970s with case fatality rates as high as 55%.[19] A significant decrease in EONS due to GBS occurred, especially in neonates greater than or equal to 34 weeks' gestation, following the publication of national guidelines for the use of intrapartum antibiotic prophylaxis to prevent neonatal GBS infection.[20,21] Intrapartum antibiotic prophylaxis has decreased overall GBS rates, but it is also associated with an increase in the incidence of EONS due to *E coli*[16] and an increase in newborn exposure to antibiotics that may have adverse consequences.[22]

Preterm neonates, especially very low-birth-weight (VLBW) neonates, suffer attack rates greater than 10 times higher than those born at term with associated mortality in more than one third.[23] Morbidities include increased respiratory distress, chronic lung disease, white-matter damage, neurodevelopmental impairment, and increased risk of death, especially with Gram-negative infections.[23,24] Compared with term neonates, VLBW neonates demonstrate an increased percentage of EONS caused by Gram-negative pathogens.[25] EONS associated with Gram-negative infection is more likely to result in death within 72 hours of birth (29%) than Gram-positive infection (6%).[25] Extremely low-birth-weight (ELBW) neonates (<1000 g) are even more vulnerable because EONS accounts for more than 50% of deaths that occur within the first 48 hours of life.[26]

An adaptive immune response, including the selection and amplification of specific clones of lymphocytes (B cells and T cells) that result in immunologic memory, generally requires 5 to 7 days to develop. Moreover, the neonatal adaptive immune response is functionally distinct from the adult response at multiple levels.[5] As a result, neonates are thought to largely depend on the function of innate immunity for protection from infection during the first days of life. The innate response, defined as that which is present at birth before microbial exposure, consists of a preformed immune response mediated by barriers, sentinel immune cells, pathogen recognition systems, inflammatory response proteins, host defense proteins and peptides, as well as passively acquired immunoglobulin from the mother.

An overview of the current state of knowledge regarding innate immunity of the newborn must take into consideration the research approaches that have thus far been used to study this area. In vitro studies have largely focused on cord blood, although in some cases similar patterns or age-dependent maturation/normalization have been documented in newborn peripheral blood. In vivo studies of nonhuman vertebrates have largely focused on newborn mice. The neonatal mouse model has 2 potential limitations: (1) mice are not humans and the murine innate immune system is particularly divergent[27] and (2) the postnatal age at which the mice are studied is a matter of variation and debate. Although all approaches have limitations, they provide valuable information toward characterizing in vivo function. This article discusses neonatal innate host defense systems and their relationship to susceptibility to and progression of EONS.

INNATE HOST DEFENSE SYSTEMS
Maternal Innate Defenses

In utero infection is a significant risk factor for the development of EONS. In particular, approximately 80% of preterm deliveries at less than 30 weeks' gestation have evidence of intrauterine infection.[28] Ascending infection induces maternal immune responses in utero that may also influence mobilization of fetal neutrophils (polymorphonuclear cells [PMNs]) found in infected amniotic fluid[29] and the development of the fetal and neonatal inflammatory response.[30] Immune responses to intra-amniotic infection likely begin with Toll-like receptors (TLRs) expressed on maternal trophoblast cells (**Fig. 1**).[28] Human trophoblast cells express all 10 TLRs and, on stimulation, produce inflammatory cytokines found in infected amniotic fluid.[28,31] In particular, elevated amniotic fluid interleukin (IL)-6 concentrations are commonly found during intra-amniotic infection[31] and are associated with rapid parturition[32] and acceleration of fetal lung maturation.[33] In addition to the TLR-mediated innate immune sensing capabilities of trophoblasts, the amnion, chorion, placenta, amniotic fluid, cervical mucosa, and vagina are replete with antimicrobial proteins and peptides (APPs) that possess key host defense functions and are upregulated with infection.[34–36] Thus, ascending bacterial infection that underlies EONS triggers early innate immune activation of maternal and fetal tissues that mobilize host defense effectors to the amniotic fluid.

Epithelial and Mucosal Barriers

Host barriers provide the first means of protection from microbial invasion. There are 2 critical barrier regions: the mucosa (respiratory and intestinal) and the skin. Although in utero, the fetus is protected within the normally sterile environment provided by the amnion and amniotic fluid that is replete with APPs.[4] At birth, vernix enhances skin barrier function for late-preterm and term neonates but is largely absent in preterm neonates born before 28 weeks' gestation. Vernix is a complex material comprised of water (80.5%), lipids (10.3%), and proteins (9.1%) produced by fetal sebaceous glands during the last trimester.[37] The vernix provides a barrier to water loss, improves temperature control, and serves as a shield containing antioxidants and innate immune factors, such as APPs.[38] Furthermore, vernix is important for maintenance of the pH balance of the skin and thus sets the stage for appropriate colonization with commensal organisms instead of pathogens.[38]

The outermost layer of the skin, the stratum corneum, prevents microbial invasion, maintains temperature, and reduces the risk of dehydration through prevention of transcutaneous water loss.[39] The immature and incompletely developed stratum corneum of preterm newborns takes at least 1 to 2 weeks after birth to become fully functional[40] and may take up to 8 weeks to develop in extremely preterm neonates, significantly increasing the risk for barrier dysfunction.[41] Neonates have an increased density of hair follicles compared with adults, which provides a larger reservoir for skin commensal organisms, such as Staphylococcus epidermidis.[42,43] Additionally, the risk for a microbial breech of the cutaneous barrier rises in the presence of intravenous

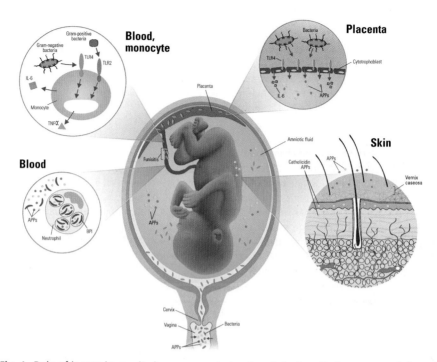

Fig. 1. Role of innate immunity in responses to in utero infection. Early-onset sepsis is typically caused by an ascending maternal lower genital tract infection. APPs within the vagina and amniotic fluid help to reduce bacterial burden and are up-regulated during infection. Pathogen detection begins with placental trophoblast cell TLRs that up-regulate APP and inflammatory cytokine production. Neonatal monocytes are simultaneously stimulated via TLR-mediated pathogen detection with subsequent cytokine production that in turn activates innate immune function (neutrophils and macrophages) and induces the hepatic production of acute phase reactants. Innate immunity within the skin and vernix (APPs) facilitates appropriate commensal microbial colonization associated with erythema toxicum.

catheters essential for critical care. The response of the dermal innate immune system to host commensal organisms is exemplified by the common newborn rash erythema toxicum. Recent evidence suggests that this common newborn condition is an immune-mediated manifestation of the bacterial colonization of the skin.[42,43] Because the skin is arid, it is a more formidable barrier for microbial invasion than that of the moist mucosal surfaces. In extremely preterm infants, however, humidification systems are used to decrease insensible water loss and these may delay cornification of the skin and thus predispose to microbial growth.

Mucosal barriers contain multiple components that serve to prevent infection, including acidic pH; mucus; cilia; destructive enzymes; APPs; opsonins, such as surfactant proteins; sentinel immune cells, such as macrophages, dendritic cells (DCs), PMNs, and T cells; and commensal organisms.[44] After birth, the gut is quickly colonized and contains a significant repository of microorganisms.[45] Although not believed to contribute significantly to the development of EONS, intestinal barrier integrity is paramount for prevention of spread of microorganisms out of the intestinal compartment and likely plays a role in the development of necrotizing enterocolitis.[46] Factors known to disrupt the neonatal intestinal barrier are antibiotic treatment, hypoxia, and remote infection and have been recently reviewed.[3,47]

Ascending infection, with or without chorioamnionitis, or acquisition of microbes during passage through the birth canal representd the common origins of EONS.[14] The portal of pathogen entry into a neonate is primarily through the respiratory tract. In utero, amniotic fluid and pulmonary APPs, surfactant proteins A and D, alveolar macrophages, PMNs, and trophoblast-based TLRs serve as the first line of defense (see **Fig. 1**). After birth, respiratory mucosal function can be impaired by surfactant deficiency, altered mucus production, intubation and mechanical ventilation associated with decreased mucociliary clearance, and airway irritation. The surface and submucosal gland epithelium of the conducting airways is a constitutive primary participant in innate immunity through the production of mucus and mucociliary clearance of pathogens and debris.[48] Premature neonates have relatively more goblet cells than more mature neonates, leading to a decrease in mucociliary clearance. Additional insult to the neonatal respiratory system may result from physical damage to lung parenchyma via atelectrauma, barotrauma, or chemical injury (eg, oxygen or aspiration). Intubation is also associated with the progressive accumulation of colonizing bacteria and bacterial endotoxin in respiratory fluids with concomitant mobilization to the airway of endotoxin-modulating host defense proteins.[49] Neonates with surfactant deficiency lack host defense proteins with valuable immune function, such as surfactant proteins A and D, that are absent in commercially available exogenous surfactants due to destruction during preparation.[50] There is an age-dependent maturation in the ability of respiratory epithelium to elaborate APPs (human cathelicidin [LL-37] and β-defensins) such that respiratory epithelium of preterm newborns mounts a deficient antimicrobial peptide response.[51] These deficiencies as well as those related to cellular function in combination with invasive procedures lead to a reduction in respiratory barrier function that increases the risk for early infection.

Pathogen Recognition Systems

The development of an immune response by local immune sentinel cells, including macrophages, endothelium, epithelium, PMNs, and DCs, is dependent on the identification of invading pathogens or the presence of tissue damage that results in elaboration of exogenous or endogenous danger signals. Evolution of pattern recognition receptors (PRRs) capable of recognizing damage/danger-associated molecular patterns (DAMPs) (cytokines, intracellular proteins, or mediators released by dying or damaged cells) in addition to pathogen-associated molecular patterns (PAMPs) (eg, bacterial cell wall components, flagellin, and nucleic acids) allow for specificity in the innate immune response. PRRs are present on the cell surface, within intracellular vesicles, and in the cytoplasm of multiple cell types. Examples include the TLRs, nucleotide-binding oligomerization domain (NOD)-like receptors, retinoic-acid–inducible protein I (RIG-I)-like receptors, and integrins.[52,53] As described later, with respect to multiple microbial stimuli, engagement of neonatal PRRs on neonatal blood leukocytes often leads to a pattern of response that is distinct from that in older individuals with impaired neonatal production of proinflammatory/T-helper type 1 (T_H1)-polarizing cytokines that may increase the risk for development and progression of infection.

Activation of TLRs by microbial or synthetic agonists results in downstream production of cytokines, chemokines, and complement and coagulation proteins as well as initiation of antimicrobial effector mechanisms, including enhanced phagocytic function.[54] There are 10 TLRs in humans that respond to specific molecular triggers.[54,55] Molecular identification of particular pathogens and subsequent signaling can occur via simultaneous stimulation of multiple TLRs, allowing for tremendous diversity in specific pathogen detection and response.[55,56] Because TLRs play an essential role in recognition and response to pathogens, alterations in their expression, structure, and signaling pathways can impair host defense and increase host vulnerability to infection.[53]

Basal expression and cellular distribution of TLRs is similar in monocytes derived from term umbilical cord blood and peripheral blood monocytes obtained from adults.[57] Cord blood monocyte TLR4 expression has been found to increase with gestational age.[58] In a study of patients with EONS, peripheral blood cells from preterm and full-term neonates demonstrated up-regulation of TLR2 and TLR4 messenger RNA during Gram-positive and Gram-negative bacteremia, respectively.[59]

Hypomorphic mutations or decreased expression of proteins that enhance TLR activation may increase the risk for progression of early neonatal infection.[60–62] Examples of ancillary proteins needed for optimal TLR-mediated pathogen recognition include lipopolysaccharide-binding protein (LBP) that extracts lipopolysaccharide (LPS) monomers from Gram-negative bacteria and delivers them to the endotoxin receptor (CD14/MD2/TLR4) on the monocyte surface and CD14, both of which are normally up-regulated during neonatal sepsis and are required for LPS-mediated signaling through TLR4.[63–65]

In addition to TLRs and their coreceptors, other intracellular signaling mechanisms are important for the detection of pathogens. Examples of cytosolic receptors include the nucleotide oligomerization domain leucine-rich repeat-containing family or NOD-like receptors (NLRs), which detect peptidoglycan in the cytosol, as well as the RIG-I–like receptors, which sense double-stranded RNA of viral origin and induce production of type I interferons (IFNs).[53] Intracellular bacteria, including *Listeria monocytogenes*, can be recognized by NLRs.[66] Polymorphisms in NLR domains are associated with dysregulated inflammatory pathology, including neonatal-onset multisystem inflammatory disease (cryopyrin),[67] but NLR alleles have not yet demonstrated any correlation with sepsis susceptibility.[68] Much remains to be learned about the functional expression of NLRs in neonates.

Recognition of a PAMP or DAMP by PRRs activates a complex series of intracellular cascades that trigger gene activation.[53] Polymorphisms or mutations in TLRs and downstream signaling molecules, such as myeloid differentiation factor 88 (MyD88), nuclear factor κB essential modulator (NEMO), and IL-1 receptor–associated kinase 4 (IRAK-4), are associated with increased risk for infection in adults[69–74] and in children.[75–78] Children with IRAK-4 deficiency manifest decreasing susceptibility to pyogenic infection with age, suggesting that the TLR pathway is of greatest importance early in life, in line with findings in murine models.[79,80] In contrast to adults, specific characterization of neonatal PRR intracellular signaling intermediates, their regulation, and response to infection have been incompletely characterized.[81] Newborn umbilical cord PMNs were found to have lower MyD88 expression and reduced p38 phosphorylation after ex vivo stimulation with endotoxin, potentially contributing to diminished responses.[82] Decreased MyD88, IRF5, and p38 phosphorylation was noted in endotoxin-stimulated monocytes isolated from umbilical cord and peripheral venous blood that exhibited gestational age-specific diminution.[83,84] Deficient expression of TLR second messenger proteins in preterm newborns likely contributes to the increased risk of infection compared with more mature neonates.

Another important neonatal PRR is the β_2-integrin complement receptor type 3 (CR3) that functions as a pathogen sensor on the surface of phagocytes in addition to its role in binding complement. CR3 (also known as MAC-1 and CD11b/CD18) binds LPS, in cooperation with or independent of CD14, as well as other microbial surface components and triggers up-regulation of inducible nitric oxide synthase and nitric oxide production.[85] Engagement of CR3 on PMNs activates reactive oxygen intermediate (ROI) production and phagocytosis. Accordingly, decreased expression of L-selectin and CR3 on stimulated neonatal PMNs impairs neonatal PMNs and monocyte activation and accumulation at sites of inflammation.[86,87] This decreased expression persists for at least the first month of life in term infants, possibly contributing to an increased risk for infection.[88] The expression of CR3 (CD11b) may be reduced further in preterm neonates compared with term neonates.[89] In umbilical cord blood from neonates less than 30 weeks' gestation, PMN CR3 content was similar to levels found in those with type 1 leukocyte adhesion deficiency (failure to express CD18).[86,87] Thus, decreased leukocyte CR3 surface expression increases the likelihood of suboptimal pathogen detection and cellular activation, particularly in preterm neonates.

Innate Cellular Immunity

Antigen-presenting cells

After compromising barriers, invading pathogens come into contact with sentinel immune cells, including monocytes, macrophages, and DCs (see the article by Wynn and Wong elsewhere in this issue for further exploration of this topic). After detection of microorganisms via the PRRs, these APCs amplify cellular recruitment through production of inflammatory mediators (complement, cytokines, coagulation factors, and extracellular matrix proteins[90]), phagocytose and kill pathogens, and present foreign antigens to cells of the adaptive immune system. Initial pathogen detection and innate response by APCs are critical for the development of an effective host immune response.

Responses after stimulation of PRRs in neonatal blood monocytes are generally reduced compared with adults.[57,91] In response to many stimuli, including most TLR agonists, human neonatal cord blood mononuclear cells tested in vitro exhibit a marked polarization, with impaired production of T_H1-polarizing cytokines, such as tumor necrosis factor (TNF)-α, IFN-γ, and IL-12p70, and increased production of T_H2/T_H17 and anti-inflammatory cytokines, such as IL-6, IL-10, IL-17, and IL-23.[4,92] Elevated concentrations in neonatal cord blood mononuclear cells of intracellular cAMP, a secondary messenger that inhibits production of T_H1-polarizing cytokines, seems to contribute to this skewed cytokine pattern.[93] Proposed benefits of this skew are immune tolerance to avoid potentially harmful alloimmune reactions between fetus and mother, avoidance of excessive inflammation on initial microbial colonization, and induction of epithelial APPs to avoid microbial penetration and infection.[4,94] A consequence of impairment in T_H1-polarizing cytokine production by neonatal mononuclear cells, however, is a reduced ability to defend against infection with microorganisms, in particular intracellular pathogens, such as Listeria spp,[95] Mycobacteria spp,[96] and herpes simplex virus.[97]

Presentation of foreign epitopes by antigen-presenting cells (APCs), including monocytes, macrophages, and DCs, to cells of the adaptive immune system is less efficient in neonates compared with adults. Neonatal monocytes and DCs demonstrate impaired expression of major histocompatibility complex class II[98,99] and of costimulatory molecules, including CD40 and CD86,[100] resulting in reduced antigen presentation to naïve CD4+ T cells. Neonatal DCs require increased stimulation for activation[101] and demonstrate poor stimulation of T-cell proliferation as well as a predilection for the induction of immune tolerance via impaired LPS-induced IL-12p70 production.[102] Still, neonatal cord blood DCs stimulated with LPS can effectively induce cytotoxic lymphocyte responses.[103] A reduction in APC function impairs development of effective adaptive immunity, placing further burden on innate immune function for pathogen clearance.

In addition to altered cytokine production and reduced antigen presentation, monocyte phagocytic and chemotactic function are also reduced during neonatal sepsis relative to adults and neonatal baseline values.[104,105] The number of peripheral mono-cytes decreases during sepsis (between 60 and 120 hours after presentation), likely secondary to extravasation and differentiation into macrophages and DCs. Located just below epithelial borders, macrophages encounter pathogens immediately after entry. Like monocytes, macrophages play an important role in the amplification of the immune response through the production of cytokines and chemokines, phagocytosis and killing, and antigen presentation to naïve CD4$^+$ T cells. Neonatal macrophages are poorly responsive to several TLR agonists[106] and IFN-γ.[94] During infection, neonatal macrophages exhibit decreased production of reactive nitrogen intermediates.[107]

In summary, neonatal APCs, including monocytes, macrophages, and DCs, exhibit deficits in pathogen recognition, activation after stimulation, phagocytic function, bacte-ricidal function, and amplification of the immune response that may increase the risk for the development and progression of EONS. Certain stimuli, however, such as GBS, *Mycobacterium bovis* (bacille Calmette-Guérin [BCG]), and TLR8 agonists, can effec-tively activate neonatal APCs in vitro.[108–110] The molecular rules that govern which stimuli do or do not effectively activate human neonatal APCs is a topic of active research with important translational implications for neonatal adjuvant development.

Neutrophils

Neutrophils or PMNs are the primary mediators of neonatal innate cellular defense. Antimicrobial mechanisms used by PMNs have been reviewed in detail.[111] Many quantitative and qualitative PMN deficits have been described for neonates compared with adults.[94,112] PMNs are activated and increased in number with onset of early during sepsis in term and preterm neonates.[113,114] Mature neonatal bone marrow PMN reserves are rapidly depleted during infection,[115] which results in a release of immature band forms (described as a left shift), the proportion of which can be used to aid in assessing the probability of sepsis.[116] Neonates who develop sepsis-associated neutropenia are more likely to have Gram-negative sepsis and exhibit a higher mortality.[114,117,118] Conflicting reports exist regarding the risk of EONS in VLBW newborns with neutropenia associated with other causes, such as maternal preeclampsia.[118–121] ELBW newborns experience the highest frequency of neutrope-nia among all neonatal groups. Neutropenia in ELBW newborns, however, is most often not secondary to sepsis. Furthermore, ELBW newborns with neutropenia do not suffer increased subsequent mortality due to sepsis compared with non-neutro-penic ELBW newborns.[122]

In addition to the quantitative PMN deficits, multiple qualitative defects of neonatal PMN function are noted. The process of PMN recruitment and extravasation to sites of inflammation is less efficient in neonates compared with older age groups and likely contributes to their increased susceptibility to early infection. Specifically, PMNs from preterm and term neonates exhibit reduced basal chemotaxis and random migration[123] that is exacerbated in septic and postoperative newborns.[124] Impaired signaling downstream of chemokine-receptor binding may be partially responsible for this finding.[125] The propensity toward very high production of IL-6, a cytokine with anti-inflammatory properties that reduces PMN migration to inflammatory sites, may also contribute to the inability of newborns to mount an adequate PMN response in the context of sepsis.[92,126] In septic neonates, bacterial evasion mechanisms may also contribute to poor chemotaxis.[127] Emerging data suggest that IL-8 priming of PMNs that occurs during labor significantly improves PMN chemotaxis over that seen with caesarean delivery and even adult controls.[128] Modifications in PRRs after labor may also contribute to the improvement in cellular chemotaxis. TLR4 is up-regu-lated on monocytes and PMNs from term neonates after labor and PMN migration is improved after exposure to a TLR4 agonist.[129–131] Decreased neonatal expression or up-regulation of surface adhesion molecules on PMNs (LFA-1 [preterm neonates], CR3 [term and preterm neonates], and L-selectin [term and preterm neonates]) during sepsis limits rolling and subsequent diapedesis.[86,87] Basal PMN deformation is reduced, and this impairment is exacerbated in the immature band forms found commonly during infection, which reduces the ability to migrate between endothelial cells to sites of infection.[132] Aggregation defects lead to vascular accumulation of newborn PMNs after stimulation and contribute to decreased extravasation, rapid depletion of bone marrow reserves, vascular crowding,[132] and an increased likelihood of microvascular ischemia.[112,133]

Similar basal degranulation capabilities are present in PMNs from premature and term neonates, but content differs compared with adults. Compared with other innate immune cells, PMNs represent the most abundant and reliable source of APPs. PMNs of term neonates contain similar amounts of myeloperoxidase and defensins but reduced lactoferrin, elastase, and bactericidal/permeability-increasing protein (BPI) relative to adult PMNs.[134,135] Neonatal PMN respiratory burst activity is also distinct compared with adult PMN function. For example, hydroxyl radical production by term PMNs is reduced, particularly under stressed or septic conditions.[112,134] In contrast, superoxide production may actually exceed that of adult PMNs but is suppressed during sepsis, contributing to poor microbicidal activity.[136–138]

When the target is fully opsonized, ex vivo phagocytosis of bacteria by PMNs from late-preterm and term neonates is equivalent to adult controls whereas that from VLBW function remains depressed.[112,139,140] Neonatal PMNs exhibit delayed apoptosis, sustained capacity for activation (CD11b up-regulation) and cytotoxic function (ROI production), as well as extracellular release of destructive enzymes or ROI.[112] These mechanisms contribute to local tissue and endothelial damage with resultant increases in inflammatory cytokine production.[141–144] Novel PMN bactericidal mechanisms have been recently identified in studies of adult cells. TLR4-mediated activation of platelets by Gram-negative bacterial endotoxin or LPS induces platelet-PMN binding with subsequent extracellular release of neutrophil extracellular traps (NETs) that contain DNA.[145] NETs also contain APP and hydrolytic enzymes that result in bacterial killing even after PMN death.[146,147] Formation of NETs after stimulation was absent in preterm ($\leq$30 weeks) and nearly absent in term neonates.[148] Overall, the constellation of neonatal PMN functional deficits may increase the risk for development and rapid dissemination of infection.

Mast cells

Mast cells may possess diverse immune functions, including production of vasoactive substances, cytokines, phagocytosis of pathogens, and antigen presentation.[149] These capabilities suggest the potential for mast cells to make a significant contribution to neonatal innate host defenses. Mast cells likely participate in the initial response to pathogens and may contribute to a neonate's predilection for immune tolerance through the actions of histamine. Neonatal mast cells secrete significantly more histamine after stimulation compared with adults.[150] Production of histamine is well known to facilitate vasodilation but also is capable of modification of subsequent immune responses. Specifically, neonatal mast cell histamine production alters DC cytokine production (increased IL-10 and decreased IL-12) and subsequent T-cell polarizing activity (T_H2 phenotype).[151] Recently, mast cell involvement was demonstrated in the common newborn rash, erythema toxicum, where mast cell recruitment, degranulation, and tryptase expression were noted.[152]

Inflammatory Response Proteins

Complement

Noncellular elements of the innate immune response include inflammatory response proteins, such as complement, acute phase reactants (APRs), cytokines, chemokines, coagulation proteins, and vasoactive substances. Actions of complement include opsonization and killing of pathogens, alteration of vascular tone to facilitate recruitment and activation of leukocytes, initiation of the coagulation cascade, and proinflammatory cytokine production.[7] Neonates exhibit gestational age-related decreases in complement proteins, assays of hemolytic function, and complement-mediated opsonic capabilities compared with adults (**Fig. 2A**).[153–156] In particular, neonates have low levels of C9,[157] which is critical for the formation of the membrane attack complex (MAC) and is associated with increased susceptibility to *Neisseria* infection in older populations. Neonatal *Neisseria* infections are most commonly ophthalmologic and rarely become systemic despite this deficiency. Moreover, human neonatal cord blood complement levels are sufficient to enhance GBS-induced TNF production in vitro (via alternative complement pathway activation and engagement of monocyte CR3).[108–110] Nevertheless, reduced complement levels may contribute to the rapid proliferation of bacteria when assayed in human cord blood in vitro.[158]

During bacterial infection the alternative complement pathway is the primary route of complement activation in preterm and term neonates.[159,160] Significant increases in alternative pathway components have been found in the plasma from newborns with

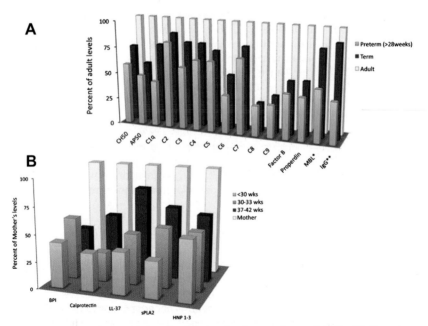

Fig. 2. Comparison of neonatal and adult levels of opsonins and APPs. (*A*) Complement functional assays and complement proteins, mannose-binding lectin, and IgG concentrations in preterm neonates, term neonates, and adults. (*Data from Refs.*[44,264,265]) (*B*) Serum antimicrobial protein and peptide levels in preterm neonates, term neonates, and maternal levels. HNP, human neutrophil peptide; MBL, mannose-binding lectin. (*Reproduced from* Strunk T, Doherty D, Richmond P, et al. Reduced levels of antimicrobial proteins and peptides in human cord blood plasma. Arch Dis Child Fetal Neonatal Ed 2009;94:F230; with permission.)

sepsis, including factor B, C3a desArg, C3bBbP (a C3 convertase), and sC5b-9 (MAC), with C3a desArg reaching levels seen in infected adults.[159] In these studies, markers of classical pathway activation were not elevated during sepsis and suggest that anti-body-mediated complement activation does not play a significant role in neonatal sepsis even in term neonates who have received ample passive immunization via placental anti-body transfer.[160] Because mannose-binding lectin (MBL) is capable of activating the alternative pathway and decreased MBL levels are associated with an increased risk of sepsis during the first month of life (term and preterm), it is likely that MBL plays an important role in complement activation and thus innate host defense (see **Fig. 2**A).[161,162]

Multiple aspects of innate cellular recruitment, activation, and function are attrib-uted to the actions of complement-receptor binding.[163–166] For example, neonatal leukocyte expression of complement receptors (CR1 and CR3) increases during sepsis, resulting in enhanced pathogen recognition, phagocytosis, and production of ROI as well as enhanced endothelial adhesion, rolling, and migration. Additional effects of complement protein-receptor binding include aggregation of platelets and endothelial activation (production of chemokines, cytokines, and vasoactive substances). Blunted up-regulation of CR3 and deficiencies of C5aR on neonatal PMNs after stimulation likely contribute to poor complement-mediated chemotaxis and transmigration compared with adult PMNs[167,168]

Cytokines and chemokines
Activation and amplification of host immune cells during infection is mediated in part by production of cytokines and chemokines after stimulation of PRRs. IL-1β, IL-6, IL-12, IL-18, IFN-γ, and TNF-α are among the elevated proinflammatory cytokines commonly found during neonatal sepsis.[169] Important aspects of the cytokine response after TLR stimulation in neonates are diminished. In particular, decreased production of T_H1-polarizing cytokines (IL-1β, TNF-α, IFN-γ, and IL-12[57,170–172]) with enhanced production of T_H2-polarizing cytokines relative to adults likely contribute to neonatal susceptibility to infection.[8,57,79,80,83,170] Decreased neonatal cytokine production during infection compared with adults is likely related to decreased intra-cellular mediators of TLR signaling.[83] Plasma adenosine, an endogenous plasma metabolite that rises with hypoxia and stress, is elevated in newborn blood plasma and inhibits production of TNF-α by monocytes with preservation of IL-6 synthesis.[93] Adenosine binds the G protein-coupled adenosine 3 receptor expressed on neonatal leukocytes, thereby triggering intracellular accumulation of cAMP, a second messenger that inhibits production of T_H1-polarizing cytokines while preserving that of T_H2-polarizing cytokines, including IL-6.[4,93] The skewed polarization of neonatal cytokine responses against T_H1 polarizing cytokines may reduce the risk of immune reactions that could trigger preterm birth or excessive postnatal inflammation during colonization with commensal flora but may also contribute to neonatal susceptibility to infection with intracellular pathogens.

Exceptions to the impairment in TLR-mediated neonatal production of T_H1-polar-izing cytokines are agonists of TLR8. Synthetic TLR8 agonists, including imidazoqui-nolines and single-stranded RNAs, induce marked neonatal production of TNF-α to adult levels revealing a signaling pathway that is fully functional at birth.[109] These observations raise the possibility that TLR8 agonists may have unique efficacy as stand alone immune response modifiers in newborns or as neonatal vaccine adju-vants, a major unmet medical need.[173]

In addition to altered signaling capacity and the effects of adenosine on cytokine production after TLR stimulation, alterations in the genes coding for cytokines and their receptors have the potential to contribute to a neonate's increased susceptibility to EONS. After the discovery of specific cytokine or cytokine receptor polymorphisms and their association with an increased risk for infection in older populations, neonates have been evaluated with mixed results.[174–180] Large, population-based studies are necessary to more completely characterize the impact of genetic variation in cytokines and their receptors on the risk for development of neonatal infection.

Development of an effective inflammatory response is necessary to successfully respond to an infectious challenge. Uncontrolled proinflammatory responses, however, may lead to host tissue injury through excessive cellular activation. A recent evaluation in mice given a large intraperitoneal dose (10 mg/kg) of endotoxin revealed an increase (>3-fold) in the relative systemic inflammatory response (serum TNF-α, Monocyte chemotactic protein-1 [CCL2] [MCP-1], and IL-6) in neonatal mice compared with adult mice.[181] Another murine evaluation reported reduced IL-6 (3 fold) and elevated TNF-α (3 fold) in 1-day-old neonates compared with adults in vivo 2 hours after subcutaneous LPS exposure.[182] The finding of elevated endotoxin-induced serum TNF-α in neonatal mice relative to adult mice is in contrast to previous reports in humans[57,170–172] and mice,[79,80] may reflect specific features of the model or the timing of cytokine sampling, and will require further investigation.

Acute phase reactants
The production of inflammatory cytokines early during infection is associated with increased hepatic production of innate immune proteins, known as APRs. Predominantly induced by IL-6, the primary function of these components is to reduce host bacterial load through improved cellular recruitment, opsonin function, and direct antimicrobial activity. Examples include MBL, LBP, pentraxins (C-reactive protein [CRP] and serum amyloid A [SAA]), and fibronectin.[4,63,64,169,183–186] APRs have been studied in neonates with sepsis primarily to assess for diagnostic usefulness rather than immunologic function. In particular, elevated plasma concentrations of CRP and LBP are often associated with EONS.[64,187] Despite APR increases and the presence of maternally derived immunoglobulin, neonates exhibit impaired opsonizing activity compared with adults, which likely increases the risk for progression of infection.[188]

The coagulation cascade is intimately tied to inflammation, including complement activation, and is important in preventing microbial spread beyond the local environment. A microvascular procoagulant state develops via stimulation of monocytes, PMNs, platelets, and endothelium, resulting in expression of tissue factor.[189,190] Tissue factor-mediated activation of the coagulation cascade results in activation of thrombin-antithrombin complex, plasminogen activator inhibitor, and plasmin-a2-antiplasmin complex[191] as well as inactivation of protein S and depletion of anticoagulant proteins including antithrombin III and protein C.[192,193] Activated platelets may be consumed in clot formation or may also be removed from the circulation by the liver,[194] potentially resulting in thrombocytopenia, particularly during Gram-negative and fungal infections.[195–197] Systemic activation of coagulation is associated with consumption of clotting factors and increased risk of bleeding, inflammation, and disseminated intravascular coagulation (DIC).[198] Inflammatory dysregulation and its effects on the coagulation system are demonstrated by the association of altered ratios of serum pro- and anti-inflammatory cytokines and the development of DIC in neonates.[170]

Passive immunity
Neonates have passively acquired antibodies via placental transfer with a significant increase beginning at approximately 20 weeks' gestation. As a result, preterm neonates have lower IgG levels compared with term neonates (see **Fig. 2**A), in particular IgG1 and IgG2 subclasses.[199] Examination of the impact of low immunoglobulin in

preterm neonates 24 to 32 weeks' gestational age (serum levels <400 mg/dL total IgG at birth) revealed an increased risk for development of late-onset infection but not mortality compared with those with levels greater than 400 mg/dL after controlling for gestational age. There was a 15% increase in late-onset neonatal sepsis risk in these infants for every 100 mg/dL decrease in serum IgG below baseline that was not reduced with IVIG infusion.[200,201] In children or adults with deficient serum IgG1 (<100 mg/dL),[202,203] there are also significant infectious consequences.[204]Despite functional immune system limitations of innate and adaptive immunity, most premature neonates do not develop overwhelming bacterial sepsis, even in the absence of significant levels of passively acquired immunoglobulins. Reliance on other means of innate immune defense likely provides premature neonates with some degree of microbial control mechanisms.

Antimicrobial Proteins and Peptides

APPs represent the most phylogenetically ancient means of innate immune defense against microbial invasion. Present in nearly every organism, including bacteria, plants, insects, nonmammalian vertebrates, and mammals, these small, often cationic peptides are capable of killing microbes of multiple types, including viruses, bacteria, parasites, and fungi largely by disruption of the pathogen membrane.[205] Constitutive expression of APPs occurs in humans on barrier areas with consistent microbial exposure, such as skin and mucosa (see **Fig. 1**). After microbial stimulation, release of preformed APPs and inducible expression are thought to contribute to early host defense.[206] There is no evidence to date for the development of microbial resistance to APPs that target fundamental components of the microbial cell wall. Some APPs can bind and neutralize microbial components, such as endotoxin, precluding engagement with TLRs and other PRRs and thereby reducing inflammation.

BPI is a 55-kDa protein present present in the respiratory tract, PMN primary granules, and blood plasma (see **Fig. 1**). BPI exerts selective cytotoxic, antiendotoxic, and opsonic activity against Gram-negative bacteria.[158] Lactoferrin is the major whey protein in mammalian milk (in particular, high concentrations in colostrum) and is important in innate immune host defenses. An 80-kDa protein, lactoferrin is also present in tears and saliva and has antimicrobial activity via binding iron (depriving microorganisms of this key nutrient) and by direct membrane perturbing activity. Lysozyme is present in tears, tracheal aspirates, skin, and in PMN primary and secondary granules and contributes to degradation of peptidoglycan of bacterial cell walls. Secretory phospholipase 2 (sPLA2) can destroy Gram-positive bacteria through hydrolysis of their membrane lipids.[207] PMN elastase is a serine protease released by activated PMNs with microbicidal function and is believed to play a role in the inflammatory damage seen with PMN recruitment, particularly in the lung.[89,208] Cathelicidin and the defensins are other APPs that possess antimicrobial properties.[209] LL-37, the only known human cathelicidin, is present in the amniotic fluid, vernix, skin, saliva, respiratory tract, and leukocytes (PMNs, B cells, T cells, monocytes, and macrophages) (see **Fig. 2**B). α-defensins are cysteine-rich 4 kDa peptides expressed in the amniotic fluid, vernix, spleen, cornea, thymus, paneth cells, and leukocytes (PMNs, monocytes, macrophages, and lymphocytes). β-defensins are found in skin, gastrointestinal tract (salivary gland, tonsil, gastric antrum, stomach, liver, pancreas, small intestine, and colon), reproductive organs and urinary tract (placenta, uterus, testes, and kidney), respiratory tract, breast milk and mammary gland, and thymus. In addition to microbicidal action, APPs possess a wide range of immunomodulatory functions on multiple cell types from the innate and adaptive immune system.[206,210,211] Immunomodulatory effects on macrophages, DCs, monocytes, mast cells, PMNs, and epithelia attributed to APPs include altered cytokine and chemokine production, improved cellular chemotaxis and recruitment, improved cell function (maturation, activation, phagocytosis, and ROI production), enhancement of wound healing (neovascularization and mitogenesis), and decreased apoptosis.

Plasma and intracellular contributions

The cytosolic granules of PMNs are rich in APPs that can be released on stimulation into the extracellular space, including α-defensins, lactoferrin, lysozyme, LL-37, sPLA$_2$, and BPI. After release into the phagolysosome after phagocytosis or extracellularly into the surrounding tissue or blood, APPs contribute to microbial killing and binding of bacterial toxins, such as LPS. Many APPs (LL-37, α/β-defensins, and BPI) can potentially reduce the intensity of the inflammatory response associated with the presence of bacterial toxins. Recently, gestational age-related decreases in the cord blood concentration of several APPs (LL-37, BPI, calprotectin, sPLA$_2$, and α-defensins) were described in comparison to maternal serum levels (see **Fig. 2B**).[212] Plasma APP deficiencies may contribute to the increased risk of infection associated with prematurity, and their absence may increase the risk of excessive levels of bacterial toxins. Up-regulation of APPs (defensins) occurs in blood of infected adults[213] and children (defensins and lactoferrin).[214] The effect of sepsis on the production of plasma APPs in neonates has not been investigated in detail. PMNs from term neonates produce similar concentrations of defensins but reduced BPI and elastase compared with adults.[112,134,135] Although term neonates demonstrate up-regulation of plasma BPI during infection, premature neonates showed a decreased ability to mobilize BPI on stimulation,[215] which may contribute to their risk for infection with Gram-negative bacteria. Polymorphisms in BPI increase the risk for Gram-negative sepsis in children, but the impact of these polymorphisms in neonates is unknown.[216]

Skin

APPs present in amniotic fluid, in vernix, and on newborn skin, including lysozyme, LL-37, ubiquitin, α/β-defensins, and psoriasin, have antimicrobial efficacy against common neonatal pathogens, such as *Staphylococcus aureus*, *E coli*, *Klebsiella spp*, and GBS.[217–219] Expression of LL-37 and β-defensin 2 are elevated on neonatal skin compared with adult skin.[220] A role for β-defensins in defense against vertical HIV transmission has been suggested by a recent single-nucleotide polymorphism study.[221] The common benign newborn skin lesions of erythema toxicum are associated with induction of LL-37 production[42] demonstrating up-regulation after colonization of the skin with commensal flora, including coagulase-negative Staphylococci.[42,43] The increased concentration of APPs on neonatal skin compared with adults and their up-regulation in response to colonization likely serves to improve immune protection for the fragile skin barrier (see **Fig. 1**).[217,222]

Airway

Airway protection is conferred in utero in part via amniotic APPs. In the absence of microbial invasion of the amniotic cavity, levels of calprotectin and BPI exhibit gestational age-dependent expression with much lower concentrations of amniotic fluid BPI levels in midtrimester (14–18 week) fetuses.[223] Significant increases (>10-fold) in amniotic fluid APPs (BPI, α-defensins, and calprotectin) occur in the presence of intraamniotic microbial infection and preterm labor (see **Fig. 1**).[223]

β-defensins 1–3, LL-37, lactoferrin, lysozyme, and BPI have been measured in neonatal tracheal aspirates. Reduced basal β-defensin concentrations in tracheal aspirates from preterm neonates may contribute to the risk of early pulmonary infection.[51] Mobilization of APPs is evident by increases in airway fluid concentrations of BPI, LL-37, and β-defensins that occur with mechanical ventilation, pneumonia, or systemic infection.[49,206,224] Reduced lactoferrin and lysozyme concentrations have been described in tracheal aspirates of neonates with BPD and may contribute to chronic cellular inflammation due to poor clearance of bacteria.[225]

Gastrointestinal tract

APPs are present in meconium and are constitutively secreted by gastrointestinal epithelium (predominantly Paneth cells). Up-regulation of APPs occurs on stimulation in neonatal intestine after microbial colonization[226] and with the development of necrotizing enterocolitis (NEC).[227] Premature neonates have fewer Paneth cells and express less APPs compared with more mature neonates that may increase their risk for poor intestinal barrier function or the development of NEC.[206] Human milk is an important postnatal source of APPs, including lactoferrin, α/β defensins, and LL-37[228] that inhibit the growth of bacteria and may be inactivated by human milk fortifier.[229] No newborn formula preparation contains human-derived, bovine-derived, or synthetic APPs at this time. Although unlikely to have a significant impact on EONS because onset precedes significant oral intake, human milk–derived APPs likely participate in the reduction of late-onset infection seen in neonates fed human milk.[230]

Efforts to Reduce EONS Mortality and Enhance Innate Defenses

Successful obstetric interventions directed at reducing the incidence and impact of EONS have included antimicrobial treatment of mothers with GBS colonization,[231] premature rupture of membranes,[232,233] preterm premature rupture of membranes,[234,235] and intra-amniotic infection.[236,237] (For a complete review on attempts to enhance neonatal immunity, see the article by Tarnow-Mordi and colleagues elsewhere in this issue).[3,237]

Activated protein C (aPC) administration demonstrated a modest reduction in mortality when given to adults with sepsis.[238] Despite reduced plasma levels of aPC in septic neonates,[239] however, evaluations of aPC in children and infants with sepsis revealed no difference in mortality compared with placebo but identified an increase in the risk for bleeding in infants less than 60 days of age.[240]

Based on suboptimal neonatal PMN function, the presence of limited bone marrow PMN reserves, and the poor outcomes associated with septic neutropenia, cytokine therapy and granulocyte transfusions have been evaluated as prophylaxis to reduce the development of sepsis and as treatment to enhance neonatal immunity and sepsis survival. Despite being well tolerated and increasing the number of effective circulating PMNs, however, granulocyte transfusions do not improve sepsis survival.[241] Treatment with colony-stimulating factor therapy (G-CSF and GM-CSF) in a subgroup (97 neonates) with documented culture-positive sepsis (largely due to Gram-negative infection and GBS) and neutropenia (absolute neutrophil count <1700/μL), however, significantly reduced the risk of death (relative risk 0.34; 95% CI 0.12, 0.92). Therefore, colony-stimulating factors may be beneficial under these specific circumstances although further studies focused on this subpopulation and outcome are needed.[242,243]

FUTURE DIRECTIONS AND TRANSLATIONAL OPPORTUNITIES
Biomarkers

Recent discoveries in neonatal immunology have brought to light some new diagnostic opportunities. New proteomic approaches can enhance detection of subclinical intra-amniotic infection, chorioamnionitis, and EONS through identification of specific inflammatory factors, including IL-6 and select defensins, and have helped to more completely characterize the immune response to in utero infection.[244,245] Multiple biomarkers of inflammation, including cytokines (IL-1β, IL-6, IL-8 [chemokine], IL-10, and IL-18), APRs (CRP, procalcitonin, SAA, and LBP), cell surface markers and molecules (E-selectin, P-selectin, vascular cell adhesion molecule-1, CD11b, CD64, HLA-DR, and CD69), receptors (IL-2 soluble receptor and urokinase plasminogen-activated receptor), and enzymes (neutrophil elastase and urokinase plasminogen activator) have been explored to enhance diagnostic accuracy.[169,187,208,246] (For review of existing and novel diagnostic laboratory tests to aid in identification of septic neonates, see the article by Benitz elsewhere in this issue).

Novel Anti-infectives

The characterization of the properties of APPs has prompted significant biopharmaceutical development and investigation.[247] None of these therapies has been examined or approved for use in neonates at present but hold promise for improvement of innate immune function. For example, development and use of skin preparations that contain APPs (synthetic or natural) may provide fragile neonatal skin with improved barrier function and capacity to protect against early microbial invasion with a resultant decrease in infectious risk. Administration of recombinant BPI congeners (eg, $rBPI_{21}$) with endotoxin-neutralizing activity may reduce the deleterious actions of LPS via neutralization, reduce proinflammatory cytokines, and improve bacterial clearance via direct microbicidal activity.[158] Other APPs may also have potential to reduce sepsis mortality when administered systemically and are under evaluation.[248] Pretreatment with LL-37 was recently evaluated in neonatal rats given systemic LPS.[249] Low-dose systemic pretreatment with LL-37 reduced inflammation (decreased CRP levels) and mortality compared with sham but higher doses led to increased mortality. As with all new investigational agents, safety concerns need to be thoroughly investigated in preclinical neonatal animal models before systemic administration to human neonates. Recently, administration of enteral bovine lactoferrin to preterm human newborns was associated with a reduction in the incidence of late-onset sepsis (bacterial and fungal).[250]

Timely abrogation of the inflammatory response helps to prevent the spread of inflammation beyond the local environment to a systemic level where dangerous consequences can occur.[12] Simultaneous increases in anti-inflammatory cytokines, such as IL-4, IL-10, IL-11, and IL-13, occur during sepsis and counter the actions of the proinflammatory cytokines.[169,251–256] Cytokine and receptor antagonists also prevent ligand-receptor coupling and reduce the effects of inflammatory cytokines. Examples of these regulatory molecules elevated during sepsis include TNFR2, IL-6sR, sIL2, and IL-1ra.[197,253,257] Despite apparent benefit in preclinical adult models of sepsis, anticytokine therapies aimed at reducing proinflammatory cytokines have been evaluated in infected human adults with minimal benefit and potential harm, likely reflecting the importance of TNF and other inflammatory cytokines to host defense.[258] In neonates, reduction of excessive or sustained inflammation could theoretically decrease the frequency and intensity of devastating postsepsis sequelae, including chronic lung disease,[259] retinopathy of prematurity,[260] and white matter damage.[13]

Pulmonary infection or intubation and subsequent ventilator-associated lung injury increases the likelihood of respiratory mucosal damage and loss of barrier integrity. Intubated preterm newborns demonstrate accumulation of endotoxin in airway fluids corresponding to duration of intubation, raising the possibility that endotoxin contributes to pulmonary inflammation and its consequences.[49] In this context, improvement of pulmonary mucosal immune function through the administration of anti-infective proteins, such as surfactant proteins A and D, β-defensins, or endotoxin antagonists, may help to reduce local and systemic inflammation associated with pneumonia. Administration of recombinant surfactant protein D reduced pulmonary and systemic inflammation after administration of intratracheal LPS in a preterm animal model.[261] Caution is indicated as recent data showed that some APPs may bind SP-D, reducing its benefit, and may increase the risk for infection.[262]

Immune Adjuvants

Sepsis survival benefit after innate immune priming via specific TLR agonists has been demonstrated in a neonatal preclinical model.[80] Priming with select TLR agonists resulted in improved cellular recruitment and function as well as decreased bacteremia and significantly improved sepsis survival over sham-primed septic neonates. Further evaluation, including assessment of safety, is necessary before such positive immunomodulation reaches phase I trials in humans. Vaccination with BCG, a live attenuated strain of *Mycobacterium bovis* with TLR2/4 agonist activity, was associated with an improvement in survival in low-birth-weight neonates (not related to tuberculosis infection) compared with those who did not receive the vaccine and may represent an existing example of the benefits and safety of innate immune priming.[263]

SUMMARY

Neonatal EONS continues to take a devastating global toll. The innate immune system is distinct at birth and, although usually adequate, does leave newborns at increased risk of infection. Unique differences exist between newborns and older individuals with respect to capacity, quantity, and quality of innate host responses to pathogens. Characterization of the age-dependent maturation of neonatal innate immune function has identified novel translational approaches that may lead to improved diagnostic, prophylactic, and therapeutic approaches.

ACKNOWLEDGMENTS

We thank Patrick Bibbins at Children's Hospital Boston for creating **Fig. 1**. OL acknowledges the mentorship of Drs. Michael Wessels, Peter Elsbach, Jerrold Weiss, Phillip Pizzo, Eva Guinan, and Raif Geha.

REFERENCES

1. Lawn JE, Cousens S, Zupan J. 4 million neonatal deaths: when? where? why? Lancet 2005;365(9462):891–900.
2. Martinot A, Leclerc F, Cremer R, et al. Sepsis in neonates and children: definitions, epidemiology, and outcome. Pediatr Emerg Care 1997;13(4):277–81.
3. Wynn JL, Neu J, Moldawer LL, et al. Potential of immunomodulatory agents for prevention and treatment of neonatal sepsis. J Perinatol 2009;29(2):79–88.
4. Levy O. Innate immunity of the newborn: basic mechanisms and clinical correlates. Nat Rev Immunol 2007;7(5):379–90.
5. Adkins B, Leclerc C, Marshall-Clarke S. Neonatal adaptive immunity comes of age. Nat Rev Immunol 2004;4(7):553–64.
6. Kollmann TR, Crabtree J, Rein-Weston A, et al. Neonatal innate TLR-mediated responses are distinct from those of adults. J Immunol 2009;183(11):7150–60.
7. Rittirsch D, Flierl MA, Ward PA. Harmful molecular mechanisms in sepsis. Nat Rev Immunol 2008;8(10):776–87.

8. Hotchkiss RS, Karl IE. The pathophysiology and treatment of sepsis. N Engl J Med 2003;348(2):138–50.

9. Abraham E, Singer M. Mechanisms of sepsis-induced organ dysfunction. Crit Care Med 2007;35(10):2408–16.

10. Cinel I, Dellinger RP. Advances in pathogenesis and management of sepsis. Curr Opin Infect Dis 2007;20(4):345–52.

11. Jean-Baptiste E. Cellular mechanisms in sepsis. J Intensive Care Med 2007; 22(2):63–72.

12. Sriskandan S, Altmann DM. The immunology of sepsis. J Pathol 2008;214(2): 211–23.

13. Shah DK, Doyle LW, Anderson PJ, et al. Adverse neurodevelopment in preterm infants with postnatal sepsis or necrotizing enterocolitis is mediated by white matter abnormalities on magnetic resonance imaging at term. J Pediatr 2008; 153(2):170–5, 175. e171.

14. Palazzi D, Klein J, Baker C. Bacterial sepsis and meningitis. In: Remington JS, Klein OJ, Wilson CB, et al, editors. Infectious diseases of the fetus and newborn infant. 6th edition. Philadelphia: Elsevier Saunders; 2006. p. 247–95.

15. Benitz WE, Gould JB, Druzin ML. Risk factors for early-onset group B streptococcal sepsis: estimation of odds ratios by critical literature review. Pediatrics 1999;103(6):e77.

16. Bizzarro MJ, Dembry LM, Baltimore RS, et al. Changing patterns in neonatal *Escherichia coli* sepsis and ampicillin resistance in the era of intrapartum antibiotic prophylaxis. Pediatrics 2008;121(4):689–96.

17. Hyde TB, Hilger TM, Reingold A, et al. Trends in incidence and antimicrobial resistance of early-onset sepsis: population-based surveillance in San Francisco and Atlanta. Pediatrics 2002;110(4):690–5.

18. Moore MR, Schrag SJ, Schuchat A. Effects of intrapartum antimicrobial prophylaxis for prevention of group-B-streptococcal disease on the incidence and ecology of early-onset neonatal sepsis. Lancet Infect Dis 2003;3(4):201–13.

19. Anthony BF, Okada DM. The emergence of group B streptococci in infections of the newborn infant. Annu Rev Med 1977;28:355–69.

20. American Academy of Pediatrics Committee on Infectious Diseases and Committee on Fetus and Newborn. Guidelines for prevention of group B streptococcal (GBS) infection by chemoprophylaxis. Pediatrics 1992;90(5):775–8.

21. Centers for Disease Control and Prevention (CDC). Trends in perinatal group B streptococcal disease—United States, 2000–2006. MMWR Morb Mortal Wkly Rep 2009;58(5):109–12.

22. Cotten CM, Taylor S, Stoll B, et al. Prolonged duration of initial empirical antibiotic treatment is associated with increased rates of necrotizing enterocolitis and death for extremely low birth weight infants. Pediatrics 2009; 123(1):58–66.

23. Stoll BJ, Hansen NI, Higgins RD, et al. Very low birth weight preterm infants with early onset neonatal sepsis: the predominance of gram-negative infections continues in the National Institute of Child Health and Human Development Neonatal Research Network, 2002–2003. Pediatr Infect Dis J 2005;24(7):635–9.

24. Stoll BJ, Hansen N. Infections in VLBW infants: studies from the NICHD Neonatal Research Network. Semin Perinatol 2003;27(4):293–301.

25. Stoll BJ, Hansen N, Fanaroff AA, et al. Changes in pathogens causing early-onset sepsis in very-low-birth-weight infants. N Engl J Med 2002;347(4):240–7.

26. Barton L, Hodgman JE, Pavlova Z. Causes of death in the extremely low birth weight infant. Pediatrics 1999;103(2):446–51.

27. Holladay SD, Smialowicz RJ. Development of the murine and human immune system: differential effects of immunotoxicants depend on time of exposure. Environ Health Perspect 2000;108(Suppl 3):463–73.
28. Koga K, Aldo PB, Mor G. Toll-like receptors and pregnancy: trophoblast as modulators of the immune response. J Obstet Gynaecol Res 2009;35(2):191–202.
29. Sampson JE, Theve RP, Blatman RN, et al. Fetal origin of amniotic fluid polymorphonuclear leukocytes. Am J Obstet Gynecol 1997;176(1 Pt 1):77–81.
30. Gotsch F, Romero R, Kusanovic JP, et al. The fetal inflammatory response syndrome. Clin Obstet Gynecol 2007;50(3):652–83.
31. Saji F, Samejima Y, Kamiura S, et al. Cytokine production in chorioamnionitis. J Reprod Immunol 2000;47(2):185–96.
32. Kemp B, Winkler M, Maas A, et al. Cytokine concentrations in the amniotic fluid during parturition at term: correlation to lower uterine segment values and to labor. Acta Obstet Gynecol Scand 2002;81(10):938–42.
33. Kallapur SG, Willet KE, Jobe AH, et al. Intra-amniotic endotoxin: chorioamnionitis precedes lung maturation in preterm lambs. Am J Physiol Lung Cell Mol Physiol 2001;280(3):L527–36.
34. Erez O, Romero R, Tarca AL, et al. Differential expression pattern of genes encoding for anti-microbial peptides in the fetal membranes of patients with spontaneous preterm labor and intact membranes and those with preterm prelabor rupture of the membranes. J Matern Fetal Neonatal Med 2009;22(12):1103–15.
35. Leth-Larsen R, Floridon C, Nielsen O, et al. Surfactant protein D in the female genital tract. Mol Hum Reprod 2004;10(3):149–54.
36. King AE, Kelly RW, Sallenave JM, et al. Innate immune defences in the human uterus during pregnancy. Placenta 2007;28(11–12):1099–106.
37. Tollin M, Bergsson G, Kai-Larsen Y, et al. Vernix caseosa as a multi-component defence system based on polypeptides, lipids and their interactions. Cell Mol Life Sci 2005;62(19–20):2390–9.
38. Visscher MO, Narendran V, Pickens WL, et al. Vernix caseosa in neonatal adaptation. J Perinatol 2005;25(7):440–6.
39. Rutter N. Clinical consequences of an immature barrier. Semin Neonatol 2000;5(4):281–7.
40. Evans NJ, Rutter N. Development of the epidermis in the newborn. Biol Neonate 1986;49(2):74–80.
41. Kalia YN, Nonato LB, Lund CH, et al. Development of skin barrier function in premature infants. J Invest Dermatol 1998;111(2):320–6.
42. Marchini G, Lindow S, Brismar H, et al. The newborn infant is protected by an innate antimicrobial barrier: peptide antibiotics are present in the skin and vernix caseosa. Br J Dermatol 2002;147(6):1127–34.
43. Marchini G, Nelson A, Edner J, et al. Erythema toxicum neonatorum is an innate immune response to commensal microbes penetrated into the skin of the newborn infant. Pediatr Res 2005;58(3):613–6.
44. Lewis D, Wilson C. Developmental immunology and role of host defenses in fetal and neonatal susceptibility to infection. In: Remington JS, Klein OJ, Wilson CB, et al, editors. Infectious diseases of the fetus and newborn infant. 6th edition. Philadelphia: Elsevier Saunders; 2006. p. 87–210.
45. Martin CR, Walker WA. Probiotics: role in pathophysiology and prevention in necrotizing enterocolitis. Semin Perinatol 2008;32(2):127–37.
46. Sharma R, Tepas JJ 3rd, Hudak ML, et al. Neonatal gut barrier and multiple organ failure: role of endotoxin and proinflammatory cytokines in sepsis and necrotizing enterocolitis. J Pediatr Surg 2007;42(3):454–61.

47. Neu J. Gastrointestinal maturation and implications for infant feeding. Early Hum Dev 2007;83(12):767–75.
48. Bartlett JA, Fischer AJ, McCray PB Jr. Innate immune functions of the airway epithelium. Contrib Microbiol 2008;15:147–63.
49. Nathe KE, Parad R, Van Marter LJ, et al. Endotoxin-directed innate immunity in tracheal aspirates of mechanically ventilated human neonates. Pediatr Res 2009;66(2):191–6.
50. Pfister RH, Soll RF. New synthetic surfactants: the next generation? Biol Neonate 2005;87(4):338–44.
51. Starner TD, Agerberth B, Gudmundsson GH, et al. Expression and activity of beta-defensins and LL-37 in the developing human lung. J Immunol 2005; 174(3):1608–15.
52. Brown GD. Dectin-1: a signalling non-TLR pattern-recognition receptor. Nat Rev Immunol 2006;6(1):33–43.
53. Kawai T, Akira S. The roles of TLRs, RLRs and NLRs in pathogen recognition. Int Immunol 2009;21(4):317–37.
54. Kumagai Y, Takeuchi O, Akira S. Pathogen recognition by innate receptors. J Infect Chemother 2008;14(2):86–92.
55. Trinchieri G, Sher A. Cooperation of toll-like receptor signals in innate immune defence. Nat Rev Immunol 2007;7(3):179–90.
56. Krumbiegel D, Zepp F, Meyer CU. Combined toll-like receptor agonists synergistically increase production of inflammatory cytokines in human neonatal dendritic cells. Hum Immunol 2007;68(10):813–22.
57. Levy O, Zarember KA, Roy RM, et al. Selective impairment of TLR-mediated innate immunity in human newborns: neonatal blood plasma reduces monocyte TNF-alpha induction by bacterial lipopeptides, lipopolysaccharide, and imiquimod, but preserves the response to R-848. J Immunol 2004;173(7):4627–34.
58. Forster-Waldl E, Sadeghi K, Tamandl D, et al. Monocyte toll-like receptor 4 expression and LPS-induced cytokine production increase during gestational aging. Pediatr Res 2005;58(1):121–4.
59. Zhang JP, Chen C, Yang Y. [Changes and clinical significance of Toll-like receptor 2 and 4 expression in neonatal infections]. Zhonghua Er Ke Za Zhi 2007;45(2):130–3 [in Chinese].
60. Hartel C, Rupp J, Hoegemann A, et al. 159C>T CD14 genotype–functional effects on innate immune responses in term neonates. Hum Immunol 2008; 69(6):338–43.
61. Mollen KP, Gribar SC, Anand RJ, et al. Increased expression and internalization of the endotoxin coreceptor CD14 in enterocytes occur as an early event in the development of experimental necrotizing enterocolitis. J Pediatr Surg 2008; 43(6):1175–81.
62. Hubacek JA, Stuber F, Frohlich D, et al. Gene variants of the bactericidal/permeability increasing protein and lipopolysaccharide binding protein in sepsis patients: gender-specific genetic predisposition to sepsis. Crit Care Med 2001;29(3):557–61.
63. Behrendt D, Dembinski J, Heep A, et al. Lipopolysaccharide binding protein in preterm infants. Arch Dis Child Fetal Neonatal Ed 2004;89(6):F551–4.
64. Berner R, Furll B, Stelter F, et al. Elevated levels of lipopolysaccharide-binding protein and soluble CD14 in plasma in neonatal early-onset sepsis. Clin Diagn Lab Immunol 2002;9(2):440–5.
65. Blanco A, Solis G, Arranz E, et al. Serum levels of CD14 in neonatal sepsis by gram-positive and gram-negative bacteria. Acta Paediatr 1996;85(6):728–32.

66. Warren SE, Mao DP, Rodriguez AE, et al. Multiple nod-like receptors activate caspase 1 during *Listeria monocytogenes* infection. J Immunol 2008;180(11): 7558–64.
67. Goldbach-Mansky R, Dailey NJ, Canna SW, et al. Neonatal-onset multisystem inflammatory disease responsive to interleukin-1beta inhibition. N Engl J Med 2006;355(6):581–92.
68. Szebeni B, Szekeres R, Rusai K, et al. Genetic polymorphisms of CD14, toll-like receptor 4, and caspase-recruitment domain 15 are not associated with necro-tizing enterocolitis in very low birth weight infants. J Pediatr Gastroenterol Nutr 2006;42(1):27–31.
69. Bochud PY, Chien JW, Marr KA, et al. Toll-like receptor 4 polymorphisms and aspergillosis in stem-cell transplantation. N Engl J Med 2008;359(17):1766–77.
70. Wurfel MM, Gordon AC, Holden TD, et al. Toll-like receptor 1 polymorphisms affect innate immune responses and outcomes in sepsis. Am J Respir Crit Care Med 2008;178(7):710–20.
71. Agnese DM, Calvano JE, Hahm SJ, et al. Human toll-like receptor 4 mutations but not CD14 polymorphisms are associated with an increased risk of gram-negative infections. J Infect Dis 2002;186(10):1522–5.
72. Lorenz E, Mira JP, Cornish KL, et al. A novel polymorphism in the toll-like receptor 2 gene and its potential association with staphylococcal infection. Infect Immun 2000;68(11):6398–401.
73. von Bernuth H, Picard C, Jin Z, et al. Pyogenic bacterial infections in humans with MyD88 deficiency. Science 2008;321(5889):691–6.
74. Picard C, Puel A, Bonnet M, et al. Pyogenic bacterial infections in humans with IRAK-4 deficiency. Science 2003;299(5615):2076–9.
75. Zhang SY, Jouanguy E, Ugolini S, et al. TLR3 deficiency in patients with herpes simplex encephalitis. Science 2007;317(5844):1522–7.
76. Mockenhaupt FP, Cramer JP, Hamann L, et al. Toll-like receptor (TLR) polymor-phisms in African children: common TLR-4 variants predispose to severe malaria. J Commun Dis 2006;38(3):230–45.
77. Faber J, Meyer CU, Gemmer C, et al. Human toll-like receptor 4 mutations are associated with susceptibility to invasive meningococcal disease in infancy. Pe-diatr Infect Dis J 2006;25(1):80–1.
78. Ku CL, von Bernuth H, Picard C, et al. Selective predisposition to bacterial infec-tions in IRAK-4-deficient children: IRAK-4-dependent TLRs are otherwise redun-dant in protective immunity. J Exp Med 2007;204(10):2407–22.
79. Wynn JL, Scumpia PO, Delano MJ, et al. Increased mortality and altered immunity in neonatal sepsis produced by generalized peritonitis. Shock 2007;28(6):675–83.
80. Wynn JL, Scumpia PO, Winfield RD, et al. Defective innate immunity predis-poses murine neonates to poor sepsis outcome but is reversed by TLR agonists. Blood 2008;112(5):1750–8.
81. Salomao R, Brunialti MK, Gomes NE, et al. Toll-like receptor pathway signaling is differently regulated in neutrophils and peripheral mononuclear cells of patients with sepsis, severe sepsis, and septic shock. Crit Care Med 2009; 37(1):132–9.
82. Al-Hertani W, Yan SR, Byers DM, et al. Human newborn polymorphonuclear neutrophils exhibit decreased levels of MyD88 and attenuated p38 phosphory-lation in response to lipopolysaccharide. Clin Invest Med 2007;30(2):E44–53.
83. Sadeghi K, Berger A, Langgartner M, et al. Immaturity of infection control in preterm and term newborns is associated with impaired toll-like receptor signaling. J Infect Dis 2007;195(2):296–302.

84. Yan SR, Qing G, Byers DM, et al. Role of MyD88 in diminished tumor necrosis factor alpha production by newborn mononuclear cells in response to lipopolysaccharide. Infect Immun 2004;72(3):1223–9.

85. Ehlers MR. CR3: a general purpose adhesion-recognition receptor essential for innate immunity. Microbes Infect 2000;2(3):289–94.

86. McEvoy LT, Zakem-Cloud H, Tosi MF. Total cell content of CR3 (CD11b/CD18) and LFA-1 (CD11a/CD18) in neonatal neutrophils: relationship to gestational age. Blood 1996;87(9):3929–33.

87. Buhrer C, Graulich J, Stibenz D, et al. L-selectin is down-regulated in umbilical cord blood granulocytes and monocytes of newborn infants with acute bacterial infection. Pediatr Res 1994;36(6):799–804.

88. Kim SK, Keeney SE, Alpard SK, et al. Comparison of L-selectin and CD11b on neutrophils of adults and neonates during the first month of life. Pediatr Res 2003;53(1):132–6.

89. Nupponen I, Pesonen E, Andersson S, et al. Neutrophil activation in preterm infants who have respiratory distress syndrome. Pediatrics 2002;110(1 Pt 1):36–41.

90. Nathan CF. Secretory products of macrophages. J Clin Invest 1987;79(2):319–26.

91. Willems F, Vollstedt S, Suter M. Phenotype and function of neonatal DC. Eur J Immunol 2009;39(1):26–35.

92. Angelone DF, Wessels MR, Coughlin M, et al. Innate immunity of the human newborn is polarized toward a high ratio of IL-6/TNF-alpha production in vitro and in vivo. Pediatr Res 2006;60(2):205–9.

93. Levy O, Coughlin M, Cronstein BN, et al. The adenosine system selectively inhibits TLR-mediated TNF-alpha production in the human newborn. J Immunol 2006; 177(3):1956–66.

94. Marodi L. Innate cellular immune responses in newborns. Clin Immunol 2006; 118(2-3):137–44.

95. Marodi L. Down-regulation of Th1 responses in human neonates. Clin Exp Immunol 2002;128(1):1–2.

96. Ottenhoff TH, De Boer T, van Dissel JT, et al. Human deficiencies in type-1 cytokine receptors reveal the essential role of type-1 cytokines in immunity to intracellular bacteria. Adv Exp Med Biol 2003;531:279–94.

97. Whitley R, Arvin A, Prober C, et al. Predictors of morbidity and mortality in neonates with herpes simplex virus infections. The National Institute of Allergy and Infectious Diseases Collaborative Antiviral Study Group. N Engl J Med 1991;324(7):450–4.

98. Jones CA, Holloway JA, Warner JO. Phenotype of fetal monocytes and B lymphocytes during the third trimester of pregnancy. J Reprod Immunol 2002; 56(1-2):45–60.

99. Hunt DW, Huppertz HI, Jiang HJ, et al. Studies of human cord blood dendritic cells: evidence for functional immaturity. Blood 1994;84(12):4333–43.

100. Velilla PA, Rugeles MT, Chougnet CA. Defective antigen-presenting cell function in human neonates. Clin Immunol 2006;121(3):251–9.

101. Krumbiegel D, Rohr J, Schmidtke P, et al. Efficient maturation and cytokine production of neonatal DCs requires combined proinflammatory signals. Clin Dev Immunol 2005;12(2):99–105.

102. Wong OH, Huang FP, Chiang AK. Differential responses of cord and adult blood-derived dendritic cells to dying cells. Immunology 2005;116(1):13–20.

103. Salio M, Dulphy N, Renneson J, et al. Efficient priming of antigen-specific cytotoxic T lymphocytes by human cord blood dendritic cells. Int Immunol 2003; 15(10):1265–73.

104. Hallwirth U, Pomberger G, Zaknun D, et al. Monocyte phagocytosis as a reliable parameter for predicting early-onset sepsis in very low birthweight infants. Early Hum Dev 2002;67(1–2):1–9.
105. Klein RB, Fischer TJ, Gard SE, et al. Decreased mononuclear and polymorphonuclear chemotaxis in human newborns, infants, and young children. Pediatrics 1977;60(4):467–72.
106. Chelvarajan L, Popa D, Liu Y, et al. Molecular mechanisms underlying anti-inflammatory phenotype of neonatal splenic macrophages. J Leukoc Biol 2007;82(2):403–16.
107. Aikio O, Vuopala K, Pokela ML, et al. Diminished inducible nitric oxide synthase expression in fulminant early-onset neonatal pneumonia. Pediatrics 2000; 105(5):1013–9.
108. Levy O, Jean-Jacques RM, Cywes C, et al. Critical role of the complement system in group B streptococcus-induced tumor necrosis factor alpha release. Infect Immun 2003;71(11):6344–53.
109. Levy O, Suter EE, Miller RL, et al. Unique efficacy of toll-like receptor 8 agonists in activating human neonatal antigen-presenting cells. Blood 2006;108(4):1284–90.
110. Vekemans J, Amedei A, Ota MO, et al. Neonatal bacillus Calmette-Guerin vaccination induces adult-like IFN-gamma production by CD4+ T lymphocytes. Eur J Immunol 2001;31(5):1531–5.
111. Dale DC, Boxer L, Liles WC. The phagocytes: neutrophils and monocytes. Blood 2008;112(4):935–45.
112. Urlichs F, Speer C. Neutrophil function in preterm and term infants. NeoReviews 2004;5:e417–30.
113. Weinschenk NP, Farina A, Bianchi DW. Premature infants respond to early-onset and late-onset sepsis with leukocyte activation. J Pediatr 2000;137(3):345–50.
114. Engle WA, McGuire WA, Schreiner RL, et al. Neutrophil storage pool depletion in neonates with sepsis and neutropenia. J Pediatr 1988;113(4):747–9.
115. Christensen RD, Rothstein G. Exhaustion of mature marrow neutrophils in neonates with sepsis. J Pediatr 1980;96(2):316–8.
116. Christensen RD, Bradley PP, Rothstein G. The leukocyte left shift in clinical and experimental neonatal sepsis. J Pediatr 1981;98(1):101–5.
117. Squire E, Favara B, Todd J. Diagnosis of neonatal bacterial infection: hematologic and pathologic findings in fatal and nonfatal cases. Pediatrics 1979; 64(1):60–4.
118. Doron MW, Makhlouf RA, Katz VL, et al. Increased incidence of sepsis at birth in neutropenic infants of mothers with preeclampsia. J Pediatr 1994;125(3):452–8.
119. Gray PH, Rodwell RL. Neonatal neutropenia associated with maternal hypertension poses a risk for nosocomial infection. Eur J Pediatr 1999;158(1):71–3. [Epub 2008 Dec 11]. PMID: 19078971.
120. Paul DA, Leef KH, Sciscione A, et al. Preeclampsia does not increase the risk for culture proven sepsis in very low birth weight infants. Am J Perinatol 1999;16(7): 365–72.
121. Teng RJ, Wu TJ, Garrison RD, et al. Early neutropenia is not associated with an increased rate of nosocomial infection in very low-birth-weight infants. J Perinatol 2009;29(3):219–24.
122. Christensen RD, Henry E, Wiedmeier SE, et al. Low blood neutrophil concentrations among extremely low birth weight neonates: data from a multihospital health-care system. J Perinatol 2006;26(11):682–7.
123. Turkmen M, Satar M, Atici A. Neutrophil chemotaxis and random migration in preterm and term infants with sepsis. Am J Perinatol 2000;17(2):107–12.

124. Merry C, Puri P, Reen DJ. Defective neutrophil actin polymerisation and chemotaxis in stressed newborns. J Pediatr Surg 1996;31(4):481–5.
125. Meade VM, Barese CN, Kim C, et al. Rac2 concentrations in umbilical cord neutrophils. Biol Neonate 2006;90(3):156–9.
126. Xing Z, Gauldie J, Cox G, et al. IL-6 is an antiinflammatory cytokine required for controlling local or systemic acute inflammatory responses. J Clin Invest 1998; 101(2):311–20.
127. Hickey MJ, Kubes P. Intravascular immunity: the host-pathogen encounter in blood vessels. Nat Rev Immunol 2009;9(5):364–75.
128. Yektaei-Karin E, Moshfegh A, Lundahl J, et al. The stress of birth enhances in vitro spontaneous and IL-8-induced neutrophil chemotaxis in the human newborn. Pediatr Allergy Immunol 2007;18(8):643–51.
129. Zentay Z, Sharaf M, Qadir M, et al. Mechanism for dexamethasone inhibition of neutrophil migration upon exposure to lipopolysaccharide in vitro: role of neutrophil interleukin-8 release. Pediatr Res 1999;46(4):406–10.
130. Molloy EJ, O'Neill AJ, Grantham JJ, et al. Labor promotes neonatal neutrophil survival and lipopolysaccharide responsiveness. Pediatr Res 2004;56(1):99–103.
131. Shen CM, Lin SC, Niu DM, et al. Labour increases the surface expression of two toll-like receptors in the cord blood monocytes of healthy term newborns. Acta Paediatr 2009;98(6):959–62.
132. Linderkamp O, Ruef P, Brenner B, et al. Passive deformability of mature, immature, and active neutrophils in healthy and septicemic neonates. Pediatr Res 1998;44(6):946–50.
133. Mease AD, Burgess DP, Thomas PJ. Irreversible neutrophil aggregation. A mechanism of decreased newborn neutrophil chemotactic response. Am J Pathol 1981;104(1):98–102.
134. Levy O, Martin S, Eichenwald E, et al. Impaired innate immunity in the newborn: newborn neutrophils are deficient in bactericidal/permeability-increasing protein. Pediatrics 1999;104(6):1327–33.
135. Kjeldsen L, Sengelov H, Lollike K, et al. Granules and secretory vesicles in human neonatal neutrophils. Pediatr Res 1996;40(1):120–9.
136. Drossou V, Kanakoudi F, Tzimouli V, et al. Impact of prematurity, stress and sepsis on the neutrophil respiratory burst activity of neonates. Biol Neonate 1997;72(4):201–9.
137. Shigeoka AO, Santos JI, Hill HR. Functional analysis of neutrophil granulocytes from healthy, infected, and stressed neonates. J Pediatr 1979;95(3):454–60.
138. Wright WC Jr, Ank BJ, Herbert J, et al. Decreased bactericidal activity of leukocytes of stressed newborn infants. Pediatrics 1975;56(4):579–84.
139. Bialek R, Bartmann P. Is there an effect of immunoglobulins and G-CSF on neutrophil phagocytic activity in preterm infants? Infection 1998;26(6):375–8.
140. Falconer AE, Carr R, Edwards SW. Impaired neutrophil phagocytosis in preterm neonates: lack of correlation with expression of immunoglobulin or complement receptors. Biol Neonate 1995;68(4):264–9.
141. Allgaier B, Shi M, Luo D, et al. Spontaneous and Fas-mediated apoptosis are diminished in umbilical cord blood neutrophils compared with adult neutrophils. J Leukoc Biol 1998;64(3):331–6.
142. Hanna N, Vasquez P, Pham P, et al. Mechanisms underlying reduced apoptosis in neonatal neutrophils. Pediatr Res 2005;57(1):56–62.
143. Koenig JM, Stegner JJ, Schmeck AC, et al. Neonatal neutrophils with prolonged survival exhibit enhanced inflammatory and cytotoxic responsiveness. Pediatr Res 2005;57(3):424–9.

144. Ohman L, Tullus K, Katouli M, et al. Correlation between susceptibility of infants to infections and interaction with neutrophils of *Escherichia coli* strains causing neonatal and infantile septicemia. J Infect Dis 1995;171(1):128–33.
145. Clark SR, Ma AC, Tavener SA, et al. Platelet TLR4 activates neutrophil extracellular traps to ensnare bacteria in septic blood. Nat Med 2007;13(4): 463–9.
146. Brinkmann V, Reichard U, Goosmann C, et al. Neutrophil extracellular traps kill bacteria. Science 2004;303(5663):1532–5 [Epub 2009 Feb 12]. PMID: 19221037.
147. Fuchs TA, Abed U, Goosmann C, et al. Novel cell death program leads to neutrophil extracellular traps. J Cell Biol 2007;176(2):231–41.
148. Yost CC, Cody MJ, Harris ES, et al. Impaired neutrophil extracellular trap (NET) formation: a novel innate immune deficiency of human neonates. Blood 2009; 113(25):6419–27.
149. Marshall JS, Jawdat DM. Mast cells in innate immunity. J Allergy Clin Immunol 2004;114(1):21–7.
150. Damsgaard TE, Nielsen BW, Henriques U, et al. Histamine releasing cells of the newborn. Mast cells from the umbilical cord matrix and basophils from cord blood. Pediatr Allergy Immunol 1996;7(2):83–90.
151. Mazzoni A, Young HA, Spitzer JH, et al. Histamine regulates cytokine production in maturing dendritic cells, resulting in altered T cell polarization. J Clin Invest 2001;108(12):1865–73.
152. Nelson A, Ulfgren AK, Edner J, et al. Urticaria neonatorum: accumulation of tryptase-expressing mast cells in the skin lesions of newborns with erythema toxicum. Pediatr Allergy Immunol 2007;18(8):652–8.
153. Drossou V, Kanakoudi F, Diamanti E, et al. Concentrations of main serum opsonins in early infancy. Arch Dis Child Fetal Neonatal Ed 1995;72(3):F172–5.
154. Miller ME, Stiehm ER. Phagocytic, opsonic and immunoglobulin studies in newborns. Calif Med 1973;119(2):43–63.
155. Wolach B, Dolfin T, Regev R, et al. The development of the complement system after 28 weeks' gestation. Acta Paediatr 1997;86(5):523–7.
156. Notarangelo LD, Chirico G, Chiara A, et al. Activity of classical and alternative pathways of complement in preterm and small for gestational age infants. Pediatr Res 1984;18(3):281–5.
157. Lassiter HA, Watson SW, Seifring ML, et al. Complement factor 9 deficiency in serum of human neonates. J Infect Dis 1992;166(1):53–7.
158. Levy O, Sisson RB, Kenyon J, et al. Enhancement of neonatal innate defense: effects of adding an N-terminal recombinant fragment of bactericidal/permeability-increasing protein on growth and tumor necrosis factor-inducing activity of gram-negative bacteria tested in neonatal cord blood ex vivo. Infect Immun 2000;68(9):5120–5.
159. Zilow EP, Hauck W, Linderkamp O, et al. Alternative pathway activation of the complement system in preterm infants with early onset infection. Pediatr Res 1997;41(3):334–9.
160. Zilow G, Zilow EP, Burger R, et al. Complement activation in newborn infants with early onset infection. Pediatr Res 1993;34(2):199–203.
161. Frakking FN, Brouwer N, van Eijkelenburg NK, et al. Low mannose-binding lectin (MBL) levels in neonates with pneumonia and sepsis. Clin Exp Immunol 2007;150(2):255–62.
162. Dzwonek AB, Neth OW, Thiebaut R, et al. The role of mannose-binding lectin in susceptibility to infection in preterm neonates. Pediatr Res 2008;63(6):680–5.

163. Nupponen I, Andersson S, Jarvenpaa AL, et al. Neutrophil CD11b expression and circulating interleukin-8 as diagnostic markers for early-onset neonatal sepsis. Pediatrics 2001;108(1):E12.
164. Berger M, O'Shea J, Cross AS, et al. Human neutrophils increase expression of C3bi as well as C3b receptors upon activation. J Clin Invest 1984;74(5):1566–71.
165. Snyderman R, Goetzl EJ. Molecular and cellular mechanisms of leukocyte chemotaxis. Science 1981;213(4510):830–7.
166. Vogt W. Anaphylatoxins: possible roles in disease. Complement 1986;3(3): 177–88.
167. Anderson DC, Rothlein R, Marlin SD, et al. Impaired transendothelial migration by neonatal neutrophils: abnormalities of Mac-1 (CD11b/CD18)-dependent adherence reactions. Blood 1990;76(12):2613–21.
168. Nybo M, Sorensen O, Leslie R, et al. Reduced expression of C5a receptors on neutrophils from cord blood. Arch Dis Child Fetal Neonatal Ed 1998;78(2):F129–32.
169. Ng PC. Diagnostic markers of infection in neonates. Arch Dis Child Fetal Neonatal Ed 2004;89(3):F229–35.
170. Ng PC, Li K, Wong RP, et al. Proinflammatory and anti-inflammatory cytokine responses in preterm infants with systemic infections. Arch Dis Child Fetal Neonatal Ed 2003;88(3):F209–13.
171. Bozza FA, Salluh JI, Japiassu AM, et al. Cytokine profiles as markers of disease severity in sepsis: a multiplex analysis. Crit Care 2007;11(2):R49.
172. Hodge G, Hodge S, Haslam R, et al. Rapid simultaneous measurement of multiple cytokines using 100 microl sample volumes–association with neonatal sepsis. Clin Exp Immunol 2004;137(2):402–7.
173. Demirjian A, Levy O. Safety and efficacy of neonatal vaccination. Eur J Immunol 2009;39(1):36–46.
174. Ahrens P, Kattner E, Kohler B, et al. Mutations of genes involved in the innate immune system as predictors of sepsis in very low birth weight infants. Pediatr Res 2004;55(4):652-6.
175. Reiman M, Kujari H, Ekholm E, et al. Interleukin-6 polymorphism is associated with chorioamnionitis and neonatal infections in preterm infants. J Pediatr 2008;153(1):19–24.
176. Gopel W, Hartel C, Ahrens P, et al. Interleukin-6-174-genotype, sepsis and cerebral injury in very low birth weight infants. Genes Immun 2006;7(1):65–8.
177. Baier RJ, Loggins J, Yanamandra K. IL-10, IL-6 and CD14 polymorphisms and sepsis outcome in ventilated very low birth weight infants. BMC Med 2006;4:10.
178. Schueller AC, Heep A, Kattner E, et al. Prevalence of two tumor necrosis factor gene polymorphisms in premature infants with early onset sepsis. Biol Neonate 2006;90(4):229–32.
179. Treszl A, Kocsis I, Szathmari M, et al. Genetic variants of TNF-[FC12]a, IL-1beta, IL-4 receptor [FC12]a-chain, IL-6 and IL-10 genes are not risk factors for sepsis in low-birth-weight infants. Biol Neonate 2003;83(4):241–5.
180. Chauhan M, McGuire W. Interleukin-6 (-174C) polymorphism and the risk of sepsis in very low birth weight infants: meta-analysis. Arch Dis Child Fetal Neonatal Ed 2008;93(6):F427–9.
181. Zhao J, Kim KD, Yang X, et al. Hyper innate responses in neonates lead to increased morbidity and mortality after infection. Proc Natl Acad Sci U S A 2008;105(21):7528–33.
182. Cusumano V, Mancuso G, Genovese F, et al. Neonatal hypersusceptibility to endotoxin correlates with increased tumor necrosis factor production in mice. J Infect Dis 1997;176(1):168–76.

183. Wong HR, Doughty LA, Wedel N, et al. Plasma bactericidal/permeability-increasing protein concentrations in critically ill children with the sepsis syndrome. Pediatr Infect Dis J 1995;14(12):1087–91.
184. Romeo MG, Tina LG, Sciacca A, et al. [Decreased plasma fibronectin (pFN) level in preterm infants with infections]. Pediatr Med Chir 1995;17(6):563–6 [in Italian].
185. Kalayci AG, Adam B, Yilmazer F, et al. The value of immunoglobulin and complement levels in the early diagnosis of neonatal sepsis. Acta Paediatr 1997;86(9):999–1002.
186. Dyke MP, Forsyth KD. Decreased plasma fibronectin concentrations in preterm infants with septicaemia. Arch Dis Child 1993;68(5 Spec No):557–60.
187. Benitz WE, Han MY, Madan A, et al. Serial serum C-reactive protein levels in the diagnosis of neonatal infection. Pediatrics 1998;102(4):E41.
188. Madden NP, Levinsky RJ, Bayston R, et al. Surgery, sepsis, and nonspecific immune function in neonates. J Pediatr Surg 1989;24(6):562–6.
189. Rivers RP, Cattermole HE, Wright I. The expression of surface tissue factor apoprotein by blood monocytes in the course of infections in early infancy. Pediatr Res 1992;31(6):567–73.
190. Markiewski MM, Nilsson B, Ekdahl KN, et al. Complement and coagulation: strangers or partners in crime? Trends Immunol 2007;28(4):184–92.
191. Aronis S, Platokouki H, Photopoulos S, et al. Indications of coagulation and/or fibrinolytic system activation in healthy and sick very-low-birth-weight neonates. Biol Neonate 1998;74(5):337–44.
192. Roman J, Velasco F, Fernandez F, et al. Coagulation, fibrinolytic and kallikrein systems in neonates with uncomplicated sepsis and septic shock. Haemostasis 1993;23(3):142–8.
193. Lauterbach R, Pawlik D, Radziszewska R, et al. Plasma antithrombin III and protein C levels in early recognition of late-onset sepsis in newborns. Eur J Pediatr 2006;165(9):585–9.
194. Grewal PK, Uchiyama S, Ditto D, et al. The Ashwell receptor mitigates the lethal coagulopathy of sepsis. Nat Med 2008;14(6):648–55.
195. Guida JD, Kunig AM, Leef KH, et al. Platelet count and sepsis in very low birth weight neonates: is there an organism-specific response? Pediatrics 2003;111(6 Pt 1):1411–5.
196. Sola MC, Del Vecchio A, Rimsza LM. Evaluation and treatment of thrombocytopenia in the neonatal intensive care unit. Clin Perinatol 2000;27(3):655–79.
197. Spear ML, Stefano JL, Fawcett P, et al. Soluble interleukin-2 receptor as a predictor of neonatal sepsis. J Pediatr 1995;126(6):982–5.
198. Hathaway WE, Mull MM, Pechet GS. Disseminated intravascular coagulation in the newborn. Pediatrics 1969;43(2):233–40.
199. Malek A, Sager R, Schneider H. Maternal-fetal transport of immunoglobulin G and its subclasses during the third trimester of human pregnancy. Am J Reprod Immunol 1994;32(1):8–14.
200. Fanaroff AA, Korones SB, Wright LL, et al. A controlled trial of intravenous immune globulin to reduce nosocomial infections in very-low-birth-weight infants. National Institute of Child Health and Human Development Neonatal Research Network. N Engl J Med 1994;330(16):1107–13.
201. Sandberg K, Fasth A, Berger A, et al. Preterm infants with low immunoglobulin G levels have increased risk of neonatal sepsis but do not benefit from prophylactic immunoglobulin G. J Pediatr 2000;137(5):623–8.
202. Ballow M, Cates KL, Rowe JC, et al. Development of the immune system in very low birth weight (less than 1500 g) premature infants: concentrations of

plasma immunoglobulins and patterns of infections. Pediatr Res 1986;20(9):
899–904.

203. Conway SP, Dear PR, Smith I. Immunoglobulin profile of the preterm baby. Arch Dis Child 1985;60(3):208–12.

204. Bonagura VR, Marchlewski R, Cox A, et al. Biologic IgG level in primary immunodeficiency disease: the IgG level that protects against recurrent infection. J Allergy Clin Immunol 2008;122(1):210–2.

205. Ganz T. Defensins: antimicrobial peptides of innate immunity. Nat Rev Immunol 2003;3(9):710–20.

206. Yoshio H, Lagercrantz H, Gudmundsson GH, et al. First line of defense in early human life. Semin Perinatol 2004;28(4):304–11.

207. Schrama AJ, de Beaufort AJ, Poorthuis BJ, et al. Secretory phospholipase A(2) in newborn infants with sepsis. J Perinatol 2008;28(4):291–6.

208. Kingsmore SF, Kennedy N, Halliday HL, et al. Identification of diagnostic biomarkers for infection in premature neonates. Mol Cell Proteomics 2008;7(10):1863–75.

209. Ayabe T, Ashida T, Kohgo Y, et al. The role of Paneth cells and their antimicrobial peptides in innate host defense. Trends Microbiol 2004;12(8):394–8.

210. Holzl MA, Hofer J, Steinberger P, et al. Host antimicrobial proteins as endogenous immunomodulators. Immunol Lett 2008;119(1-2):4–11.

211. Selsted ME, Ouellette AJ. Mammalian defensins in the antimicrobial immune response. Nat Immunol 2005;6(6):551–7.

212. Strunk T, Doherty D, Richmond P, et al. Reduced levels of antimicrobial proteins and peptides in human cord blood plasma. Arch Dis Child Fetal Neonatal Ed 2009;94(3):F230–1.

213. Ihi T, Nakazato M, Mukae H, et al. Elevated concentrations of human neutrophil peptides in plasma, blood, and body fluids from patients with infections. Clin Infect Dis 1997;25(5):1134–40.

214. Thomas NJ, Carcillo JA, Doughty LA, et al. Plasma concentrations of defensins and lactoferrin in children with severe sepsis. Pediatr Infect Dis J 2002;21(1):34–8.

215. Nupponen I, Turunen R, Nevalainen T, et al. Extracellular release of bactericidal/permeability-increasing protein in newborn infants. Pediatr Res 2002; 51(6):670–4.

216. Michalek J, Svetlikova P, Fedora M, et al. Bactericidal permeability increasing protein gene variants in children with sepsis. Intensive Care Med 2007; 33(12):2158–64.

217. Dorschner RA, Lin KH, Murakami M, et al. Neonatal skin in mice and humans expresses increased levels of antimicrobial peptides: innate immunity during development of the adaptive response. Pediatr Res 2003;53(4):566–72.

218. Yoshio H, Tollin M, Gudmundsson GH, et al. Antimicrobial polypeptides of human vernix caseosa and amniotic fluid: implications for newborn innate defense. Pediatr Res 2003;53(2):211–6.

219. Baker SM, Balo NN, Abdel Aziz FT. Is vernix caseosa a protective material to the newborn? A biochemical approach. Indian J Pediatr 1995;62(2):237–9.

220. Larson AA, Dinulos JG. Cutaneous bacterial infections in the newborn. Curr Opin Pediatr 2005;17(4):481–5.

221. Ricci E, Malacrida S, Zanchetta M, et al. Role of beta-defensin-1 polymorphisms in mother-to-child transmission of HIV-1. J Acquir Immune Defic Syndr 2009; 51(1):13–9.

222. Walker VP, Akinbi HT, Meinzen-Derr J, et al. Host defense proteins on the surface of neonatal skin: implications for innate immunity. J Pediatr 2008; 152(6):777–81.

223. Espinoza J, Chaiworapongsa T, Romero R, et al. Antimicrobial peptides in amniotic fluid: defensins, calprotectin and bacterial/permeability-increasing protein in patients with microbial invasion of the amniotic cavity, intra-amniotic inflammation, preterm labor and premature rupture of membranes. J Matern Fetal Neonatal Med 2003;13(1):2–21.

224. Schaller-Bals S, Schulze A, Bals R. Increased levels of antimicrobial peptides in tracheal aspirates of newborn infants during infection. Am J Respir Crit Care Med 2002;165(7):992–5.

225. Revenis ME, Kaliner MA. Lactoferrin and lysozyme deficiency in airway secretions: association with the development of bronchopulmonary dysplasia. J Pediatr 1992;121(2):262–70.

226. Kai-Larsen Y, Bergsson G, Gudmundsson GH, et al. Antimicrobial components of the neonatal gut affected upon colonization. Pediatr Res 2007;61(5 Pt 1):530–6.

227. Salzman NH, Polin RA, Harris MC, et al. Enteric defensin expression in necrotizing enterocolitis. Pediatr Res 1998;44(1):20–6.

228. Armogida SA, Yannaras NM, Melton AL, et al. Identification and quantification of innate immune system mediators in human breast milk. Allergy Asthma Proc 2004;25(5):297–304.

229. Chan GM, Lee ML, Rechtman DJ. Effects of a human milk-derived human milk fortifier on the antibacterial actions of human milk. Breastfeed Med 2007;2(4):205–8.

230. Newburg DS, Walker WA. Protection of the neonate by the innate immune system of developing gut and of human milk. Pediatr Res 2007;61(1):2–8.

231. Schrag SJ, Zell ER, Lynfield R, et al. A population-based comparison of strategies to prevent early-onset group B streptococcal disease in neonates. N Engl J Med 2002;347(4):233–9.

232. Cararach V, Botet F, Sentis J, et al. Administration of antibiotics to patients with rupture of membranes at term: a prospective, randomized, multicentric study. Collaborative Group on PROM. Acta Obstet Gynecol Scand 1998;77(3):298–302.

233. Pylipow M, Gaddis M, Kinney JS. Selective intrapartum prophylaxis for group B streptococcus colonization: management and outcome of newborns. Pediatrics 1994;93(4):631–5.

234. Segel SY, Miles AM, Clothier B, et al. Duration of antibiotic therapy after preterm premature rupture of fetal membranes. Am J Obstet Gynecol 2003;189(3): 799–802.

235. Johnston MM, Sanchez-Ramos L, Vaughn AJ, et al. Antibiotic therapy in preterm premature rupture of membranes: a randomized, prospective, double-blind trial. Am J Obstet Gynecol 1990;163(3):743–7.

236. Hopkins L, Smaill F. Antibiotic regimens for management of intraamniotic infection. Cochrane Database Syst Rev 2002;3:CD003254.

237. Cohen-Wolkowiez M, Benjamin DK Jr, Capparelli E. Immunotherapy in neonatal sepsis: advances in treatment and prophylaxis. Curr Opin Pediatr 2009;21(2): 177–81.

238. Dellinger RP, Levy MM, Carlet JM, et al. Surviving sepsis campaign: international guidelines for management of severe sepsis and septic shock: 2008. Intensive Care Med 2008;34(1):17–60.

239. Venkataseshan S, Dutta S, Ahluwalia J, et al. Low plasma protein C values predict mortality in low birth weight neonates with septicemia. Pediatr Infect Dis J 2007;26(8):684–8.

240. Nadel S, Goldstein B, Williams MD, et al. Drotrecogin alfa (activated) in children with severe sepsis: a multicentre phase III randomised controlled trial. Lancet 2007;369(9564):836–43.

241. Mohan P, Brocklehurst P. Granulocyte transfusions for neonates with confirmed or suspected sepsis and neutropaenia. Cochrane Database Syst Rev 2003;4: CD003956.

242. Carr R, Modi N, Dore C. G-CSF and GM-CSF for treating or preventing neonatal infections. Cochrane Database Syst Rev 2003;3:CD003066.

243. Carr R, Brocklehurst P, Dore CJ, et al. Granulocyte-macrophage colony stimulating factor administered as prophylaxis for reduction of sepsis in extremely preterm, small for gestational age neonates (the PROGRAMS trial): a single-blind, multicentre, randomised controlled trial. Lancet 2009;373(9659):226–33.

244. Buhimschi CS, Bhandari V, Hamar BD, et al. Proteomic profiling of the amniotic fluid to detect inflammation, infection, and neonatal sepsis. PLoS Med 2007; 4(1):e18.

245. Buhimschi CS, Bhandari V, Han YW, et al. Using proteomics in perinatal and neonatal sepsis: hopes and challenges for the future. Curr Opin Infect Dis 2009;22(3):235–43.

246. Ng PC, Li G, Chui KM, et al. Quantitative measurement of monocyte HLA-DR expression in the identification of early-onset neonatal infection. Biol Neonate 2006;89(2):75–81.

247. Hancock RE, Sahl HG. Antimicrobial and host-defense peptides as new anti-infective therapeutic strategies. Nat Biotechnol 2006;24(12):1551–7.

248. Hirsch T, Metzig M, Niederbichler A, et al. Role of host defense peptides of the innate immune response in sepsis. Shock 2008;30(2):117–26.

249. Fukumoto K, Nagaoka I, Yamataka A, et al. Effect of antibacterial cathelicidin peptide CAP18/LL-37 on sepsis in neonatal rats. Pediatr Surg Int 2005;21(1): 20–4.

250. Manzoni P, Rinaldi M, Cattani S, et al. Bovine lactoferrin supplementation for prevention of late-onset sepsis in very low-birth-weight neonates: a randomized trial. JAMA 2009;302(13):1421–8.

251. Brubaker JO, Montaner LJ. Role of interleukin-13 in innate and adaptive immunity. Cell Mol Biol (Noisy-le-grand) 2001;47(4):637–51.

252. Koj A. Termination of acute-phase response: role of some cytokines and anti-inflammatory drugs. Gen Pharmacol 1998;31(1):9–18.

253. Sikora JP, Chlebna-Sokol D, Krzyzanska-Oberbek A. Proinflammatory cytokines (IL-6, IL-8), cytokine inhibitors (IL-6sR, sTNFRII) and anti-inflammatory cytokines (IL-10, IL-13) in the pathogenesis of sepsis in newborns and infants. Arch Immunol Ther Exp (Warsz) 2001;49(5):399–404.

254. Opal SM, Esmon CT. Bench-to-bedside review: functional relationships between coagulation and the innate immune response and their respective roles in the pathogenesis of sepsis. Crit Care 2003;7(1):23–38.

255. Trepicchio WL, Bozza M, Pedneault G, et al. Recombinant human IL-11 attenuates the inflammatory response through down-regulation of proinflammatory cytokine release and nitric oxide production. J Immunol 1996;157(8):3627–34.

256. Wang P, Wu P, Siegel MI, et al. Interleukin (IL)-10 inhibits nuclear factor kappa B (NF kappa B) activation in human monocytes. IL-10 and IL-4 suppress cytokine synthesis by different mechanisms. J Biol Chem 1995;270(16):9558–63.

257. Dollner H, Vatten L, Linnebo I, et al. Inflammatory mediators in umbilical plasma from neonates who develop early-onset sepsis. Biol Neonate 2001;80(1):41–7.

258. Cunnington A, Nadel S. New therapies for sepsis. Curr Top Med Chem 2008; 8(7):603–14.

259. Bancalari E. Changes in the pathogenesis and prevention of chronic lung disease of prematurity. Am J Perinatol 2001;18(1):1–9.

260. Chawla D, Agarwal R, Deorari AK, et al. Retinopathy of prematurity. Indian J Pediatr 2008;75(1):73–6.
261. Ikegami M, Carter K, Bishop K, et al. Intratracheal recombinant surfactant protein d prevents endotoxin shock in the newborn preterm lamb. Am J Respir Crit Care Med 2006;173(12):1342–7.
262. Doss M, White MR, Tecle T, et al. Interactions of alpha-, beta-, and theta-defensins with influenza A virus and surfactant protein D. J Immunol 2009;182(12): 7878–87.
263. Roth A, Jensen H, Garly ML, et al. Low birth weight infants and Calmette-Guerin bacillus vaccination at birth: community study from Guinea-Bissau. Pediatr Infect Dis J 2004;23(6):544–50.
264. Lau YL, Chan SY, Turner MW, et al. Mannose-binding protein in preterm infants: developmental profile and clinical significance. Clin Exp Immunol 1995;102(3): 649–54.
265. Fanaroff AA, Korones SB, Wright LL, et al. Incidence, presenting features, risk factors and significance of late onset septicemia in very low birth weight infants. The National Institute of Child Health and Human Development Neonatal Research Network. Pediatr Infect Dis J 1998;17(7):593–8.

Diagnosis and Management of Clinical Chorioamnionitis

Alan T.N. Tita, MD, PhD*, William W. Andrews, PhD, MD

KEYWORDS

• Chorioamnionitis • Infection • Pregnancy • Management

Chorioamnionitis is a common complication of pregnancy associated with significant maternal, perinatal, and long-term adverse outcomes. Adverse maternal outcomes include postpartum infections and sepsis whereas adverse infant outcomes include stillbirth, premature birth, neonatal sepsis, chronic lung disease, and brain injury leading to cerebral palsy and other neurodevelopmental disabilities. Research in the past 2 decades has expanded understanding of the mechanistic links between intra-amniotic infection and preterm delivery as well as morbidities of preterm and term infants. Recent and ongoing clinical research into better methods for diagnosing, treating, and preventing chorioamnionitis is likely to have a substantial impact on short and long-term outcomes in the neonate.

DEFINITION

Chorioamnionitis or intra-amniotic infection is an acute inflammation of the membranes and chorion of the placenta, typically due to ascending polymicrobial bacterial infection in the setting of rupture of membranes (ROM). Chorioamnionitis can occur with intact membranes, and this seems especially common for the very small fastidious genital mycoplasmas, such as *Ureaplasma* species and *Mycoplasma hominis*, found in the lower genital tract of more than 70% of women.[1] Only rarely is hematogeneous spread implicated in chorioamnionitis, as occurs with *Listeria monocytogenes*.[2] When characteristic clinical signs are present, the condition is referred to as clinical chorioamnionitis or clinical intra-amniotic infection. Although there is

Dr Tita was a Women's Reproductive Health Research Scholar supported by Grant No. 5K12 HD01258-09 from the Eunice Kennedy Shriver NICHD, National Institutes of Health at the time of manuscript preparation.
Division of Maternal-Fetal Medicine, Department of Obstetrics and Gynecology, School of Medicine, University of Alabama at Birmingham, 619 19th South, Birmingham, AL 3524, USA
* Corresponding author.
E-mail address: alan.tita@obgyn.uab.edu

significant overlap between clinical and histologic chorioamnionitis, the latter is a more common diagnosis based on pathologic findings on microscopic examination of the placenta that encompasses clinically unapparent (subclinical) chorioamnionitis and clinical chorioamnionitis. Funisitis, also a histopathologic diagnosis, is the extension of infection or inflammation to the umbilical cord. The definition of chorioamnionitis varies according to key diagnostic criteria, which can be clinical (presence of typical clinical findings), microbiologic (culture of microbes from appropriately collected amniotic fluid or chorioamnion), or histopathologic (microscopic evidence of infection or inflammation on examination of the placenta or chorioamnionic specimens).

EPIDEMIOLOGY (INCIDENCE AND RISK FACTORS)

Overall, 1% to 4% of all births in the United States are complicated by chorioamnionitis[2]; however, the frequency of chorioamnionitis varies markedly by diagnostic criteria, specific risk factors, and gestational age.[3-7] Chorioamnionitis (clinical and histologic combined) complicates as many as 40% to 70% of preterm births with premature ROM or spontaneous labor[8] and 1% to 13% of term births.[9-11] Twelve percent of primary cesarean births at term involve clinical chorioamnionitis, with the most common indication for cesarean in these cases being failure to progress usually after ROM.[12]

Several studies have reported risk factors for chorioamnionitis, including longer duration of ROM, prolonged labor, nulliparity, African American ethnicity, internal monitoring of labor, multiple vaginal examinations, meconium-stained amniotic fluid, smoking, alcohol or drug abuse, immunocompromised states, epidural anesthesia, colonization with group B streptococcus (GBS), bacterial vaginosis, sexually transmissible genital infections, and vaginal colonization with ureaplasma.[3-7,13-18] A strong association between untreated GBS bacteriuria and chorioamnionitis may reflect the high concentration of GBS in the genital tract.[19] After adjusting for potential confounding variables and depending on the specific confounders considered, some of the risk factors for chorioamnionitis identified in older studies no longer demonstrate an association in recent studies. Select factors independently associated with chorioamnionitis and their strength of association are summarized in **Table 1**.[3-7,13-17] Contrary to most obstetric conditions, chorioamnionitis in a previous pregnancy may not be associated with an increased risk of chorioamnionitis in a subsequent pregnancy.[20] Although preterm premature rupture of membranes (PPROM) is a major risk factor for clinical chorioamnionitis, together with preterm labor, PPROM frequently is the consequence of subclinical chorioamanionitis.[21]

MECHANISMS OF CHORIOAMNIONITIS AND ITS ASSOCIATED COMPLICATIONS

The pathogenesis of chorioamnionitis is marked by the passage of infectious organisms to the chorioamnion or umbilical cord of the placenta (**Figs. 1** and **2**).[21,22] This passage occurs most commonly by retrograde or ascending infection from the lower genital tract (cervix and vagina) (see **Fig. 1**). Hematogenous/transplacental passage and iatrogenic infection complicating amniocentesis or chorionic villous sampling are less common routes of infection. Anterograde infection from the peritoneum via the fallopian tubes has also been postulated.[22] The presence of infectious agents in the chorioamnion engenders a maternal and fetal inflammatory response characterized by the release of a combination of proinflammatory and inhibitory cytokines and chemokines in the maternal and fetal compartments (see **Fig. 2**). The inflammatory response may produce clinical chorioamnionitis or lead to prostaglandin release, ripening of the cervix, membrane injury, and labor at term or premature birth at earlier gestational ages. Aside from the risk of direct fetal infection and sepsis, the fetal

Table 1
Selected risk factors and their relative risks for chorioamnionitis

Risk Factor	Relative Risk	References
Prolonged ROM (including PPROM)		
≥12 Hours	5.8	13
>18 Hours	6.9	15
Prolonged labor		
Second stage >2 hours	3.7	15
Active labor >12 hours	4.0	14
Multiple digital examinations with ROM		
≥3 Examinations	2 to 5	13,14
Nulliparity	1.8	14
GBS colonization	1.7 to 7.2	14,16,19
Bacterial vaginosis	1.7	17
Alcohol and tobacco use	7.9	15
Meconium-stained amniotic fluid	1.4–2.3	7,14
Internal monitoring	2.0	13
Epidural anesthesia	4.1	15

inflammatory response may induce cerebral white matter injury, which may result in cerebral palsy and other short and long-term neurologic deficits (see **Fig. 2**).

Host defense mechanisms preventing intra-amniotic infection remain poorly elucidated, but specific local host factors likely play an important role. The cervical mucous plug and the placenta and membranes provide a barrier to infection of the amniotic

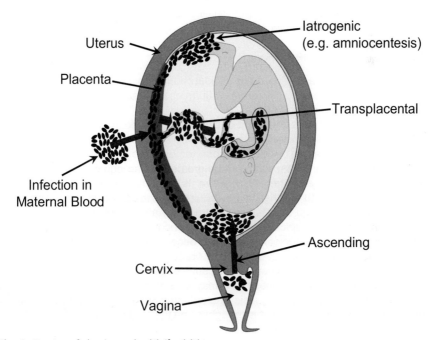

Fig. 1. Routes of chorioamnionitis/funisitis.

Chorioamnionitis/Funisitis

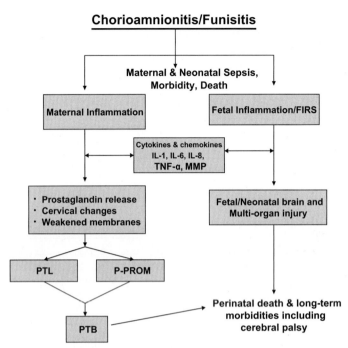

Fig. 2. Pathogenesis of chorioamnionitis: maternal and fetal response and complications. FIRS, fetal inflammatory response syndrome; IL, interleukin; MMP, matrix metalloproteinase; PTB, preterm birth; TNF, tumor necrosis factor.

fluid and fetus. Peroxide-producing lactobacilli in the birth canal may induce changes in the flora that impair the virulence of pathogenic organisms.

CLINICAL SIGNS AND SYMPTOMS

The key clinical findings associated with clinical chorioamnionitis include fever, uterine fundal tenderness, maternal tachycardia (>100/min), fetal tachycardia (>160/min), and purulent or foul amniotic fluid.[2,4]

Maternal fever is the most important clinical sign of chorioamnionitis. Temperature greater than 100.4°F is considered abnormal in pregnancy. Although isolated low-grade fever (<101°F) may be transient in labor, temperature greater than 100.4°F persisting more than 1 hour or any temperature greater than or equal to 101°F warrants evaluation and appropriate intervention. Fever is present in 95% to 100% of cases of clinical chorioamnionitis and typically is required for the diagnosis (discussed later). Fever in the setting of epidural anesthesia, particularly among nulliparous women with prolonged labor (so-called epidural fever), is often encountered and poses a diagnostic quagmire vis-à-vis chorioamnionitis.[23] This is because (1) in addition to fever, the 2 conditions share other major risk factors (low parity and prolonged labor); (2) epidural anesthesia masks signs of chorioamnionitis, such as fundal tenderness; and (3) medications given during epidural anesthesia may induce maternal or fetal tachycardia and, therefore, confound the diagnosis of chorioamnionitis.[24] The exact mechanism of epidural fever is unknown, but it is thought to be the result of epidural sympathetic blockade of thermoregulatory processes, such as sweating.[24] In one study, maternal fever was more common among the epidural group when placental inflammation was present (35% vs 17%) but not in the absence of inflammation (11% vs 9%). This suggests that the pathologic basis for epidural fever is chorioamnionitis.[23] In sum, the concept of epidural fever remains controversial and warrants additional studies.

Maternal tachycardia (>100 beats per minute [bpm]) and fetal tachycardia (>160 bpm) occur frequently in chorioamnionitis, reported in 50% to 80% and 40% to 70% of cases, respectively. Tachycardia may be present in the absence of chorioamnionitis and requires careful assessment for alternative origins. Medications, such as ephedrine, antihistamines, and β-agonists, may raise maternal or fetal heart rate. The combination of maternal fever and maternal or fetal tachycardia is strongly suggestive, however, of intrauterine infection and should be treated accordingly.

Aside from the objective measurements of maternal fever and tachycardia, other signs of chorioamnionitis are highly subjective. Uterine fundal tenderness and a foul odor to the amniotic fluid are reported in only 4% to 25% of cases of chorioamnionitis.[4] Fundal tenderness is difficult to interpret in the context of the pain of labor and may be masked by analgesics, including epidural, or confounded by the pain associated with placental abruption. Purulence or foul odor of amniotic fluid is more likely present with severe or prolonged infection and may be organism-specific but may or may not be appreciated by clinicians.

Chorioamnionitis that is subclinical by definition does not present the clinical signs (discussed previously) but may manifest as preterm labor or, even more commonly, as PPROM. In addition, premature ROM at term (membrane rupture at ≥37 weeks' gestation but before onset of uterine contractions), which occurs in 8% or less of term births, is associated with an increased risk of chorioamnionitis.[25]

DIAGNOSIS OF CHORIOAMNIONITIS
Clinical

As suggested by the name, clinical chorioamnionitis is diagnosed solely based on clinical signs because access to uncontaminated amniotic fluid or placenta for culture is invasive and usually avoided. Typically, the presence of temperature greater than 100.4° is required in addition to 2 other signs (uterine tenderness, maternal or fetal tachycardia, and foul/purulent amniotic fluid).[2,4,26] Individual clinical criteria have variable sensitivity and low specificity for chorioamnionitis (**Table 2**). Because of the low specificity of clinical findings, consideration of other potential sources of fever and other causes of clinical symptoms is essential for the diagnosis of chorioamnionitis.[26] In the absence of other causes, the combination of 3 clinical criteria provides a highly accurate diagnosis of chorioamnionitis. The presence of risk factors of chorioamnionitis, especially ROM, further strengthens the diagnosis.

Laboratory Tests

Findings from laboratory or bedside testing may aid in ruling in or out the diagnosis of chorioamnionitis, particularly when the clinical signs and symptoms are equivocal (see **Table 2**).[2,27–32] Recent research on proteomic analysis for diagnosing intra-amniotic infection see the article by Irina Buhimschi and Catalin Buhimschi elsewhere in this issue for further exploration on this topic.

Complete blood cell count
Maternal leukocytosis (variously defined as white blood cell count >12,000/μL or >15,000/μL) or the presence of a left shift or bandemia (>9%) often supports the diagnosis of chorioamnionitis. Leukocytosis is reported in approximately 70% to 90% of cases of clinical chorioamnionitis. Isolated leukocytosis in the absence of other signs or symptoms, however, is of limited value because it may be induced by several other

Table 2
Clinical and amniotic fluid laboratory diagnosis of chorioamnionitis

Test	Result Suggesting Chorioamnionitis	Comments
Clinical parameters		Generally nonspecific[4]
Fever	Temperature >100.4°F twice or >101°F once	95%–100% sensitive[4]
Maternal tachycardia	>100/min	50%–80% sensitive
Fetal tachycardia	>160/min	40%–70% sensitive
Fundal tenderness	Tenderness on palpation	4%–25% sensitive
Vaginal discharge	Foul-smelling discharge	5%–22% sensitive
Amniotic fluid parameters		
Culture	Microbial growth	Diagnostic gold standard
Gram stain	Bacteria or white blood cells (>6/High Power Field)	24% sensitive, 99% specific[31]
Glucose level	<15 mg/dL	Affected by maternal hyperglycemia 57% sensitive, 74% specific[31]
IL-6	>7.9 ng/mL	81% sensitive, 75% specific[31]
Matrix metalloproteinase	Positive result	90% sensitive and 80% specific[30]
White blood cell count	>30/cubic mm	57% sensitive, 78% specific[31]
Leukocyte esterase	Positive (dipsticks)	85%–91% sensitive, 95%–100% specific[26,32]

conditions, including labor and steroid use. Therefore, routine monitoring of complete blood cell count in high-risk women (eg, those with PPROM) in the absence of clinical signs of chorioamnionitis is not useful.

Other blood tests

Other laboratory parameters, including high levels of C-reactive protein (CRP), lipopo-lysacharide-binding protein, soluble intercellular adhesion molecule 1, and interleukin (IL)-6, are associated with a higher risk of chorioamnionitis in the setting of PPROM or preterm delivery.[33–37] Their usefulness for the diagnosis or prediction of choriamnioni-tis, however, as part of routine clinical practice is not established.

Amniotic fluid testing

Tests on amniotic fluid, usually obtained by amniocentesis, have been used for the diagnosis of chorioamnionitis (see **Table 2**).[26,30–32] Culture of amniotic fluid is the most reliable test but is of limited use because culture results may not be available for up to 3 days. In addition, because of the invasive nature of the procedure, amnio-centesis is not performed in the majority of cases of chorioamnionitis, which occur during labor. Some clinicians use amniocentesis to confirm clinically suspected cho-rioamnionitis to determine whether or not preterm delivery is warranted (thus avoiding iatrogenic prematurity). Amniocentesis is also used in some centers to identify subclin-ical chorioamnionitis in women with spontaneous preterm labor and preterm ROM at early gestational ages. The value of this practice, however, has recently been questioned.[38]

Histologic chorioamnionitis captures subclinical and clinical chorioamnionitis; thus, it is not surprising that overall histologic chorioamnionitis at term is up to 3 times as frequent as clinical chorioamnionitis confirmed by amniotic fluid culture.[39] This is in part because cultures for genital mycoplasmas, the most common organisms associated with chorioamnionitis, are not very sensitive. Subclinical chorioamnionitis and noninfectious inflammation also contribute to this discrepancy. Histologic chorioamnionitis is defined by the presence of acute histologic changes on examination of the amnionic membrane and chorion of the placenta, and funisitis is characterized by leukocyte infiltration of the umbilical vessel wall or Wharton jelly.[8] Acute histologic changes are typically characterized according to the number of polymorphonuclear leukocytes per high power field or by detailed systems of staging/grading involving documentation of polymorphonuclear leukocyte location, density, and degeneration to estimate intensity and progression of chorioamnionitis.[40] Consequently, depending on the criteria used and maternal characteristics (including ethnicity and type of labor), the prevalence of chorioamnionitis based on placental pathology varies widely. Using varying thresholds of polymorphonuclear leukocytes per high-power field, the prevalence ranged from 7% to 85% in term and 4% to 63% in preterm deliveries in one study.[40] Overall, histologic chorioamnionitis is a sensitive (83%–100%) but not a specific (23%–52%) predictor of chorioamnionitis when the diagnosis is based on culture-positive amniotic fluid.[41] Alternatively, clinical chorioamnionitis is not uniformly confirmed on pathologic evaluation. In one study, only 62% of women with clinically diagnosed chorioamnionitis had histologic evidence of chorioamnionitis, leading to the speculation that noninflammatory causes, such as epidural fever and abruption, accounted for some of the cases.[42] For these reasons, placental pathology should be performed to confirm suspected chorioamnionitis even if amniotic fluid culture is negative. The pathologic finding of funisitis (inflammation of the umbilical cord) is even more concerning than chorioamnionitis alone because it represents a fetal response to infection. Although chorioamnionitis is present in nearly all cases of funisitis, funisitis is present in only up to 60% of cases of chorioamnionitis.[43]

Organisms Causing Chorioamnionitis

Chorioamnionitis is a polymicrobial infection most often due to ascending genital microbes[2,44]; more than 65% of positive amniotic fluid cultures involve 2 or more organisms. The genital mycoplasmas, *Ureaplasma urealyticum* and *M hominis* (genital mycoplasmas), constitute the most frequent microbes, occurring in up to 47% and 30%, respectively, of cases of culture-confirmed chorioamnionitis.[44,45] Their role in the pathogenesis of chorioamnionitis and neonatal complications, once controversial, is increasingly accepted.[46] These fastidious organisms provoke a robust inflammatory reaction affecting maternal and fetal compartments, particularly in preterm gestations.[45–47] They are commonly isolated from amniotic fluid in the setting of preterm birth or premature ROM with or without clinical chorioamnionitis.[46] Although genital mycoplasmas are found in the lower genital tract (vagina or cervix) of more than 70% of women, their presence in the upper genital tract (uterus or fallopian tubes) and chorioamnion of pregnant women is rare (<5%) in the absence of labor or ROM.[46–48]

Other common isolates in women with chorioamnionitis include anaerobes, such as *Gardnerella vaginalis* (25%) and bacteroides (30%), and aerobes, including GBS (15%) and gram-negative rods, including *Escherichia coli* (8%).[44] These organisms are commonly part of the vaginal flora (especially in women with bacterial vaginosis) or the enteric flora (*E coli* and other gram-negative rods, enterococci, and anaerobes). An entity of aerobic vaginitis (distinguished from bacterial vaginosis in that it represents a strong host immune response to aerobic vaginal flora typically comprised of GBS and *E coli*) has been associated with ascending chorioamnionitis, PPROM, and preterm birth.[49] Occasionally, chorioamnionitis is the result of hematogenous spread of bacterial or viral infection to the placenta. *Listeria monocytogenes* infection of the fetus, which presents a pattern of early-onset and late-onset neonatal sepsis similar to GBS, is presumed due to a hematogenous route rather than an ascending infection.[50] More research is needed to clarify the significance of individual microbes and their potential interactions in the pathogenesis of chorioamnionitis. For clinical decision making and management, however, knowing the exact organisms involved in chorioamnionitis is not generally useful.

Other tests on amniotic fluid (see **Table 2**) are limited in their overall predictive abilities for chorioamnionitis, although the tests for IL-6 and matrix metalloproteinase are more promising because of higher sensitivity and specificity.[30–32] The use of vaginal pool fluid after premature ROM for these assessments (eg, glucose level) is rudimentary and warrants further investigation.[51]

Differential Diagnosis

Several other conditions should be considered in the differential diagnosis of chorioamnionitis. In intrapartum patients with epidural and low-grade fever without tachycardia (maternal or fetal) or other clinical signs of intrauterine inflammation, epidural-associated fever is a strong consideration. Extrauterine infections can cause fever and abdominal pain, during or in absence of labor, including urinary tract infection (pyelonephritis), influenza, appendicitis, and pneumonia. Noninfectious conditions associated with abdominal pain (usually in absence of fever) include thrombophlebitis, round ligament pain, colitis, connective tissue disorders, and placental abruption.

Complications of Chorioamnionitis

Clinical chorioamnionitis carries adverse consequences affecting women and their infants (see **Fig. 2**).

Maternal Complications

Chorioamnionitis leads to a 2- to 3-fold increased risk for cesarean delivery and a 2- to 4-fold increase in endomyometritis, wound infection, pelvic abscess, bacteremia, and postpartum hemorrhage.[12,52–55] The increase in postpartum hemorrhage seems due to dysfunctional uterine muscle contractions as a result of inflammation.[53,54] Ten percent of women with chorioamnionitis have positive blood cultures (bacteremia) most commonly involving GBS and *E coli*.[2] Fortunately, however, septic shock, disseminated intravascular coagululation, adult respiratory distress syndrome, and maternal death are only rarely encountered.[56]

Fetal Complications

Fetal exposure to infection may lead to fetal death, neonatal sepsis, and many other postnatal complications (see **Fig. 2**). The fetal response to infection—termed, *fetal inflammatory response syndrome* (FIRS)—may cause or aggravate some of these complications. FIRS is the fetal counterpart of the systemic inflammatory response syndrome (SIRS). Because clinical parameters analogous to those defining SIRS are difficult to ascertain in the fetus, FIRS was originally defined by elevation of cord blood IL-6 in the setting of preterm labor and PPROM[57,58] but can also occur in term gestations. The histopathologic hallmarks of FIRS are funisitis and chorionic vasculitis.[59] FIRS is now recognized as representing the fetal immune response to infection or injury mediated by the release of cytokines and chemokines, such as interleukins, tumor necrosis factor α, CRP, and matrix melloproteinases.[58] FIRS has also been linked to preterm labor culminating in perinatal death (see **Fig. 2**) and is associated, particularly in preterm neonates, with multiorgan injury, including chronic lung disease, periventricular leukomalacia, and cerebral palsy,[60–62] Although FIRS may occur in the setting of noninfectious inflammation, its magnitude tends to be significantly more robust with documented infection.[63] Although somewhat controversial, fetal exposure to genital mycoplasmas (*U urealyticum* and *M hominis*) has been associated with a fetal and neonatal SIRS, pneumonia and bronchopulmonary dysplasia.[64–67]

Neonatal and Long-Term Complications

Neonates exposed to intrauterine infection and inflammation may show adverse effects at or shortly after birth. Adverse outcomes may include perinatal death, asphyxia, early-onset neonatal sepsis, septic shock, pneumonia, intraventricular hemorrhage (IVH), cerebral white matter damage, and long-term disability, including cerebral palsy.[9,68–72] In one study of term infants, neonatal pneumonia, sepsis, and perinatal death did not occur in the absence of chorioamnionitis but occurred, respectively, in 4%, 8%, and 2% of term deliveries associated with chorioamnionitis. In this study, respiratory distress occurred in 2% of term infants in absence of chorioamnionitis and 20% when chorioamnionitis was present.[68] Preterm infants have an even higher rate of complications of chorioamnionitis than term infants, including perinatal death (25% vs 6% preterm vs term), neonatal sepsis (28% vs 6%), pneumonia (20% vs 3%), grades 3 or 4 IVH (24% vs 8%), and respiratory distress (62% vs 35%).[69] Overall, chorioamnionitis is associated with up to 40% of cases of early-onset neonatal sepsis. Chorioamnionitis is also well established as a risk factor for long-term neurodevelopmental disability, especially when it occurs before term.[2,73–77] In term and near-term infants it is associated with a 4-fold increase in the frequency of cerebral palsy.[74,75]

Management of Chorioamnionitis

Prompt initiation of antibiotic therapy is essential to prevent maternal and fetal complications in the setting of clinical chorioamnionitis.[2] Time to delivery after institution of antibiotic therapy has been shown to not affect morbidities; therefore, cesarean section to expedite delivery is not indicated for chorioamnionitis unless there are other obstetric indications.[12,52,76]

Antibiotics

Evidence from randomized trials and observational studies demonstrate that immediate intrapartum use of broad-spectrum antibiotics significantly reduces maternal and fetal complications of chorioamnionitis.[77–81] The frequency of neonatal sepsis is reduced by up to 80% with intrapartum antibiotic treatment.[78,79] In a small randomized trial, neonatal sepsis occurred in none of 26 deliveries with intrapartum use of antibiotics compared with 21% of the 19 infants treated immediately postpartum.[77]

The optimal antibiotic regimen for treatment of clinical chorioamnionitis has not been well studied and current recommendations are based largely on clinical consensus.[81] Intravenous administration of ampicillin every 6 hours and gentamicin every 8 to 24 hours until delivery is the typical regimen.[81,82] If cesarean delivery is performed, clindamycin every 8 hours (or metronidazole) is often added for anaerobic coverage. Optimal treatment should also include administration of a single intravenous additional dose of antibiotics after delivery (<5% failure rate)[83]; further oral antibiotic treatment is not beneficial in most cases.[84]

Although genital mycoplasmas are the most commonly isolated organisms associated with chorioamnionitis, the standard antibiotic regimens used for clinical chorioamnionitis do not provide optimal coverage against these organisms. Clindamycin does provide coverage against *M hominis* but none of the 3 standard antibiotics is effective against ureaplasma species, which is the most common group associated with infection. The standard regimen effectively treats maternal infection (>95% success rate) and reduces neonatal sepsis, and there are currently no published trials suggesting that specific coverage against ureaplasma (with macrolide antibiotics) provides additional benefits in the setting of chorioamnionitis.

Supportive measures

Supportive measures include the use of antipyretics (acetaminophen). This is particularly important during the intrapartum period because fetal acidosis in the setting of fever is associated with a marked increase in the incidence of neonatal encephalopathy.[85] Maternal fever even in the absence of documented fetal acidosis is associated with adverse neonatal outcomes, in particular neonatal encephalopathy, although it is unclear to what extent the etiology of the fever rather than the fever itself is causative.[86] Treating intrapartum fever with antipyretics may also be helpful in reducing fetal tachycardia, thereby avoiding the tendency to perform cesarean for a nonreassuring fetal status.

Prevention of Chorioamnionitis

Expectant management of PPROM is a major cause of clinical chorioamnionitis—up to 70% of those who subsequently develop contractions or labor have chorioamnionitis.[8] Prophylactic or latency antibiotics, typically ampicillin and erythromycin, have been demonstrated in large clinical trials (ORACLE I and II) and systematic reviews as conferring benefits, including reduction in a primary composite of neonatal death, chronic lung disease, or major cerebral abnormality on ultrasound. Antibiotics also reduce the incidence of clinical or pathologic chorioamnionitis and neonatal sepsis and prolong time to delivery among women with preterm ROM managed expectantly but not among those in active preterm labor with intact membranes (in whom maternal infection was reduced).[87–89] Amoxicillin/clavulanate antibiotic combinations should be avoided for this indication because of a potential association with an increased risk of necrotizing enterocolitis.[87–89] Furthermore, in the ORACLE II trial, the use of antibiotics for women with spontaneous preterm labor with intact membranes was associated with an unexpected increase in cerebral palsy in infants.[90,91] The findings were limited by potential selection bias (only 70% followed-up) and use of maternal report to ascertain outcomes (no direct examination). The investigators speculated that the findings could be due to chance or to maintenance of the fetus in a milieu with suppressed (not eradicated) subclinical infection given the low dose and oral route of antibiotics.[90,91] Another large trial conducted by the National Institute of Child Health and Human Development Maternal-Fetal Medicine Units Network in the late 1990s suggested a benefit of erythromycin in reducing adverse perinatal outcomes, including perinatal death and morbidity and maternal infection.[92] No long-term follow-up data from this study are reported. The usual standard in the United States, therefore, remains the administration of broad-spectrum antibiotics, typically involving a macrolide (erythromycin or azithromycin) and ampicillin for 7 to 10 days via intravenous (2 days) followed by oral routes.[93] Induction of labor and delivery for PPROM after 34 weeks' gestation is recommended because, compared with expectant management, expeditious delivery is associated with reduced maternal infection and need for neonatal intensive care without any increase in perinatal morbidity and mortality.[25,94,95] There is currently wide variation in practice, however, and additional trials are ongoing to firmly establish the benefit of induction of labor before 37 weeks in cases of PPROM.[25,96–98] In the setting of prolonged ROM (>18 hours) at term, prophylactic antibiotics are not indicated if the mother is not colonized with GBS; however, the CDC recommends starting GBS prophylaxis if GBS status is unknown.[99] In one randomized trial, the use of intrapartum prophylactic antibiotics (ampicillin/sulbactam) for meconium-stained fluid was associated with a reduction in the risk of chorioamnionitis.[100]

SUMMARY

Chorioamnionitis is a common infection of pregnancy, typically occurring in the setting of prolonged ROM or labor. It may be diagnosed clinically, based on signs, such as maternal fever; microbiologically, based on amniotic fluid culture obtained by amniocentesis; or by histopathologic examination of the placenta and umbilical cord. Chorioamnionitis is associated with postpartum maternal infections and potentially devastating fetal complications, including premature birth, neonatal sepsis, and cerebral palsy. The main preventative strategy is administration of antibiotics to women with PPROM, which reduces the incidence of clinical chorioamnionitis, prolongs the time to delivery, and improves neonatal outcomes. Optimal management of clinical chorioamnionitis includes antibiotic therapy and delivery. Shortening the time between diagnosis and delivery, however, by performance of cesarean section in the setting of broad-spectrum antibiotic administration has been shown not to improve outcomes.

REFERENCES

1. Eschenbach DA. Ureaplasma urealyticum and premature birth. Clin Infect Dis 1993;17(Suppl 1):S100–6.
2. Gibbs RS, Duff P. Progress in pathogenesis and management of clinical intraamniotic infection. Am J Obstet Gynecol 1991;164:1317.
3. Soper DE, Mayhall CG, Dalton HP. Risk factors for intraamniotic infection: a prospective epidemiologic study. Am J Obstet Gynecol 1989;161:562.
4. Newton ER. Chorioamnionitis and intraamniotic infection. Clin Obstet Gynecol 1993;36:795.
5. Newton ER, Prihoda TJ, Gibbs RS. Logistic regression analysis of risk factors for intra-amniotic infection. Obstet Gynecol 1989;73:571.
6. Piper JM, Newton ER, Berkus MD, et al. Meconium: a marker for peripartum infection. Obstet Gynecol 1998;91:741.
7. Tran SH, Caughey AB, Musci TJ. Meconium-stained amniotic fluid is associated with puerperal infections. Am J Obstet Gynecol 2003;189:746.
8. Yoon BH, Romero R, Moon JB, et al. Clinical significance of intra-amniotic inflammation in patients with preterm labor and intact membranes. Am J Obstet Gynecol 2001;185(5):1130–6.
9. Alexander JM, McIntire DM, Leveno KJ. Chorioamnionitis and the prognosis for term infants. Obstet Gynecol 1999;94(2):274–8.
10. Seong HS, Lee SE, Kang JH, et al. The frequency of microbial invasion of the amniotic cavity and histologic chorioamnionitis in women at term with intact membranes in the presence or absence of labor. Am J Obstet Gynecol 2008; 199(4):375.e1–5.

11. Blume HK, Li CI, Loch CM, et al. Intrapartum fever and chorioamnionitis as risks for encephalopathy in term newborns: a case-control study. Dev Med Child Neurol 2008;50(1):19–24.

12. Rouse DJ, Landon M, Leveno KJ, et al. The Maternal-Fetal Medicine Units cesarean registry: chorioamnionitis at term and its duration-relationship to outcomes. Am J Obstet Gynecol 2004;191:211.

13. Soper DE, Mayhall CG, Froggatt JW. Characterization and control of intraamniotic infection in an urban teaching hospital. Am J Obstet Gynecol 1996;175(2):304–9 [discussion: 309–10].

14. Seaward PG, Hannah ME, Myhr TL, et al. International Multicentre Term Prelabor Rupture of Membranes Study: evaluation of predictors of clinical chorioamnionitis and postpartum fever in patients with prelabor rupture of membranes at term. Am J Obstet Gynecol 1997;177(5):1024–9.

15. Rickert VI, Wiemann CM, Hankins GD, et al. Prevalence and risk factors of chorioamnionitis among adolescents. Obstet Gynecol 1998;92(2):254–7.

16. Yancey MK, Duff P, Clark P, et al. Peripartum infection associated with vaginal group B streptococcal colonization. Obstet Gynecol 1994;84(5):816–9.

17. Newton ER, Piper J, Peairs W. Bacterial vaginosis and intraamniotic infection. Am J Obstet Gynecol 1997;176(3):672–7.

18. Abele-Horn M, Peters J, Genzel-Boroviczény O, et al. Vaginal Ureaplasma urealyticum colonization: influence on pregnancy outcome and neonatal morbidity. Infection 1997;25(5):286–91.

19. Anderson BL, Simhan HN, Simons KM, et al. Untreated asymptomatic group B streptococcal bacteriuria early in pregnancy and chorioamnionitis at delivery. Am J Obstet Gynecol 2007;196(6):524.e1–5.

20. Dinsmoor MJ, Gibbs RS. Previous intra-amniotic infection as a risk factor for subsequent peripartal uterine infections. Obstet Gynecol 1989;74(3 Pt 1):299–301.

21. Goldenberg RL, Andrews WW, Hauth JC. Choriodecidual infection and preterm birth. Nutr Rev 2002;60(5 Pt 2):S19–25.

22. Fahey JO. Clinical management of intra-amniotic infection and chorioamnionitis: a review of the literature. J Midwifery Womens Health 2008;53(3):227–35.

23. Dashe JS, Rogers BB, McIntire DD, et al. Epidural analgesia and intrapartum fever: placental findings. Obstet Gynecol 1999;93(3):341–4.

24. Apantaku O, Mulik V. Maternal intra-partum fever. J Obstet Gynaecol 2007;27(1):12–5.

25. ACOG Committee on Practice Bulletins-Obstetrics. ACOG Practice Bulletin No. 80: premature rupture of membranes. Clinical management guidelines for obstetrician-gynecologists. Obstet Gynecol 2007;109(4):1007–19.

26. Riggs JW, Blanco JD. Pathophysiology, diagnosis, and management of intra-amniotic infection. Semin Perinatol 1998;22(4):251–9.

27. Gomez R, Ghezzi F, Romero R, et al. Premature labor and intra-amniotic infection. Clinical aspects and role of the cytokines in diagnosis and pathophysiology. Clin Perinatol 1995;22:281.

28. Harirah H, Donia SE, Hsu CD. Amniotic fluid matrix metalloproteinase-9 and interleukin-6 in predicting intra-amniotic infection. Obstet Gynecol 2002;99:80.

29. Gauthier DW, Meyer WJ. Comparison of gram stain, leukocyte esterase activity, and amniotic fluid glucose concentration in predicting amniotic fluid culture results in preterm premature rupture of membranes. Am J Obstet Gynecol 1992;167:1092.

30. Kim KW, Romero R, Park HS, et al. A rapid matrix metalloproteinase-8 bedside test for the detection of intraamniotic inflammation in women with preterm premature rupture of membranes. Am J Obstet Gynecol 2007;197(3):292.e1–5.
31. Romero R, Yoon BH, Mazor M, et al. A comparative study of the diagnostic performance of amniotic fluid glucose, white blood cell count, interleukin-6, and gram stain in the detection of microbial invasion in patients with preterm premature rupture of membranes. Am J Obstet Gynecol 1993;169(4): 839–51.
32. Hoskins IA, Marks F, Ordorica SA, et al. Leukocyte esterase activity in amniotic fluid: normal values during pregnancy. Am J Perinatol 1990;7(2):130–2.
33. Maeda K, Matsuzaki N, Fuke S, et al. Value of the maternal interleukin 6 level for determination of histologic chorioamnionitis in preterm delivery. Gynecol Obstet Invest 1997;43(4):225–31.
34. Steinborn A, Sohn C, Scharf A, et al. Serum intercellular adhesion molecule-1 levels and histologic chorioamnionitis. Obstet Gynecol 2000;95(5):671–6.
35. Zou L, Zhang H, Zhu J, et al. The value of the soluable intercellular adhesion molecule-1 levels in matermal serum for determination of occult chorioamnionitis in premature rupture of membranes. J Huazhong Univ Sci Technolog Med Sci 2004;24(2):154–7.
36. Wu HC, Shen CM, Wu YY, et al. Subclinical histologic chorioamnionitis and related clinical and laboratory parameters in preterm deliveries. Pediatr Neonatol 2009;50(5):217–21.
37. van de Laar R, van der Ham DP, Oei SG, et al. Accuracy of C-reactive protein determination in predicting chorioamnionitis and neonatal infection in pregnant women with premature rupture of membranes: a systematic review. Eur J Obstet Gynecol Reprod Biol 2009;147(2):124–9.
38. Andrews WW, Cliver SP, Biasini F, et al. Early preterm birth: association between in utero exposure to acute inflammation and severe neurodevelopmental disability at 6 years of age. Am J Obstet Gynecol 2008;198(4):466.e1–466.e11.
39. Dong Y, St. Clair PJ, Ramzy I, et al. A microbiologic and clinical study of placental inflammation at term. Obstet Gynecol 1987;70:175.
40. Holzman C, Lin X, Senagore P, et al. Histologic chorioamnionitis and preterm delivery. Am J Epidemiol 2007;166(7):786–94.
41. Pettker CM, Buhimschi IA, Magloire LK, et al. Value of placental microbial evaluation in diagnosing intra-amniotic infection. Obstet Gynecol 2007;109(3):739–49.
42. Smulian JC, Shen-Schwarz S, Vintzileos AM, et al. Clinical chorioamnionitis and histologic placental inflammation. Obstet Gynecol 1999;94:1000.
43. Holcroft CJ, Askin FB, Patra A, et al. Are histopathologic chorioamnionitis and funisitis associated with metabolic acidosis in the preterm fetus? Am J Obstet Gynecol 2004;191(6):2010–5.
44. Sperling RS, Newton E, Gibbs RS. Intraamniotic infection in low-birth-weight infants. J Infect Dis 1988;157(1):113–7.
45. Waites KB, Katz B, Schelonka RL. Mycoplasmas and ureaplasmas as neonatal pathogens. Clin Microbiol Rev 2005;18(4):757–89.
46. Cassell GH, Waites KB, Watson HL, et al. Ureaplasma urealyticum intrauterine infection: role in prematurity and disease in newborns. Clin Microbiol Rev 1993;6(1):69–87.
47. Yoon BH, Romero R, Park JS, et al. Microbial invasion of the amniotic cavity with Ureaplasma urealyticum is associated with a robust host response in fetal, amniotic, and maternal compartments. Am J Obstet Gynecol 1998;179(5):1254–60.

48. Witt A, Berger A, Gruber CJ, et al. Increased intrauterine frequency of Ureaplasma urealyticum in women with preterm labor and preterm premature rupture of the membranes and subsequent cesarean delivery. Am J Obstet Gynecol 2005; 193(5):1663–9.
49. Donders GG, Vereecken A, Bosmans E, et al. Definition of a type of abnormal vaginal flora that is distinct from bacterial vaginosis: aerobic vaginitis. BJOG 2002;109(1):34–43.
50. Silver HM. Listeriosis during pregnancy. Obstet Gynecol Surv 1998;53(12): 737–40.
51. Buhimschi CS, Sfakianaki AK, Hamar BG, et al. A low vaginal "pool" amniotic fluid glucose measurement is a predictive but not a sensitive marker for infection in women with preterm premature rupture of membranes. Am J Obstet Gynecol 2006;194:309.
52. Hauth JC, Gilstrap LC 3rd, Hankins GD, et al. Term maternal and neonatal complications of acute chorioamnionitis. Obstet Gynecol 1985;66:59.
53. Mark SP, Croughan-Minihane MS, Kilpatrick SJ. Chorioamnionitis and uterine function. Obstet Gynecol 2000;95:909.
54. Satin AJ, Maberry MC, Leveno KJ, et al. Chorioamnionitis: a harbinger of dystocia. Obstet Gynecol 1992;79:913.
55. Newton ER, Schroeder BC, Knape KG, et al. Epidural analgesia and uterine function. Obstet Gynecol 1995;85:749.
56. Moretti M, Sibai BM. Maternal and perinatal outcome of expectant management of premature rupture of membranes in the midtrimester. Am J Obstet Gynecol 1988;159(2):390–6.
57. Gomez R, Romero R, Ghezzi F, et al. The fetal inflammatory response syndrome. Am J Obstet Gynecol 1998;179(1):194–202.
58. Gotsch F, Romero R, Kusanovic JP, et al. The fetal inflammatory response syndrome. Clin Obstet Gynecol 2007;50(3):652–83.
59. Pacora P, Chaiworapongsa T, Maymon E, et al. Funisitis and chorionic vasculitis: the histological counterpart of the fetal inflammatory response syndrome. J Matern Fetal Neonatal Med 2002;11:18–25.
60. Yoon BH, Romero R, Kim KS, et al. A systemic fetal inflammatory response and the development of bronchopulmonary dysplasia. Am J Obstet Gynecol 1999; 181(4):773–9.
61. Mittendorf R, Covert R, Montag AG, et al. Special relationships between fetal inflammatory response syndrome and bronchopulmonary dysplasia in neonates. J Perinat Med 2005;33(5):428–34.
62. Bashiri A, Burstein E, Mazor M. Cerebral palsy and fetal inflammatory response syndrome: a review. J Perinat Med 2006;34(1):5–12.
63. Lee SE, Romero R, Jung H, et al. The intensity of the fetal inflammatory response in intraamniotic inflammation with and without microbial invasion of the amniotic cavity. Am J Obstet Gynecol 2007;197(3):294.e1–6.
64. Aaltonen R, Vahlberg T, Lehtonen L, et al. Ureaplasma urealyticum: no independent role in the pathogenesis of bronchopulmonary dysplasia. Acta Obstet Gynecol Scand 2006;85(11):1354–9.
65. Aaltonen R, Heikkinen J, Vahlberg T, et al. Local inflammatory response in choriodecidua induced by Ureaplasma urealyticum. BJOG 2007;114(11):1432–5.
66. Goldenberg RL, Andrews WW, Goepfert AR, et al. The Alabama Preterm Birth Study: umbilical cord blood Ureaplasma urealyticum and Mycoplasma hominis cultures in very preterm newborn infants. Am J Obstet Gynecol 2008; 198(1):43.e1–5.

67. Jacobsson B, Aaltonen R, Rantakokko-Jalava K, et al. Quantification of Urea-plasma urealyticum DNA in the amniotic fluid from patients in PTL and pPROM and its relation to inflammatory cytokine levels. Acta Obstet Gynecol Scand 2009;88(1):63–70.

68. Yoder PR, Gibbs RS, Blanco JD, et al. A prospective, controlled study of maternal and perinatal outcome after intra-amniotic infection at term. Am J Obstet Gynecol 1983;145:695.

69. Morales WJ, Washington SR 3rd, Lazar AJ. The effect of chorioamnionitis on perinatal outcome in preterm gestation. J Perinatol 1987;7:105.

70. Lau J, Magee F, Qiu Z, et al. Chorioamnionitis with a fetal inflammatory response is associated with higher neonatal mortality, morbidity, and resource use than chorioamnionitis displaying a maternal inflammatory response only. Am J Obstet Gynecol 2005;193:708.

71. Aziz N, Cheng YW, Caughey AB. Neonatal outcomes in the setting of preterm premature rupture of membranes complicated by chorioamnionitis. J Matern Fetal Neonatal Med 2009;22:780–4.

72. Ramsey PS, Lieman JM, Brumfield CG, et al. Chorioamnionitis increases neonatal morbidity in pregnancies complicated by preterm premature rupture of membranes. Am J Obstet Gynecol 2005;192:1162.

73. Cornette L. Fetal and neonatal inflammatory response and adverse outcome. Semin Fetal Neonatal Med 2004;9:459.

74. Wu YW, Escobar GJ, Grether JK, et al. Chorioamnionitis and cerebral palsy in term and near-term infants. JAMA 2003;290:2677.

75. Nelson KB, Ellenberg JH. Antecedents of cerebral palsy. I. Univariate analysis of risks. Am J Dis Child 1985;139:1031.

76. Gilstrap LC 3rd, Cox SM. Acute chorioamnionitis. Obstet Gynecol Clin North Am 1989;16:373.

77. Gibbs RS, Dinsmoor MJ, Newton ER, et al. A randomized trial of intrapartum versus immediate postpartum treatment of women with intra-amniotic infection. Obstet Gynecol 1988;72:823.

78. Sperling RS, Ramamurthy RS, Gibbs RS. A comparison of intrapartum versus immediate postpartum treatment of intra-amniotic infection. Obstet Gynecol 1987;70:861.

79. Gilstrap LC 3rd, Leveno KJ, Cox SM, et al. Intrapartum treatment of acute chorioamnionitis: impact on neonatal sepsis. Am J Obstet Gynecol 1988;159:579.

80. Maberry MC, Gilstrap LC 3rd. Intrapartum antibiotic therapy for suspected intra-amniotic infection: impact on the fetus and neonate. Clin Obstet Gynecol 1991; 34:345.

81. Hopkins L, Smaill F. Antibiotic regimens for management of intraamniotic infection. Cochrane Database Syst Rev 2002;3:CD003254.

82. Locksmith GJ, Chin A, Vu T, et al. High compared with standard gentamicin dosing for chorioamnionitis: a comparison of maternal and fetal serum drug levels. Obstet Gynecol 2005;105:473.

83. Edwards RK, Duff P. Single additional dose postpartum therapy for women with chorioamniotis. Obstet Gynecol 2003;102:957.

84. Dinsmoor MJ, Newton ER, Gibbs RS. A randomized, double-blind, placebo-controlled trial of oral antibiotic therapy following intravenous antibiotic therapy for postpartum endometritis. Obstet Gynecol 1991;77:60.

85. Impey LW, Greenwood CE, Black RS, et al. The relationship between intrapartum maternal fever and neonatal acidosis as risk factors for neonatal encephalopathy. Am J Obstet Gynecol 2008;198:49.

86. Impey L, Greenwood C, MacQuillan K, et al. Fever in labour and neonatal encephalopathy: a prospective cohort study. BJOG 2001;108(6):594–7.

87. Kenyon SL, Taylor DJ, Tarnow-Mordi W, ORACLE Collaborative Group. Broad-spectrum antibiotics for preterm, prelabour rupture of fetal membranes: the ORACLE I randomised trial. ORACLE Collaborative Group. Lancet 2001; 357(9261):979–88.

88. Kenyon SL, Taylor DJ, Tarnow-Mordi W, ORACLE Collaborative Group. Broad-spectrum antibiotics for spontaneous preterm labour: the ORACLE II randomised trial. ORACLE Collaborative Group. Lancet 2001;357(9261):989–94.

89. Kenyon S, Boulvain M, Neilson J. Antibiotics for preterm rupture of the membranes: a systematic review. Obstet Gynecol 2004;104(5 Pt 1):1051–7.

90. Kenyon S, Pike K, Jones DR, et al. Childhood outcomes after prescription of antibiotics to pregnant women with preterm rupture of the membranes: 7-year follow-up of the ORACLE I trial. Lancet 2008;372:1310–8.

91. Kenyon S, Pike K, Jones DR, et al. Childhood outcomes after prescription of antibiotics to pregnant women with spontaneous preterm labour: 7-year follow-up of the ORACLE II trial. Lancet 2008;372:1319–27.

92. Mercer BM, Miodovnik M, Thurnau GR, et al. Antibiotic therapy for reduction of infant morbidity after preterm premature rupture of the membranes. A randomized controlled trial. National Institute of Child Health and Human Development Maternal-Fetal Medicine Units Network. JAMA 1997;278(12):989–95.

93. American College of Obstetricians and Gynecologists. Practice bulletin number 47, October 2003: prophylactic antibiotics in labor and delivery. Obstet Gynecol 2003;102(4):875–82.

94. Simhan HN, Canavan TP. Preterm premature rupture of membranes: diagnosis, evaluation and management strategies. BJOG 2005;112(Suppl 1):32–7.

95. Dare MR, Middleton P, Crowther CA, et al. Planned early birth versus expectant management (waiting) for prelabour rupture of membranes at term (37 weeks or more). Cochrane Database Syst Rev 2006;1:CD005302.

96. Ramsey PS, Nuthalapaty FS, Lu G, et al. Contemporary management of preterm premature rupture of membranes (PPROM): a survey of maternal-fetal medicine providers. Am J Obstet Gynecol 2004;191(4):1497–502.

97. Morris JM, Roberts CL, Crowther CA, et al. Protocol for the immediate delivery versus expectant care of women with preterm prelabour rupture of the membranes close to term (PPROMT) Trial [ISRCTN44485060]. BMC Pregnancy Childbirth 2006;6:9.

98. van der Ham DP, Nijhuis JG, Mol BW, et al. Induction of labour versus expectant management in women with preterm prelabour rupture of membranes between 34 and 37 weeks (the PPROMEXIL-trial). BMC Pregnancy Childbirth 2007;7:11.

99. Schrag S, Gorwitz R, Fultz-Butts K, et al. Prevention of perinatal group B streptococcal disease. Revised guidelines from the CDC. MMWR 2002;51(No. RR-11): 1–22.

100. Adair CD, Ernest JM, Sanchez-Ramos L, et al. Meconium-stained amniotic fluid-associated infectious morbidity: a randomized, double-blind trial of ampicillin-sulbactam prophylaxis. Obstet Gynecol 1996;88(2):216–20.

The Role of Proteomics in the Diagnosis of Chorioamnionitis and Early-Onset Neonatal Sepsis

Irina A. Buhimschi, MD[a],*, Catalin S. Buhimschi, MD[b]

KEYWORDS

- Newborn • Sepsis • Biomarkers • Proteomics
- DAMPs • RAGE

PROTEOMICS
General Principles

Proteomics is a newly developed field of research that has emerged to complement genomics. Although several definitions are available, most scientists agree that proteomics studies provide insight into the functional expression of proteins present in a tissue, cell, or organism at a given moment. Moreover, there is a general perception that data derived from proteomics experimentation are more clinically relevant and easier to translate into diagnostic tools and therapies than genomics results, which rely on DNA or mRNA studies.

Part of this work was supported from National Institutes of Heath/Eunice Kennedy Shriver National Institute of Child Health and Human Development Grant RO1 HD 047321 (IAB) and March of Dimes Basil O'Connor Award (IAB). IAB and CSB are co-inventors on patent applications regarding the use of proteomics analysis of amniotic fluid, cord blood, and urine to determine the risk of intra-amniotic inflammation, neonatal sepsis, and preeclampsia, respectively. The authors have not served as consultants or received any honoraria from any third party as related to the information included in this article.

[a] Department of Obstetrics, Gynecology and Reproductive Sciences, Yale University School of Medicine, 333 Cedar Street, LLCI 804, New Haven, CT 06520, USA
[b] Division of Maternal Fetal Medicine, Department of Obstetrics, Gynecology and Reproductive Sciences, Yale University School of Medicine, 333 Cedar Street, LLCI 804, New Haven, CT 06520, USA
* Corresponding author.
E-mail address: irina.buhimschi@yale.edu

Like other "omics" approaches, proteomics is viewed as a nonreductionist approach to identification of protein biomarkers. Proteomics should be viewed as complementary to traditional approaches with potential to greatly enhance their reach. In hypothesis-driven research, the view that one or a group of specific proteins could be diagnostic markers is heavily dependent on prior knowledge, which links a precise protein or factor to a specific disease process. Proteomics, however, enables a reverse pathway. Proteomics allows an unbiased perspective by discovering that a group of named intact proteins or unnamed proteins fragments are characteristic to a diseased but not to a nondiseased state of the same organism. Such relationships are nonintuitive and draw a picture of the dysregulated biologic phenomena that otherwise could not have been predicted through the classical reductionist approach.

Several lessons have been learned from the human genome project: there are only approximately 30,000 genes in the human genome, which encode for more than 500,000 proteins; 99.9% of humans are identical at gene level; one of the most notable characteristics of the human genome is the startling amount of non-coding DNA it possesses; and only 1% to 1.5% of the human genome is coding DNA, devoted to genes encoding proteins.[1] Based on these observations, the major advantage of proteomics over DNA-RNA–based technologies is that proteomics investigates directly functional molecules and not the source code. Evidence in support of this assertion is that protein abundance and activity do not correlate with mRNA amount.[2] This suggests that post-transcriptional regulation of gene expression, which cannot be predicted by linear genetics, is a frequent phenomenon in higher-level organisms. The recent discovery of small silencing RNAs provides another explanation of the divergence between information coded into the RNA versus proteins. Thus, in the context of this biologic complexity, it should not be surprising that the results of proteomics versus genomics experimentation could be divergent yet complementary.[3]

Proteomics involves a diversity of techniques first aimed at separating and then identifying the proteins of interest. Practical aspects of proteomics experimentation, however, can be hugely complex. Proteins are heterogeneous and complex entities. They vary widely in concentration, molecular weight, isoelectric point, and hydrophobicity. They differ from individual to individual and change dynamically over time while interacting with each other, DNA or RNA, metal ions, and hormones. Protein fragmentation, association, and aggregation can create nonstandard endogenous ligands with biologic activity that is divergent from that of the precursor encoded by the original mRNA.[4] To place everything into perspective, if there is one genome per individual, it is estimated that the number of possible human proteomes is in the thousands.[5] These proteomes further change dynamically with food and drugs and over time.

In contrast to genomics, which relies mostly on standardized and automated techniques, proteomics requires experimental fine tuning, which has to be optimized depending on tested hypotheses and goals. The more complex a sample, the more challenging it is to reveal the differentially expressed proteins, especially if these proteins are less abundant. The nature of the human body fluid proteome, with its large dynamic range of protein concentrations, presents problems with detection and with quantitation. Seeing or not seeing a polypeptide from the realm of signals depends on the copy number, quantity of sample loaded, and "white noise" of the method of detection.[6] In human plasma, the ratio of albumin to signaling molecules is approximately 10^{12}. For instance, albumin and glucagon have 9 orders of magnitude difference. A significant experimental proteomic challenge is that regular silver-stained two dimensional (2-D) gel electrophoresis can display only 4 orders of magnitude in plasma proteins. In this context, most proteomic techniques display just the tip of the iceberg.

This challenge becomes especially important when studying disease processes given that not all biologic compartments are expected to be equally affected.

Faced with such challenges, the authors' group has advocated the idea of hypothesis-driven proteomics, proposing that three experimental design choices should be made a priori of proteomics experimentation. These are (1) choice of the disease, (2) choice of the biologic sample, and (3) choice of proteomics technique/data analysis. All three choices are critical and necessary to maximize the likelihood that the biomarkers extracted at the end of the exploratory phase have the required biologic and clinical relevance to allow them to pass the challenge phase against the clinically implemented gold standard (**Fig. 1**). The principles of experimental design required for successful completion of proteomic research in reproductive sciences have been recently reviewed.[7,8]

Proteomics Techniques

Protein separation from complex protein mixtures is possible through several high-throughput technologies. These experimental techniques make use of intrinsic properties of proteins: molecular weight (gel electrophoresis and mass spectrometry), isoelectric point (isoelectric focusing and ion-exchange chromatography), hydrophobicity (reverse-phase or hydrophobic interaction chromatography), or unusual affinities for metals and specific antibodies (affinity chromatography). It is generally

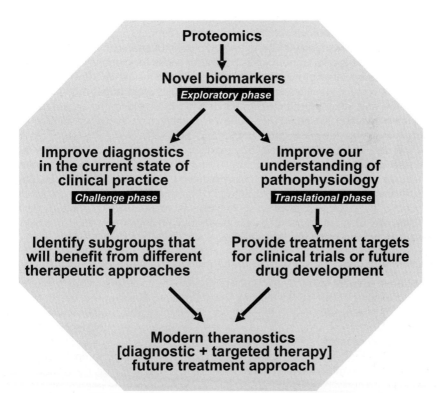

Fig. 1. Basic paradigm of proteomics workflow in the authors' laboratory. (*From* Buhimschi IA, Buhimschi CS. Proteomics of the amniotic fluid in assessment of the placenta. Relevance for preterm birth. Placenta 2008;29:S95–101; with permission.)

recognized that there is a trade-off between using multiple complementary techniques successively, thus being able to visualize a larger part of the proteome, and the excessive manipulation of the biologic sample with potential of introducing experimental artifacts. Therefore, emphasis has been placed on proteomics platforms that simultaneously combine at least two of the previously enumerated separation modalities. Some of these are 2-D polyacrylamide gel electrophoresis (2-D–PAGE), surface-enhanced laser desorption/ionization time of flight (SELDI-TOF), and multidimensional protein identification technology (MudPIT). Use of different labels applied in complex biologic mixtures at the proteome level raises the sensitivity and accuracy for identification of differentially expressed targets. Two such technologies are 2-D differential gel electrophoresis (2-D–DIGE), developed on a 2-D–PAGE platform, and isotope-coded affinity tag, developed on a mass spectrometry platform.

In essence, two opposing approaches to proteomics discovery are available. At this time most proteomics platforms enable just one. One approach relies on generating proteomic patterns from biologic samples using high-throughput mass spectrometry platforms. This approach minimizes the need to establish the identity of the discriminatory biomarkers (proteomics pattern-centered approach).[9] The second proteomic strategy focuses on protein identification by digesting them into peptides. This process is followed by sequencing using tandem mass spectrometry and database searching (proteomics identification-centered approach).[10] As both have advantages and limitations, understanding each method in the context of the disease of interest, of the biologic sample available for analysis, and of the expectations is important and the essence of the third choice (proteomics technique/data analysis). For instance, in pattern-centered proteomics, additional bioinformatic tools and experimentation are needed to determine identity of the extracted protein biomarkers. Although this information is not needed for correct classification of cases for diagnostics purpose, the identity of dysregulated proteins may provide powerful insight into novel therapeutic targets. Conversely, identification-centered proteomics approaches are at best semiquantitative and, recently, extensive emphasis has been placed on algorithms, such as multiple reaction monitoring, to improve quantification in high-resolution mass spectrometry approaches.[11] More important, however, is the limitation resulting from the data output. Most often, this represents a list of protein identities found increased or decreased over an arbitrary cutoff. As these identities are converged into unique identifiers, they are ultimately matched to genes indexed in databases. Thus, this approach annuls the advantage of proteomics in providing an accurate snapshot of the proteome. It would entirely miss biomarkers derived through proteolyic cleavage of a precursor because the fragment and the precursor would be converged into the same unique identifier.

Principles of Proteomics Approaches in the Authors' Laboratory

The authors' laboratory used a combined pattern-centered and identification-centered approach placing SELDI-TOF at the front-end as choice of technique for the proteomics exploratory phase. SELDI-TOF is mostly a pattern-centered proteomics technique, which combines chromatography with mass spectrometry. This offers technical advantages, such as ease and speed of screening, ability to use very small amounts of crude biologic fluids, and rapidly screening large numbers of biologic samples. Using this approach aims to minimize the biologic noise and errors in clinical classification due to imperfect diagnostic gold standards or arbitrary cutoffs. The separation ability of SELDI-TOF is enhanced by the use of the various active surfaces placed on aluminum-based ProteinChip arrays (Bio-Rad, Hercules, CA, USA). The active surfaces contain chemicals that allow the capture of subsets of proteins while repelling others.

The bound proteins are laser desorbed and ionized for mass spectroscopy analysis. The differential mass spectral patterns reflect the protein expression bound on the chip surface and allow the comparison between various samples.[12–14] At the end of the exploratory phase, a bioinformatic algorithm (mass restricted [MR] scoring) is applied and a combination of protein biomarkers that fulfill all set criteria are extracted from the SELDI-TOF tracings.[7,8,15–17] Proteins of interest are next identified using peptide mass fingerprinting or tandem mass spectrometry in conjunction with the PCI 1000 ProteinChip interface (Bio-Rad).

When successful, the exploratory phase was followed by a proteomics challenge phase on a different set and larger number of biologic specimens from consecutively enrolled patients with varying grades of disease severities and confounding morbidities.[16,18] The purpose of the challenge phase was to validate the initial biomarker combination and to provide a robust diagnostic tool with potential to improve classification of cases in the current state of clinical practice. This tool is provided in the form of a proteomics score based on relative abundance of select biomarkers as identified by their mass on SELDI-TOF tracings. In parallel, the translational phase was pursued, which begins with strategies aimed at identifying the biomarkers composing the proteomics score. As deemed necessary for each project, other complementary proteomics approaches (2-D–PAGE, 2-D–DIGE, and SELDI-immunocapture) were used. The choice of proteomics platform for identification was based on the type of biologic sample and the abundance of the biomarkers of interest at the initial SELDI-TOF screen.[15–17] Once identification was unambiguously established, a wide range of mechanistic experiments was undertaken to determine the biologic relevance of the newly identified markers. A schematic representation of the proteomics approach in the authors' laboratory is illustrated in **Fig. 1**.[7,8]

As choice of disease, the authors' group mainly focused on entities responsible for preterm birth and neonatal morbidity, such as spontaneous preterm birth, intrauterine infection, and inflammation as well as preeclampsia. These conditions are especially difficult to tackle with respect to development of new diagnostics due to patient heterogeneity, difficulty in obtaining serial biologic samples from the fetus, and imperfect gold standards for presence or absence of disease. By using the approach (discussed previously), several proteomic profiles could be extracted with biologic and clinical significance. Two of the profiles have been prospectively validated and, because of their high accuracy in delineating specific subgroups of preterm birth, are currently used in the authors' laboratory as research gold standards. The two prospectively validated profiles are the amniotic fluid proteomic fingerprint (the MR score)[18–22] and the urine proteomic score (UPS) of preeclampsia.[16] In addition to the UPS profile, the authors reported another SELDI-TOF profile composed of 4 peaks in cerebrospinal fluid, which carried the ability to identify subclinical intracranial bleeding in women with severe preeclampsia.[23] Its analogous presence in amniotic fluid was indicative of decidual hemorrhage related to abruption.[24] The presence of the same biomarkers in different biologic fluids related to different diseases speaks for the compartmentalization of biomarkers in each disease process and to the importance of choosing a relevant biologic sample for proteomics analysis. By using 2-D–DIGE in conjunction with SELDI-TOF and a hierarchical bioinformatics algorithm, the authors identified a distinct subgroup of patients at risk for preterm birth in the absence of intra-amniotic inflammation or bleeding (Q-profile),[25] thus providing first-hand evidence of an alternative pathway leading to prematurity for which no other marker existed. The differentially expressed proteins associated with the Q-profile were determined to be involved in noninflammatory processes, such as protein metabolism, signal transduction, and transport.[25] Lastly, the authors recently provided the first comprehensive mapping of human cord blood and identified potential markers that can be used to characterize at birth presence and susceptibility to early-onset neonatal sepsis (EONS).[17] This work is ongoing.

PROTEOMICS BIOMARKERS FOR IMPROVED DIAGNOSIS OF INTRAUTERINE INFECTION, INFLAMMATION, AND EONS
Clinical Relevance of Intrauterine Infection, Inflammation, and EONS

Neonatal sepsis is a global public health challenge and a significant contributor to morbidity and death. Early- and late-onset sepsis occur with increased frequency in neonates born prematurely.[26–28] Because the mortality rate of untreated sepsis can be as high as 50%, most clinicians believe that the hazard of untreated sepsis is too great to wait for confirmation based on positive culture results. Therefore, treatment is commonly begun in the absence of documented infection. In data published by the Yale Newborn Special Care Unit, which holds the longest running, single-center database of neonatal sepsis, started in 1928, mortality attributable to sepsis remains at 11%.[29] This mortality rate is unchanged in recent years despite advances in neonatal care. It is extremely important to make a prompt diagnosis of sepsis, because earlier initiation of antimicrobial therapy improves outcomes.

Intrauterine infection and subsequent inflammation are important risk factors for EONS and poor neonatal outcome.[30,31] During the past two decades, it has become clear that intrauterine infection has a strong association with preterm birth.[32–34] The problem of quantifying the causal role of infection in determinism of preterm birth and EONS results from lack of a proper gold standard for infection and from the heterogeneous nature of intra-amniotic inflammation. In the past decade, it became increasingly evident that the process of intra-amniotic inflammation is not necessarily linked to an exogenous microbial attack. For instance, abruption and decidual hemorrhage fuel into the same downstream inflammatory and oxidative pathways as intra-amniotic infection through release of thrombin, heme and free iron, and globin-centered free radicals.[35]

There is a priority in identifying clinically relevant biomarkers that can predict pregnancies complicated by intra-amniotic infection, which are at a high risk for fetal damage. Proteomics provides a unique opportunity given that in the short run such markers may aid with medical decision making, including timing of delivery and steroid administration. Conversely, ruling out intra-amniotic inflammation or a vulnerable fetus may allow for safe expectant management and reduce unnecessary treatment.

Role of Proteomics in Diagnosis of Intra-amniotic Infection and Inflammation

It has become increasingly recognized that in most cases intrauterine infection in pregnancy is not clinically apparent.[18,36] Thus, clinical chorioamnionitis is an insensitive measure of the presence of inflammation, infection, or fetal sepsis.[37,38] Direct analysis of the amniotic fluid with use of amniocentesis remains the most accurate modality to diagnose intrauterine infection and to determine the extent of intra-amniotic inflammation.[39] One of the problems in establishing clinical usefulness of amniocentesis in preterm birth rests with the lack of sensitive and specific diagnostic gold standards for infection and inflammation. In addition, the turnaround time for test results to become available to clinicians is too long for clinical decision making. For example, the median time when amniotic fluid culture results are available is 7 days (range 2–24 days) after an amniocentesis procedure.[18] Meanwhile, decision of expectant management or indicated delivery has already occurred as guided by clinical manifestations and results of rapid tests, such as amniotic fluid Gram stain, white blood cell (WBC) count, glucose concentration, and lactate dehydrogenase activity. In one of the authors' studies, the results of this battery were concordant in excluding intra-amniotic inflammation in the setting of preterm birth in only 50% of cases and in confirming inflammation in 14%, which often is not sufficient to remove uncertainty required for medical decision making.[18] Although portrayed by some investigators as a simple, rapid, and accurate test of infection, the results of the amniotic fluid WBC count alone could be misleading, especially in clinical scenarios, such as contamination of the amniotic fluid with blood or bacterial-induced lysis of leukocytes.[18]

Historical data using amniotic fluid cultures detects presence of intra-amniotic infection in 10% of patients with preterm labor and intact membranes and in 38% of patients with preterm premature rupture of membranes (PPROM).[40,41] Molecular biology techniques, however, which are more sensitive than cultures, detect bacteria in up to 60% of pregnancies complicated with preterm labor.[42] A variety of microbial pathogens have been implicated as etiologic agents of intra-amniotic infection.[29,43,44] The most frequently found isolates are thought to originate primarily from the genital flora, such as *Gardnerella vaginalis*, *Mycoplasma hominis*, *Ureaplasma*, *Peptostreptococcus*, and *Bacteroides* spp.[44] Regretfully, this assumption is significantly biased by the limited number of laboratory techniques for pathogen cultivation, which normally target for identification only a handful of microbes.[45] Thus, uncultivated or difficult-to-cultivate bacteria cannot be found when relying on culture conditions alone.[21,46,47] In contrast, culture-independent methods, such as polymerase chain reaction (PCR), can detect bacterial DNA in up to 35% to 60% of pregnancies complicated by preterm birth.[42,48] Yet, their use alone as diagnostics cannot discriminate between in vivo infection and ex vivo contamination, thus may result in unnecessary early deliveries. Therefore, there is a need for better tools to diagnose intra-amniotic infection and inflammation.

In recent years, proteomics has been extensively used by the authors and others to search for biologically relevant biomarkers and to generate protein profiles characteristic of intra-amniotic inflammation and preterm birth.[15,49,50] As choice of sample for proteomics experimentation, amniotic fluid offers clear advantages over maternal blood or plasma. Given that almost 99% of neutrophils extravasated in amniotic fluid is of fetal origin, evaluation of this compartment reflects more closely the nuances of the fetal inflammatory response to infection.[51] Other biologic samples, such as maternal urine and cervicovaginal secretions, are not significantly modified in the proteome over biologic noise despite fetal sepsis.[52] Several groups have investigated the cervicovaginal proteome in search of biomarkers predictive of preterm birth.[53–55] Although the preliminary results are encouraging, a challenge phase to confirm the clinical usefulness for the proposed identities has not yet been published. Their superiority over the best-performing cervicovaginal biomarker to date (fetal fibronectin) in predicting the risk for preterm birth remains to be tested in a prospective blinded fashion.

After applying the algorithm of MR scoring to SELDI-TOF tracings obtained from amniotic fluid of women with intra-amniotic infection and inflammation versus women of similar gestational age but with normal pregnancy outcomes, the authors extracted a combination of 4 biomarkers that were necessary and sufficient for 100% correct classification of cases selected for the exploratory phase.[7,8,15] The MR score denotes the number of markers identifiable over the technical noise of the SELDI-TOF instrument. The MR score ranges from 0 (all biomarkers absent) to 4 (all biomarkers present). In the original study, an MR score of 3 or 4 (denoted MR 3-4) indicated the presence of inflammation whereas an MR score of 0 or 2 (MR 0-2) was considered to exclude it.[15] On-chip immunoassays and peptide mass fingerprinting, confirmed by Western blotting, established that the 4 biomarkers of the MR score were neutrophil defensin-2 (3.3 kDa), neutrophil defensin-1 (3.4 kDa), S100A12 (10.4 kDa), and A100A8 (10.8 kDa), all members of the innate immunity arm of antimicrobial defense.[15] The relevance of these proteins as diagnostic biomarkers of intra-amniotic inflammation was subsequently confirmed independently by other group of investigators.[49,50,56]

To establish the MR score's clinical value, it was critical to demonstrate that the MR score retains its diagnostic efficacy when tested in other populations at high risk for preterm birth and that it relates to relevant outcomes. In one series, the authors tested the ability of the MR score to predict the clinical success of rescue cerclage in women with cervical incompetence and demonstrated that an MR 3-4 in amniotic fluid at the time of surgery was highly predictive of cerclage failure.[22] Next, the authors sought to determine in a prospective and blinded fashion in a cohort of 169 consecutive women, pregnant with singletons, whether or not the MR score is reproducible and comparable with previously established or proposed markers of intra-amniotic inflammation or infection.[18] This approach was consistent with the challenge phase (as described in **Fig. 1**). The accuracy of an MR 3-4 was the highest (>90%) in detecting intra-amniotic inflammation followed by lactate dehydrogenase activity. Stepwise logistic regression analysis was further used to identify which clinical test or combination of tests optimally predicts inflammation and found the MR score performed better than any test or combination of tests (odds ratio 76, $P<.0001$). The authors observed a sequential appearance of the biomarkers as the process of intra-amniotic inflammation developed from acute to chronic, with the peaks corresponding to S100A12 and S100A8 appearing last. This finding enabled stratifying the study population based on progression and severity of inflammation (MR 0, absent; MR 1-2, mild; and MR 3-4, severe) (**Fig. 2**).[18] This classification was unique and would not have been apparent without the prospective study design of the challenge phase. As discussed later, the authors believe that such performance relates to the ability of the MR score to uniquely predict clinically relevant intra-amniotic inflammation, histologic chorioamnionitis, funisitis, and EONS.

The authors next asked the question of why the MR score was superior to all other clinical analyses of amniotic fluid in its ability to identify intra-amniotic inflammation. Using 16S ribosomal RNA sequencing and phylogenetic analysis, in collaboration with Han (Case Western Reserve University), the authors demonstrated that all specimens with MR score 3-4 but negative cultures showed presence of bacterial DNA.[21] Furthermore, most samples of amniotic fluid with MR 3-4 and positive cultures contained DNA of additional bacterial species compared with those found by cultures. In fact, 60% of species detected by culture-independent methods were missed by general laboratory cultures. The key finding of this study was that the missed prokaryotes belonged to the class of uncultivated and difficult-to-cultivate species, such as *Fusobacterium nucleatum*, *Leptotrichia/Sneathia*, *Bergeyella*, *Peptostreptococcus*, *Ureaplasma parvum*, *Bacteroides*, and *Clostridiales* spp. These results suggest that the prevalence of amniotic fluid infection and diversity of etiologic agents linked to preterm birth is underestimated.[21] Moreover, the authors' and others' data bring into perspective that a fetus may encounter pathogenic bacteria more often than previously thought.[57]

The Role of Proteomics in Diagnosis of Histologic Chorioamnionitis and Funisitis

The proximity of the placenta to the fetus, its common embryologic origin and genotype, and the availability of this reproductive tissue for research have all contributed to the significant number of studies relating various placental lesions to short- and long-term neonatal outcomes, including cerebral palsy.[58] The major disadvantage of

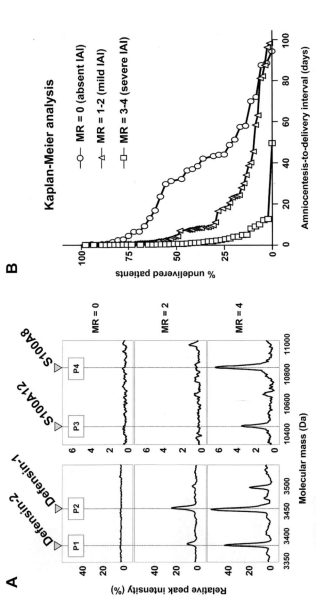

Fig. 2. (A) Representative SELDI-TOF mass spectrometry profiles of the amniotic fluid based on the severity of intra-amniotic inflammation (IAI). P1 to P4 represent the biomarkers of the MR score, which are neutrophil defensin-2 (P1: 3,377 Da), neutrophil defensin-1 (P2: 3,448 Da), S100A12 (P3: 10,444 Da), and S100A8 (P4: 10,835 Da). The X axis of the tracings represents the molecular mass in daltons; the Y axis represents the relative peak intensity. (B) Kaplan-Meier analysis illustrating the duration from amniocentesis to delivery in women with MR scores of 0, 1-2, and 3-4. (*Reproduced from* Buhimschi CS, Bhandari V, Hamar BD, et al. Proteomic profiling of the amniotic fluid to detect inflammation, infection, and neonatal sepsis PLoS Med 2007;4[1]:e18. Republication by authors permitted under Creative Commons Attribution License; with permission.)

placental pathologic examination is that histologic biomarkers are irrelevant for ante-natal therapeutic choices aimed at preventing preterm birth or adverse neonatal outcome. Valuable studies have associated short- and long-term follow-up character-istics with distinct placental lesions, however.[58–61]

Because proteomics is a young science, conclusions regarding the clinical usefulness of proteomic biomarkers in predicting the long-term outcome of the neonates are not yet possible. Until such data become available the authors took a step-by-step approach using as intermediate outcome variables results of placental examination as performed by a perinatal pathologist blinded to the MR score. The presence and severity of acute inflammation in the chorionic plate, amnion, choriodeciduas, and umbilical cord (funisitis) were determined to be significantly associated with the occurrence and the degree of intra-amniotic inflammation as determined by MR score.[18–20] The MR score also correlated significantly with the stages of chorioamnionitis ($P<.001$) and funisitis ($P<.001$) independent of the interval to delivery ($P = .16$ for MR score vs amniocentesis-to-delivery interval). The authors further found, among the biomarkers of the MR score, that the appearance of at least one of the peaks corresponding to the S100 proteins (S100A12 or S100A8) in amniotic fluid was highly indicative of bio-logically relevant funisitis (at least grade 2) or chorioamnionitis (**Fig. 3**). As a result, the authors became interested in exploring mechanistically the implication of these proteins for EONS and for processes that could possibly lead to antenatal fetal damage in the setting of intra-amniotic inflammation.

The Role of Proteomics in Diagnosis of EONS

The disconnect between EONS as a clinical entity and the responsible microorgan-isms may be even greater than for intra-amniotic infection. As a result, many newborns receive empiric antibiotic therapy based on nonspecific symptoms of suspected EONS or maternal risk factors (such as prematurity, intrapartum fever, chorioamnioni-tis, and prolonged rupture of membranes).[62] Several explanations are available to justify the well-recognized inability of neonatal blood culture to correctly diagnose EONS and why newborns are treated with empiric antibiotics even when unnecessary. The frequency of bloodstream infections fluctuates widely from 8% to 73% in the diagnosis of "suspected" EONS.[19,63] Moreover, microbiology laboratories only search for a narrow spectrum of pathogens. For example, culturing for *Ureaplasma* and *Mycoplasma* spp is not part of the routine sepsis work-up in neonates. A study that

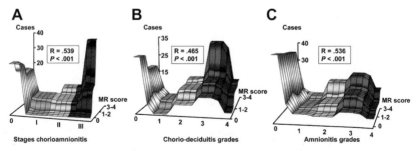

Fig. 3. 3-D representation of the relationship between histologic markers of placental inflammation on the X axis. (*A*) Stages of chorioamnionitis; (*B*) grades of choriodeciduitis; and (*C*) grades of amnionitis. Number of analyzed cases on the Y axis and the proteomics MR score on the Z axis. (*From* Buhimschi IA, Zambrano E, Pettker CM, et al. Using proteomic analysis of the human amniotic fluid to identify histologic chorioamnionitis. Obstet Gynecol 2008;111:403–12; with permission.)

evaluated the frequency of umbilical cord blood infections with these species found that 23% of newborns born at less than 32 weeks tested positive for these pathogens.[57] It is also plausible that analogous to intra-amniotic inflammation, the fetal and newborn insult may be induced by additional uncultivated and difficult-to-cultivate species. Data supporting this premise have shown that 16S ribosomal RNA PCR technology improves the accuracy of culture-based methods for diagnosis of neonatal sepsis.[64]

In the context of an unreliable gold standard for EONS, the authors turned their attention to clinical assessments and neonatal hematologic indices at less than or equal to 72 hours after birth as surrogates for early sepsis.[27,65,66] In collaboration with Bhandari (Yale University), the authors analyzed all newborns admitted to Yale Newborn Special Care unit whose mothers presented with signs and symptoms of preterm birth, had an amniocentesis to rule out infection and were enrolled in the authors' MR score challenge phase cohort (n = 104).[27] Confirmed EONS was defined as the presence of a positive blood or any other body fluid microbial culture result. Suspected EONS was noted in the presence of clinical signs of sepsis with support from laboratory hematologic results.[27] Neonates of women with MR 3-4 were more often lymphopenic and had significantly higher absolute band count and ratio of immature to total neutrophils ($P<.001$) compared with the other groups. Neonates of women with MR 3-4 (severe inflammation) had an increased incidence of EONS (odds ratio 4.4, $P = .007$) compared with neonates from mothers with MR 0 or MR 1-2. These results remained significant after adjusting for gestational age at birth. In logistic regression, the MR 3-4 was significantly associated with EONS whereas the results of amniotic fluid culture and WBC count were excluded from the equation. Of all component biomarkers of the MR score, the presence of the S100A8 had the strongest association with EONS. The association of S100A12 with chorioamnionitis and funisitis and of S100A8 with EONS suggests that these proteins may reflect a chronic process with significant relevance for antenatal fetal damage in the setting of intrauterine severe inflammation. Moreover, the authors' data may provide first-hand evidence that, similar to intra-amniotic inflammation, EONS may be a heterogeneous pathogenic entity.[67] For instance, at least some of the newborns that have nonspecific clinical manifestations of EONS (lethargy, apnea, respiratory distress, hypoperfusion, and shock) may not have had true fetal infection. It is plausible to propose that EONS could be a consequence of a pathologic process initiated in utero through chronic exposure of the fetus to a noxious prooxidative and proinflammatory intrauterine environment. In this context, early delivery of the fetus may be justified.

Pathogenic Basis and Implications of EONS Heterogeneity

Antibiotics are routinely used ante- and intrapartum in women with PPROM to extend duration of pregnancy, decrease the risk of neonatal group B streptococcal (GBS) sepsis, and reduce the risk of neonatal illness after delivery.[68–71] Due to the widespread use of antepartum antibiotics, the majority of EONS cases in preterm infants are no longer caused by GBS but rather by gram-negative bacteria with *Escherichia coli* as the most frequent pathogen.[29,72] Antibiotics, although inducing bacterial killing, do not quell an inflammatory process already under way. A study conducted by Gravett and colleagues[73] demonstrated in a primate model of intra-amniotic infection that with GBS, antibiotics eradicated infection whereas uterine activity, amniotic fluid cytokines, prostaglandins, and matrix metalloproteinases remained elevated. The observation that the combination of antibiotics and anti-inflammatory and antiprostaglandin agents suppressed inflammation and significantly prolonged gestation is valuable because it suggest that multiple pathways need to be suppressed simultaneously to obtain a successful therapeutic result. The authors' data related to fetal inflammatory syndrome and fetal adaptation to intra-amniotic inflammation suggest that the clinical manifestations of EONS could be the result of an active trafficking process, which occurs between the amniotic fluid compartment and the fetus.[19,74] It would suffice for endotoxin, other pathogen-associated molecular pattern molecules (PAMPs), lipophilic damage-associated molecular pattern proteins (DAMPs), or cytokines to "spill" from amniotic fluid into the fetal circulation to cause manifestations consistent with septic shock. In this case, passage of live bacteria to the fetus may not be a requirement for clinical manifestations of EONS.

The Role of DAMPs and Receptor of Advanced Glycation End Products in Mediating Fetal Injury

The danger theory holds that injured cells release alarm signals, which in turn activate an immune response.[75] Consistent with this premise, DAMPs (alarmins) are a pleiotropic group of intracellular proteins, which, when released in the extracellular compartment, become endogenous danger signals by activating membrane receptors and amplifying the damage.[76] DAMPs have been implicated as key mediators of a host's immune response. Evidence from adults and animal models have demonstrated significantly elevated systemic concentrations of inflammatory mediators (such as monocyte chemoattractant protein-1 and interleukin [IL]-6) after traumatic crush injury or ischemia.[77] The generalized endothelial damage at a distance from the affected areas suggests that DAMPs alone are able to initiate and sustain inflammation, even in the absence of infectious triggers. Involvement of molecules, such as high-mobility group box protein-1 (HMGB1), a prototype DAMP released by somatic cells subjected to injury or necrosis, and receptor of advanced glycation end products (RAGE) may offer a plausible explanation as to why patients with noninfectious critical illness develop a syndrome that is indistinguishable from microbial-induced sepsis.[78–80]

RAGE is a redox-sensitive receptor of the immunoglobulin family and acts as a pattern recognition receptor for DAMPs, such as HMGB1 and S100 proteins. Engagement of RAGE converts transient cellular stimulation into sustained cellular dysfunction driven by activation of nuclear factor κB.[81,82] A DAMP-RAGE activation axis has been implicated in the progression of an acute event to a chronic inflammatory state associated with tissue destruction. An important feature of the RAGE receptor is that its expression is low in normal tissues but increases transcriptionally in environments where RAGE ligands, such as DAMPs, accumulate, escalating tissue damage in a spiral positive feedback fashion.[83] In genetic animal models, deletion of RAGE and pharmacologic interventions that reduce DAMP levels or block RAGE-DAMP interactions suppress inflammation and dampen tissue damage.[84–88]

The authors' group was the first to provide evidence that activation of a DAMP-RAGE axis occurs in pregnancies complicated by intra-amniotic infection and inflammation.[89,90] This finding was spearheaded through the discovery of the proteomic biomarkers components of the MR score.[15,91] The identity of two of the proteomic biomarkers as the RAGE ligands S100A12 and S100A8[92] led to the hypothesis that intrauterine infection or inflammation induces release of DAMPs, which in turn promote fetal cellular damage via RAGE activation.[93] Evidence from the authors' research suggests this premise is relevant for newborns exposed antenatally to a noxious intrauterine environment, such as that resulting from intra-amniotic inflammation.[90] As identified by the MR score at the time of amniocentesis, many of these pregnancies had histologic evidence of chorioamnionitis and funisitis and the newborns developed signs or symptoms consistent with EONS. A link between these endpoints was provided by recent data suggesting that damage to the barrier between the hostile intrauterine environment and the fetus may occur in utero as appreciated by the degree of funisitis and chorioamnionitis.[19] In this context, the authors demonstrated that the cord blood–to–amniotic fluid IL-6 ratio (CB/AF IL-6), an indicator of the differential inflammatory response in the fetal versus the amniotic fluid compartment, correlates with the MR score in a manner dependent on the severity of histologic inflammation of the chorionic plate, choriodecidua, and umbilical cord (funisitis).[19] The authors' data suggest that inflammation-induced damage of the maternal-fetal interface may play a permissive role in trafficking of cytokines DAMPs and PAMPs between the amniotic fluid and cord blood. The authors further observed that in most EONS cases with evidence of severe intra-amniotic inflammation (88% of all EONS cases in the study), the absolute amniotic fluid IL-6 concentration was significantly higher than that measured in cord blood. This suggests that should the maternal-fetal interface become damaged, the IL-6 gradient favors spillage into the fetal compartment. Yet, in a minority of EONS newborns, the ratio was reversed. This finding provided support for the conclusion that progression of inflammation may occur in the fetal compartment independent of the amniotic fluid space. In fetuses with a reversed CB/AF IL-6 ratio, EONS confirmed by positive blood cultures reached 50%. It is likely that in the remaining 50% of the newborns, sepsis was induced by "uncultivated" bacteria in utero. Equally plausible is that these fetuses had a disproportionate activation of their innate immune response to PAMPs and DAMPs leaked into fetal circulation.[19] **Fig. 4** illustrates the proposed mechanism leading to fetal damage. Based on the existing data, the authors consider that bacterial PAMPs

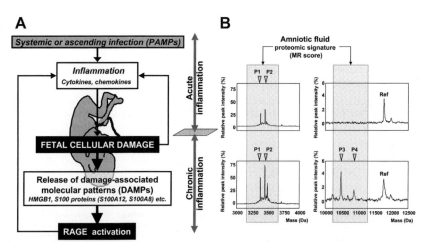

Fig. 4. (*A*) Working model for the potential roles of PAMPs, DAMPs, and RAGE in fueling cellular damage to the fetus exposed to acute and chronic intrauterine infection, inflammation, and oxidative stress. (*B*) The underlying change in the amniotic fluid MR score from an MR 0-2 to an MR 3-4 is in 93% of cases due to appearance of biomarker peaks P3 and P4 representing the DAMPs S100A12 and S100A8, respectively. The MR score is calculated as the arithmetic sum of present biomarker peaks and ranges from 0 (all 4 peaks absent) to 4 (all 4 peaks present). The upper tracings is representative of an MR 2 while the lower tracing shown an MR of 4. Pathogenically this corresponds to the transition of intra-amniotic inflammation from an acute, perhaps reversible, process to a chronic process characterized by cellular damage via RAGE activation. (*From* Buhimschi CS, Bhandari V, Han YW, et al. Using proteomics in perinatal and neonatal sepsis: hopes and challenges for the future. Curr Opin Infect Dis 2009;22:235–43; with permission.)

continue to engage signaling receptors, such as toll-like receptors, and participate in the release of cellular endogenous danger signal molecules (ie, DAMPs) that perpetuate the inflammatory cascade leading to fetal cellular damage via RAGE activation. This process may continue even after antibiotic treatment is initiated and thus perhaps even after birth. If such fetuses are correctly identified antenatally as enabled by MR score, there is a window of opportunity for targeted interventions. Such therapies may in the future include anti-DAMP, anti-RAGE, or anticytokine strategies alone or in conjunction with antibiotics as deemed necessary for each case scenario.

Data in support of EONS heterogeneity emerge from the evidence that maternal antibiotic treatment, which results in killing of maternal bacteria, may induce excess release of PAMPs. In addition, data derived from animal models of sepsis show that antibiotic-treated rats display higher plasma endotoxin levels than untreated animals despite decreased bacteremia. Moreover, different antibiotics may induce the release of different forms of endotoxin, which may be lethal for sensitized animals.[94] This may explain why attempts to prevent preterm birth with antibiotic treatment in patients with bacterial vaginosis, *Trichomonas*, or preterm labor had no effect or increased the rate of preterm birth or the risk of cerebral palsy.[69,71,95] **Fig. 5** illustrates the authors' proposed model of EONS variants.

In light of these considerations, the authors' propose the following classification of EONS. Based on this model, each newborn may require different theranostic (therapeutic/diagnostic) approaches.

EONS I: Vertical transmission of live bacteria to the fetus. This condition requires prompt pathogen identification and targeted antibiotic treatment.
EONS II: Translocation of bacterial footprints (ie, endotoxin) and DAMPs from the mother and damaged placenta to the fetus. This condition requires general cardiovascular support and could be amenable to anti-inflammatory treatment and specific endotoxin-neutralizing strategies.
EONS III: Translocation of cytokines (such as IL-6) from the mother and damaged placenta to the fetus. This condition could require circulatory support or anti-inflammatory treatment.
EONS 0: None of the above, which in the context of current clinical care often is associated with overtreatment.

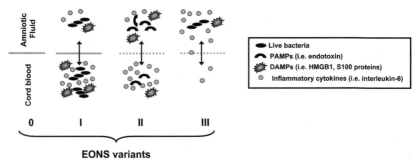

Fig. 5. Schematic representation of pathogenic variants of EONS. EONS 0 (lack thereof); EONS I (passage of a live bacterial inoculum to the fetus from the intra-amniotic compartment or via hematogenous dissemination); EONS II (passage of endotoxin, other bacterial products, or DAMPs through a damaged maternal-fetal interface represented by the interrupted gray line); and EONS III (spillage of inflammatory cytokines only through the damaged interface). Ability to differentiate among these variants is important for future therapeutic purpose.

CONCLUDING REMARKS

For the past 3 decades obstetricians, neonatologists, and developmental neurobiologists have had powerful debates regarding the best way to diagnose intra-amniotic infection and inflammation and the appropriate time to deliver a fetus exposed to a hostile intrauterine environment. In the absence of a preventative or curative therapy for intra-amniotic infection/inflammation, the answers to key questions, such as how much of an inflammatory stress can each fetus withstand or whether or not there is time to wait for a complete course of steroids when infection or inflammation is identified, remain rhetorical. Proteomics offers a unique opportunity to provide answers to these questions through functional biomarkers, which could represent targets for future therapeutic intervention.

ACKNOWLEDGMENTS

We are indebted to the nurses, fellows, residents, and faculty at Yale-New Haven Hospital, the Department of Obstetrics and Gynecology and Reproductive Sciences, and all patients who participated in our study. Special thanks to Drs Vineet Bhandari, Carolyn Salafia, Eduardo Zambrano, and Charles J. Lockwood for their insight and support with our studies.

REFERENCES

1. International Human Genome Sequencing Consortium. Initial sequencing and analysis of the human genome. Nature 2001;409(6822):860–921.
2. Anderson L, Seilhamer J. A comparison of selected mRNA and protein abundances in human liver. Electrophoresis 1997;18:533–7.
3. Ghildiyal M, Zamore PD. Small silencing RNAs: an expanding universe. Nat Rev Genet 2009;10(2):94–108.
4. Piekarska B, Rybarska J, Stopa B, et al. Supramolecularity creates nonstandard protein ligands. Acta Biochim Pol 1999;46(4):841–51.
5. Hoogland C, Mostaguir K, Sanchez JC, et al. SWISS-2DPAGE, ten years later. Proteomics 2004;4(8):2352–6.
6. Apweiler R, Aslanidis C, Deufel T, et al. Approaching clinical proteomics: current state and future fields of application in fluid proteomics. Clin Chem Lab Med 2009;47(6):724–44.
7. Buhimschi IA, Buhimschi CS. Proteomics of the amniotic fluid in assessment of the placenta. Relevance for preterm birth. Placenta 2008;29(Suppl A):S95–101.
8. Buhimschi IA. Using SELDI-TOF mass spectrometry for clinical proteomics of amniotic fluid and future theranostics. Methods Mol Biol 2010, in press.
9. Petricoin EE, Paweletz CP, Liotta LA. Clinical applications of proteomics: proteomic pattern diagnostics. J Mammary Gland Biol Neoplasia 2002;7(4):433–40.
10. Nesvizhskii AI. Protein identification by tandem mass spectrometry and sequence database searching. Methods Mol Biol 2007;367:87–119.
11. Kitteringham NR, Jenkins RE, Lane CS, et al. Multiple reaction monitoring for quantitative biomarker analysis in proteomics and metabolomics. J Chromatogr B Analyt Technol Biomed Life Sci 2009;877(13):1229–39.
12. Weinberger SR, Morris TS, Pawlak M. Recent trends in protein biochip technology. Pharmacogenomics 2000;1(4):395–416.
13. Fung ET, Enderwick C. ProteinChip clinical proteomics: computational challenges and solutions. Biotechniques 2002;32(Suppl 1):34–41.

14. Langbein S. Identification of disease biomarkers by profiling of serum proteins using SELDI-TOF mass spectrometry. Methods Mol Biol 2008;439:191–7.
15. Buhimschi IA, Christner R, Buhimschi CS. Proteomic biomarker analysis of amniotic fluid for identification of intra-amniotic inflammation. BJOG 2005;112(2):173–81.
16. Buhimschi IA, Zhao G, Funai EF, et al. Proteomic profiling of urine identifies specific fragments of SERPINA1 and albumin as biomarkers of preeclampsia. Am J Obstet Gynecol 2008;199(5):551, e1–16.
17. Buhimschi CS, Bhandari V, Dulay AT, et al. Comprehensive proteomic mapping of cord blood to identify novel biomarkers and functional protein networks characteristic of early-onset neonatal sepsis (EONS). Am J Obstet Gynecol 2008; 199(6A):S3.
18. Buhimschi CS, Bhandari V, Hamar BD, et al. Proteomic profiling of the amniotic fluid to detect inflammation, infection, and neonatal sepsis. PLoS Med 2007; 4(1):e18.
19. Buhimschi CS, Buhimschi IA, Abdel-Razeq S, et al. Proteomic biomarkers of intra-amniotic inflammation: relationship with funisitis and early-onset sepsis of the premature neonate. Pediatr Res 2007;61:318–24.
20. Buhimschi IA, Zambrano E, Pettker CM, et al. Using proteomic analysis of the human amniotic fluid to identify histologic chorioamnionitis. Obstet Gynecol 2008;111(2 Pt 1):403–12.
21. Han YW, Shen T, Chung P, et al. Uncultivated bacteria as etiologic agents of intra-amniotic inflammation leading to preterm birth. J Clin Microbiol 2009;47(1):38–47.
22. Weiner CP, Lee KY, Buhimschi CS, et al. Proteomic biomarkers that predict the clinical success of rescue cerclage. Am J Obstet Gynecol 2005;192(3):710–8.
23. Norwitz ER, Tsen LC, Park JS, et al. Discriminatory proteomic biomarker analysis identifies free hemoglobin in the cerebrospinal fluid of women with severe preeclampsia. Am J Obstet Gynecol 2005;193(3 Pt 2):957–64.
24. Buhimschi IA, Buhimschi CS, Zhao GM, et al. Mass spectrometry—a novel approach in deciphering the origin and duration of intra-amniotic bleeding. Am J Obstet Gynecol 2005;193(6):S107.
25. Buhimschi IA, Zhao G, Abdel-Razeq S, et al. Multidimensional proteomics analysis of the amniotic fluid to provide insight into the mechanisms of idiopathic preterm birth. PLoS One 2008;3(4):e2049.
26. Ng PC, Lam HS. Diagnostic markers for neonatal sepsis. Curr Opin Pediatr 2006; 18(2):125–31.
27. Smulian JC, Bhandari V, Campbell WA, et al. Value of umbilical artery and vein levels of interleukin-6 and soluble intracellular adhesion molecule-1 as predictors of neonatal hematologic indices and suspected early sepsis. J Matern Fetal Med 1997;6(5):254–9.
28. Gonzalez BE, Mercado CK, Johnson L, et al. Early markers of late-onset sepsis in premature neonates: clinical, hematological and cytokine profile. J Perinat Med 2003;31(1):60–8.
29. Bizzarro MJ, Dembry LM, Baltimore RS, et al. Changing patterns in neonatal Escherichia coli sepsis and ampicillin resistance in the era of intrapartum antibiotic prophylaxis. Pediatrics 2008;121(4):689–96.
30. Murphy DJ, Sellers S, MacKenzie IZ, et al. Case-control study of antenatal and intrapartum risk factors for cerebral palsy in very preterm singleton babies. Lancet 1995;346(8988):1449–54.
31. Martius JA, Roos T, Gora B, et al. Risk factors associated with early-onset sepsis in premature infants. Eur J Obstet Gynecol Reprod Biol 1999;85(2): 151–8.

32. Wenstrom KD, Andrews WW, Hauth JC, et al. Elevated second-trimester amniotic fluid interleukin-6 levels predict preterm delivery. Am J Obstet Gynecol 1998; 178(3):546–50.
33. Dammann O, Leviton A. Role of the fetus in perinatal infection and neonatal brain damage. Curr Opin Pediatr 2000;12:99–104.
34. Jacobsson B, Mattsby-Baltzer I, Andersch B, et al. Microbial invasion and cytokine response in amniotic fluid in a Swedish population of women with preterm prelabor rupture of membranes. Acta Obstet Gynecol Scand 2003;82:423–31.
35. Motterlini R, Foresti R, Vandegriff K, et al. Oxidative-stress response in vascular endothelial cells exposed to acellular hemoglobin solutions. Am J Physiol 1995; 269(2 Pt 2):H648–55.
36. Muglia LJ, Katz M. The enigma of spontaneous preterm birth. N Engl J Med 2010; 362(6):529–35.
37. Moberg LJ, Garite TJ, Freeman RK. Fetal heart rate patterns and fetal distress in patients with preterm premature rupture of membranes. Obstet Gynecol 1984; 64(1):60–4.
38. Hauth JC, Gilstrap LC 3rd, Hankins GD, et al. Term maternal and neonatal complications of acute chorioamnionitis. Obstet Gynecol 1985;66(1):59–62.
39. Angus SR, Segel SY, Hsu CD, et al. Amniotic fluid matrix metalloproteinase-8 indicates intra-amniotic infection. Am J Obstet Gynecol 2001;185(5):1232–8.
40. Andrews WW, Goldenberg RL, Hauth JC. Preterm labor: emerging role of genital tract infections. Infect Agents Dis 1995;4(4):196–211.
41. Goldenberg RL, Hauth JC, Andrews WW. Intrauterine infection and preterm delivery. N Engl J Med 2000;342(20):1500–17.
42. Markenson G, Martin R, Foley K, et al. The use of polymerase chain reaction to detect bacteria in amniotic fluid in pregnancies complicated with preterm labor. Am J Obstet Gynecol 1997;177(6):1471–7.
43. Larsen JW, Sever JL. Group B Streptococcus and pregnancy: a review. Am J Obstet Gynecol 2008;198(4):440–8.
44. Pettker CM, Buhimschi IA, Magloire LK, et al. Value of placental microbial evaluation in diagnosing intra-amniotic infection. Obstet Gynecol 2007;109(3):739–49.
45. Barron EJ, Jorgensen JH, Landry ML, et al. Bacteriology. In: Murray PR, editor. Manual of clinical bacteriology. 9th edition. Washington, DC: ASM Press; 2007. p. 974.
46. Dong J, Olano JP, McBride JW, et al. Emerging pathogens: challenges and successes of molecular diagnostics. J Mol Diagn 2008;10(3):185–97.
47. Kuypers MM. Microbiology. Sizing up the uncultivated majority. Science 2007; 317(5844):1510–1.
48. Hitti J, Riley DE, Krohn MA, et al. Broad-spectrum bacterial rDNA polymerase chain reaction assay for detecting amniotic fluid infection among women in premature labor. Clin Infect Dis 1997;24(6):1228–32.
49. Gravett MG, Novy MJ, Rosenfeld RG, et al. Diagnosis of intra-amniotic infection by proteomic profiling and identification of novel biomarkers. JAMA 2004; 292(4):462–9.
50. Ruetschi U, Rosen A, Karlsson G, et al. Proteomic analysis using protein chips to detect biomarkers in cervical and amniotic fluid in women with intra-amniotic inflammation. J Proteome Res 2005;4(6):2236–42.
51. Sampson JE, Theve RP, Blatman RN, et al. Fetal origin of amniotic fluid polymorphonuclear leukocytes. Am J Obstet Gynecol 1997;176(1):77–81.
52. Buhimschi IA, Buhimschi CS, Norwitz E, et al. Proteomic analysis of cervicovaginal secretions during pregnancy. Am J Obstet Gynecol 2004;191(6):S137.

53. Di Quinzio MK, Oliva K, Holdsworth SJ, et al. Proteomic analysis and character-isation of human cervico-vaginal fluid proteins. Aust N Z J Obstet Gynaecol 2007; 47(1):9–15.

54. Shaw JL, Smith CR, Diamandis EP. Proteomic analysis of human cervico-vaginal fluid. J Proteome Res 2007;6(7):2859–65.

55. Gravett MG, Thomas A, Schneider KA, et al. Proteomic analysis of cervical-vaginal fluid: identification of novel biomarkers for detection of intra-amniotic infection. J Proteome Res 2007;6(1):89–96.

56. Cobo T, Palacio M, Navarro-Sastre A, et al. Predictive value of combined amniotic fluid proteomic biomarkers and interleukin-6 in preterm labor with intact membranes. Am J Obstet Gynecol 2009;200(5):499 e1-6.

57. Goldenberg RL, Andrews WW, Goepfert AR, et al. The Alabama preterm birth study: umbilical cord blood *Ureaplasma urealyticum* and *Mycoplasma hominis* cultures in very preterm newborn infants. Am J Obstet Gynecol 2008;198(1): e1–5.

58. Redline RW. Placental pathology and cerebral palsy. Clin Perinatol 2006;33(2): 503–16.

59. Bejar R, Wozniak P, Allard M, et al. Antenatal origin of neurologic damage in newborn infants. I. Preterm infants. Am J Obstet Gynecol 1988;159(2):357–63.

60. De Felice C, Toti P, Laurini RN, et al. Early neonatal brain injury in histologic cho-rioamnionitis. J Pediatr 2001;138(1):101–4.

61. Grafe MR. The correlation of prenatal brain damage with placental pathology. J Neuropathol Exp Neurol 1994;53(4):407–15.

62. Yancey MK, Duff P, Kubilis P, et al. Risk factors for neonatal sepsis. Obstet Gyne-col 1996;87(2):188–94.

63. Buttery JP. Blood cultures in newborns and children: optimising an everyday test. Arch Dis Child Fetal Neonatal Ed 2002;87(1):F25–8.

64. Jordan JA, Durso MB, Butchko AR, et al. Evaluating the near-term infant for early-onset sepsis: progress and challenges to consider with 16S rDNA polymerase chain reaction testing. J Mol Diagn 2006;8(3):357–63.

65. Rodwell RL, Leslie AL, Tudehope DI. Early diagnosis of neonatal sepsis using a hematologic scoring system. J Pediatr 1988;112(5):761–7.

66. Rodwell RL, Taylor KM, Tudehope DI, et al. Hematologic scoring system in early diagnosis of sepsis in neutropenic newborns. Pediatr Infect Dis J 1993;12(5): 372–6.

67. Miller ME. Host defenses in the human neonate. Pediatr Clin North Am 1977; 24(2):413–23.

68. ACOG Committee on Practice Bulletins-Obstetrics. ACOG Practice Bulletin No. 80: premature rupture of membranes. Clinical management guidelines for obste-trician-gynecologists. Obstet Gynecol 2007;109(4):1007–19.

69. American College of Obstetricians and Gynecologists. ACOG Committee Opinion: number 279, December 2002. Prevention of early-onset group B strep-tococcal disease in newborns. Obstet Gynecol 2002;100(6):1405–12.

70. Kenyon SL, Taylor DJ, Tarnow-Mordi W, et al. Broad-spectrum antibiotics for preterm, prelabour rupture of fetal membranes: the ORACLE I randomised trial. ORACLE Collaborative Group. Lancet 2001;357:979–88.

71. Kenyon SL, Taylor DJ, Tarnow-Mordi W, et al. Broad-spectrum antibiotics for spontaneous preterm labour: the ORACLE II randomised trial. ORACLE Collabo-rative Group. Lancet 2001;357:989–94.

72. Stoll BJ, Hansen N, Fanaroff AA, et al. Changes in pathogens causing early-onset sepsis in very-low-birth-weight infants. N Engl J Med 2002;347:240–7.

73. Gravett MG, Adams KM, Sadowsky DW, et al. Immunomodulators plus antibiotics delay preterm delivery after experimental intraamniotic infection in a nonhuman primate model. Am J Obstet Gynecol 2007;197(5):518, e1–8.
74. Buhimschi CS, Abdel-Razeq S, Cackovic M, et al. Fetal heart rate monitoring patterns in women with amniotic fluid proteomic profiles indicative of inflammation. Am J Perinatol 2008;25(6):359–72.
75. Pétrilli V, Dostert C, Muruve DA, et al. The inflammasome: a danger sensing complex triggering innate immunity. Curr Opin Immunol 2007;19(6):615–22.
76. Lotze MT, Zeh HJ, Rubartelli A, et al. The grateful dead: damage-associated molecular pattern molecules and reduction/oxidation regulate immunity. Immunol Rev 2007;220:60–81.
77. Sonoi H, Matsumoto N, Ogura H, et al. The effect of antithrombin on pulmonary endothelial damage induced by crush injury. Shock 2009;32(6):593–600.
78. Scaffidi P, Misteli T, Bianchi ME. Release of chromatin protein HMGB1 by necrotic cells triggers inflammation. Nature 2002;418(6894):191–5.
79. Ombrellino M, Wang H, Ajemian MS, et al. Increased serum concentrations of high-mobility-group protein 1 in haemorrhagic shock. Lancet 1999;354(9188):1446–7.
80. Yang H, Tracey KJ. Targeting HMGB1 in inflammation. Biochim Biophys Acta 2010;1799(1-2):149–56.
81. Hofmann MA, Drury S, Fu C, et al. RAGE mediates a novel proinflammatory axis: a central cell surface receptor for S100/calgranulin polypeptides. Cell 1999;97(7):889–901.
82. Chavakis T, Bierhaus A, Al-Fakhri N, et al. The pattern recognition receptor (RAGE) is a counterreceptor for leukocyte integrins: a novel pathway for inflammatory cell recruitment. J Exp Med 2003;198(10):1507–15.
83. Yan SF, Ramasamy R, Naka Y, et al. Glycation, inflammation, and RAGE: a scaffold for the macrovascular complications of diabetes and beyond. Circ Res 2003;93(12):1159–69.
84. Lutterloh EC, Opal SM. Antibodies against RAGE in sepsis and inflammation: implications for therapy. Expert Opin Pharmacother 2007;8(9):1193–6.
85. Lutterloh EC, Opal SM, Pittman DD, et al. Inhibition of the RAGE products increases survival in experimental models of severe sepsis and systemic infection. Crit Care 2007;11(6):R122.
86. Yang H, Ochani M, Li J, et al. Reversing established sepsis with antagonists of endogenous high-mobility group box 1. Proc Natl Acad Sci U S A 2004;101(1):296–301.
87. Lotze MT, Tracey KJ. High-mobility group box 1 protein (HMGB1): nuclear weapon in the immune arsenal. Nat Rev Immunol 2005;5(4):331–42.
88. Wang H, Bloom O, Zhang M, et al. HMG-1 as a late mediator of endotoxin lethality in mice. Science 1999;285(5425):248–51.
89. Buhimschi IA, Zhao G, Pettker CM, et al. The receptor for advanced glycation end products (RAGE) system in women with intraamniotic infection and inflammation. Am J Obstet Gynecol 2007;196(2):181e1–181.e13.
90. Buhimschi CS, Baumbusch MA, Dulay AT, et al. Characterization of RAGE, HMGB1 and S100β in inflammation induced preterm birth and fetal tissue injury. Am J Pathol 2009;175(3):958–75.
91. Buhimschi CS, Buhimschi IA. Proteomic biomarkers of adverse pregnancy outcome in preterm birth – a theranostics opportunity. Expert Rev Obstet Gynecol 2007;2(6):743–53.
92. Heizmann CW, Ackermann GE, Galichet A. Pathologies involving the S100 proteins and RAGE. Subcell Biochem 2007;45:93–138.

93. Buhimschi CS, Rosenberg VA, Dulay AT, et al. Multidimensional system biology: genetic markers and proteomic biomarkers of adverse pregnancy outcome in preterm birth. Am J Perinatol 2008;25(3):175–87.
94. Holzheimer RG. Antibiotic induced endotoxin release and clinical sepsis: a review. J Chemother 2001;1(1):159–72.
95. Klebanoff MA, Carey JC, Hauth JC, et al. Failure of metronidazole to prevent preterm delivery among pregnant women with asymptomatic *Trichomonas vaginalis* infection. N Engl J Med 2001;345(7):487–93.

Group B Streptococcal Disease in Infants: Progress in Prevention and Continued Challenges

Jennifer R. Verani, MD, MPH*, Stephanie J. Schrag, DPhil

KEYWORDS

- *Streptococcus agalactiae* • *Streptococcus* group B
- Infant • Newborn • Sepsis • Meningitis

The burden of early onset neonatal sepsis due to group B *Streptococcus* (GBS) has declined substantially over the past 20 years as a result of widespread use of intrapartum antibiotic prophylaxis. However, GBS remains the leading cause of neonatal sepsis in the United States. And unlike other diseases prevented through measures that may decrease or even eliminate the pathogen from the population, GBS colonization among pregnant women — and therefore the risk of transmission to newborns — has remained steady over time. It is important, therefore, that obstetricians and neonatologists remain vigilant about preventing and diagnosing GBS infections.

GBS DISEASE IN INFANTS

GBS emerged in the 1970s as the leading cause of neonatal sepsis and meningitis in the United States.[1–3] Two distinct clinical syndromes among infants became apparent: early onset disease that presented within the first week of life, and late-onset disease that manifested between 1 week and 3 months.[3] Before the initiation of prevention strategies, the burden of early onset disease was much greater than that of late-onset disease, with approximately 80% of GBS disease in infants occurring within the first week of life.[4] The annual incidence of early onset disease in the United States in the early 1990s (before the widespread implementation of preventive measures) was 1.7 cases per 1000 live births. The incidence of early-onset disease, however, has declined dramatically over the past 20 years, and in recent years it

The findings and conclusions in this paper are those of the authors and do not necessarily represent the views of the Centers for Disease Control and Prevention.

Respiratory Diseases Branch, Division of Bacterial Diseases, National Center for Immunization and Respiratory Diseases, Centers for Disease Control and Prevention, 1600 Clifton Road, MS C-23, Atlanta, GA 30333, USA

* Corresponding author.

E-mail address: jverani@cdc.gov

Clin Perinatol 37 (2010) 375–392

doi:10.1016/j.clp.2010.02.002

0095-5108/10/$ – see front matter. Published by Elsevier Inc.

perinatology.theclinics.com

has remained less than 0.4 cases per 1000 live births.[5] It is noteworthy that the incidence of late-onset disease (0.4 cases per 1000 live births) has remained relatively stable over the past 20 years[6] (**Fig. 1**).

Early onset GBS infections are vertically transmitted.[7] The organism may ascend from the vagina to the amniotic fluid during the intrapartum period. Once in the amniotic fluid, the bacteria may replicate and colonize the infant's skin or mucus membranes, or may be aspirated into the lungs of the infant, leading to an invasive infection. Exposure to the bacteria also may occur during passage through the birth canal. Less commonly, GBS can cross intact membranes, leading to intrauterine infection in the fetus, which may result in stillbirth or advanced infection at the time of delivery.[8,9]

In contrast to early onset disease, late-onset GBS infection is not always acquired from the mother. Maternal colonization, does play an important role; one study found approximately 50% of infants with late-onset disease had been colonized at birth, and their mothers had been colonized with an identical serotype.[10] However, the source of infection among infants born to noncolonized women is unclear. Nosocomial transmission has been demonstrated.[11,12] Horizontal transmission from mother to infant after the perinatal period may occur, and case reports also have identified breast milk as a source of infection for late-onset disease.[13–16]

Early onset disease often presents within the first hours of life, and most cases occur within the first 24 to 48 hours. Most infants exhibit signs of respiratory distress. Cardiovascular instability and apnea also are observed frequently. The most common clinical syndrome of early onset disease is bacteremia, with or without pneumonia. Less

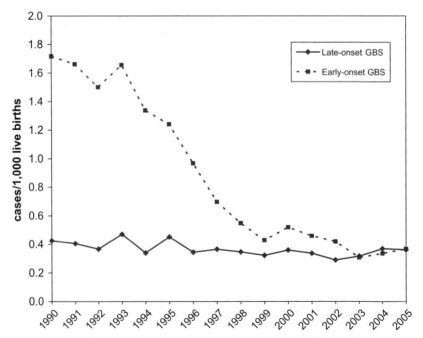

Fig. 1. Trends in early- and late-onset neonatal group B streptococcal infections in active bacterial core surveillance areas, United States, 1990–2005. (*Adapted from* Jordan HT, Farley MM, Craig A, et al. Revisiting the need for vaccine prevention of late-onset neonatal group B streptococcal disease. Pediatr Infect Dis J 2008;27:1060; with permission.)

commonly, early onset GBS infection may manifest as meningitis.[4,17,18] Early onset disease is characterized by rapid clinical deterioration.

Late-onset disease can present at any time between 1 week and 3 months of life. The median age of onset in a large review of cases in the United States was 36 days.[6] The clinical presentation of late-onset GBS infections may be similar to that of early-onset disease. Meningitis is relatively more common in infants with late-onset disease compared with early onset disease, comprising more than 25% of late-onset cases.[6,18] Sepsis, however, is the most commonly observed clinical syndrome for both early and late-onset disease. Late-onset infections also may present as septic arthritis or osteomyelitis, although such manifestations are relatively rare. The course of late-onset disease is generally less fulminant than that of early onset disease.

In the 1970s, mortality rates associated with early onset disease were reported to be 50% or higher, whereas late onset-disease had a case fatality rate of approximately 20%.[19] Advances in neonatal medical care led to improved outcomes for both clinical syndromes, with mortality rates around 4% to 6% for early and late-onset GBS infections in recent years.[6,18,20] Mortality rates among preterm infants are up to eight times higher than those of full-term infants; the risk of mortality increases with decreasing gestational age.[6,18,20,21] Despite improved survival rates, long-term sequelae resulting from GBS infections, particularly meningitis, represent a major morbidity. One long-term follow-up study of survivors of GBS meningitis found that approximately 50% of the children had some deficit, and 29% exhibited severe neurologic sequelae.[22]

RISK FACTORS FOR GBS DISEASE
Early Onset GBS Disease

The primary risk factor for early onset disease is maternal vaginal colonization with GBS. Colonization with GBS during pregnancy can be transient, intermittent, or persistent.[23–25] Colonization is asymptomatic, and the gastrointestinal tract likely serves as a reservoir for vaginal colonization.[24,26,27] In the United States, approximately 10% to 30% of pregnant woman are colonized with GBS.[28] Rates of GBS colonization are higher among black women,[27,29–32] a factor which likely contributes to the disproportionate burden of GBS disease observed among black infants.[5] HIV infection does not appear to influence likelihood of GBS colonization among pregnant women.[33] The risk for early onset disease increases with heavier colonization in the mother.[34,35] GBS bacteriuria is considered a marker of heavy maternal colonization and has been associated with an increased risk of neonatal disease.[36–38]

In the absence of any intervention, approximately 1% to 2% of infants born to colonized mothers develop early onset GBS infections.[17,39,40] Additional factors beyond maternal GBS colonization, however, play a role in risk for early onset disease. Maternal chorioamnionitis, intrapartum maternal fever (a marker of chorioamnionitis) and prolonged rupture of membranes are all strongly associated with early onset GBS disease.[10,41–43] These obstetric risk factors may reflect increased and prolonged infant exposure to GBS before delivery. Some studies have identified certain obstetric procedures, such as the use of intrauterine fetal monitoring devices[41,44] or greater than or equal to five vaginal examinations during labor,[41,45] to be associated with early onset disease.

Preterm infants, in addition to suffering worse outcomes from GBS disease, are at 3- to 30-fold greater risk of developing early onset infections compared with full-term infants, with the highest risk at lower gestational ages (**Fig. 2**).[44,46,47] The risk among preterm infants likely is related to decreased transfer of maternal antibodies.[48] Although preterm infants have a much greater risk of early onset GBS disease,

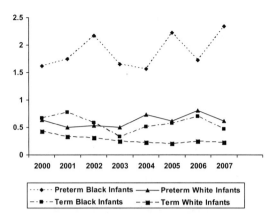

Fig. 2. Early-onset group B streptococcal incidence rates in active bacterial core surveillance areas stratified by race and term, 2000—2007. (*Adapted from* CDC. Trends in perinatal group B streptococcal disease—United States, 2000–2006. MMWR Morb Mortal Wkly Rep 2009;58:109–12.)

approximately 75% of cases occur among term infants.[28,49] This is in contrast to other pathogens causing neonatal sepsis (such as *Escherichia coli*) that predominantly affect preterm infants.

Early onset GBS disease disproportionately affects black infants, even after stratifying by term to adjust for the higher rates of preterm delivery among blacks (see **Fig. 2**).[5,46] Higher rates of maternal colonization may be a contributing factor; yet the racial disparity has persisted despite widespread use of intrapartum antibiotics. The implementation of universal screening and intrapartum antibiotic prophylaxis (IAP) has been relatively high among women of all races, and differences in implementation do not account for the observed racial disparities in infant GBS disease.[49]

Young maternal age is associated with an increased risk of early onset disease,[43,46] likely as a result of lower levels of anti-GBS antibodies in younger age groups of women.[29] Low maternal antibody levels have been shown to convey an increased risk of early onset disease in the infant.[50–52] Previous delivery of an infant with GBS disease—which may also be associated with low maternal antibody levels—is a risk factor for early onset GBS disease in subsequent pregnancies.[53–55]

Late-onset GBS Disease

The risk factors for late-onset disease are not as well characterized as those for early onset disease. Maternal colonization, while not as strongly associated as it is with early onset disease, is a risk factor for late-onset GBS sepsis.[56] As with early onset disease, prematurity has been found to be an important risk factor for late-onset GBS disease.[56] Black race is also a risk factor for late-onset disease.[46] The incidence of late-onset GBS disease is three times higher among black infants in the United States compared with white infants, and the increased risk persists after stratifying by gestational age.[6] As with early onset disease, the cause of this racial disparity is unclear.

GBS PREVENTION IN THE UNITED STATES

Clinical trials in the 1980s demonstrated that IAP could reduce the risk of early onset GBS infections in infants.[57,58] The efficacy of IAP for preventing early onset disease is nearly

90%.[59,60] Use of IAP increased throughout the 1990s, with widespread uptake following the publication of consensus guidelines for the prevention of perinatal GBS disease developed by the Centers for Disease Control and Prevention (CDC), the American College of Obstetricians and Gynecologists, and the American Academy of Pediatrics (AAP) in 1996.[40] The guidelines advocated one of two methods to identify candidates for IAP:

1. Culture-based screening for pregnant women between 35 and 37 weeks gestation to identify women colonized with GBS
2. Risk-based screening for women with intrapartum risk factors (including gestational age less than 37 weeks, temperature of at least 100.4°, or rupture of membranes for at least 18 hours).

IAP also was recommended for women with GBS bacteriuria at any point during the pregnancy, and women with a history of a previous infant with invasive GBS disease. The 1996 guidelines were implemented widely across the Untied States, with IAP administered in approximately 27% of deliveries in 1998 and 1999.[59] Early onset GBS disease declined by approximately 70% during the 1990s.[28]

In 2002, the GBS prevention guidelines were revised. The fundamental change in the updated guidelines was a recommendation for universal culture-based screening, since a population-based study had demonstrated the superiority of this approach over risk factor-based screening.[59] The risk-based approach was recommended only in cases where the maternal GBS status was unknown or unavailable at the time of delivery. The 2002 guidelines also incorporated recommendations for the prevention of GBS disease in the context of preterm labor, and for revised second-line antibiotic agents for penicillin-allergic women. The 2002 guidelines stated that IAP was not indicated in the context of planned cesarean deliveries before the onset of labor or rupture of membranes.[28]

A large population-based cohort study conducted in 2003 and 2004 demonstrated that the acceptance of universal screening as recommended in the 2002 guidelines was widespread. Van Dyke and colleagues[49] reported that the proportion of pregnant women screened before delivery increased from 48% in 1998 and1999 to 85% in 2003 and 2004. The proportion of women with an indication for IAP who actually received intrapartum antibiotics increased from 74% to 85% during the same time period (**Fig. 3**).

The study by Van Dyke and colleagues[49] also identified areas for improvement in the implementation of the GBS prevention guidelines. Although the 2002 guidelines recommended that women with threatened preterm labor should be screened on admission if GBS culture was not performed in the previous 4 weeks, among women with threatened preterm delivery and unknown GBS status, only 18% of those who progressed to delivery and 31% of those who did not progress to delivery underwent GBS screening on admission. Furthermore, despite preterm delivery being an indication for IAP in women with unknown GBS colonization status, only 63% of women who delivered preterm with unknown colonization received IAP. Suboptimal implementation also was noted in the choice of antibiotic agent for penicillin-allergic women. Only 14% of penicillin-allergic women at low risk for anaphylaxis received the recommended agent cefazolin. Clindamycin was the most commonly used agent among penicillin-allergic mothers, given to 70% of women at low risk for anaphylaxis and 84% of those at high risk. However, the effectiveness of clindamycin as an IAP agent is unknown; there are very limited data on the pharmacokinetics of clindamycin in pregnancy, and GBS is becoming increasingly resistant to clindamycin.[18,61]

Despite these limitations, the incidence of early onset disease was reduced further following the issuance of the 2002 guidelines. In recent years, the incidence has

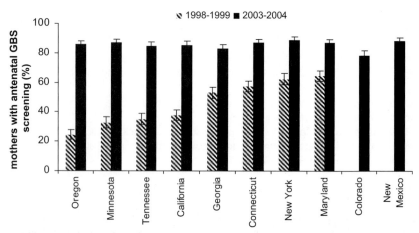

Fig. 3. Proportion of pregnant women with antenatal screening for GBS in active bacterial core surveillance areas across the United States. (*From* Van Dyke MK, Phares CR, Lynfield R, et al. Evaluation of universal antenatal screening for Group B Streptococcus. NEJM 2009;360:2630; with permission.)

remained fairly stable at 0.34 to 0.37 cases per 1000 live births.[5,18] Late-onset disease unfortunately is not impacted by IAP, and incidence rates have remained fairly stable of the past 20 years (see **Fig. 1**).

Neonatal Management Challenges in the era of GBS Prevention

As the use of IAP for prevention of GBS disease became more widespread in the 1990s, there was initially substantial apprehension about whether exposure to IAP would complicate detection of sepsis in the newborn or impact the management approach of pediatricians. The 1996 and 2002 guidelines for GBS prevention included a sample algorithm for the management of infants exposed to intrapartum antibiotics that recommended a full diagnostic evaluation and empiric treatment for infants considered to be at very high risk of sepsis, a more limited evaluation in those with a lesser risk, and observation only for infants whose mother received at least 4 hours of an appropriate antibiotics. These recommendations aimed to identify infants at high risk for early onset GBS disease, while avoiding unnecessary diagnostic evaluations in neonates. Nonetheless, the management of infants in the era of universal screening and IAP remains challenging. Studies in recent years have provided additional data that permit a refining of the neonatal management recommendations in the GBS prevention guidelines.

Presentation of Early Onset GBS Disease After Exposure to IAP

Uncertainty about how IAP might affect the clinical presentation of early onset GBS sepsis led to concerns that prevention efforts could impair the ability of pediatricians to diagnose GBS disease. Exposure to antibiotics potentially could mask the signs of sepsis in a newborn, or delay the onset until after the infant had been discharged home, resulting in true cases of early onset disease going undetected until late in the clinical course. Several studies conducted after 1996, however, have found no significant difference in the clinical presentation of early onset GBS sepsis between infants exposed to IAP and those not exposed. Although some cases of early onset disease are detected in infants with no signs of sepsis who are screened because of risk factors for GBS sepsis,[21,62–64] most infants with GBS sepsis present with signs of infection within the first 24 to 48 hours of life, a pattern unaffected by exposure to IAP.[21,62–65]

Management of Infants Exposed to IAP

During the early phase of GBS prevention efforts, there was also concern that pediatricians might react to the uncertainty of the clinical management of infants exposed to IAP by conducting excessive evaluations and treating infants unnecessarily with antibiotics.[66,67] A population-based study in Connecticut in 1996 found that infants of women who received IAP were no more likely to receive an antibiotic and did not have a significant increase in length of stay compared with infants born to women who did not receive IAP.[68] In contrast, a study conducted in 19 hospitals in Utah from 1998 to 2002 found that infants born to mothers who received any intravenous antibiotic were more likely to receive intravenous antibiotics for more than 72 hours and had significantly longer lengths of stay and hospital costs, compared with infants whose mothers did not receive any intravenous antibiotics. This study was limited by use of administrative data only, which did not permit the authors to determine whether maternal antibiotics were administered intrapartum and thus were administered for GBS prevention or some other reason.[69] Further studies on the impact of the GBS prevention guidelines on the management of at-risk infants are needed.

The 2002 guidelines recommend that infants of mothers who receive intrapartum antibiotics for suspected chorioamnionitis undergo a full diagnostic evaluation and receive empiric antibiotic therapy for possible GBS disease. Chorioamnionitis is an important risk factor for early onset GBS disease, and may indicate active infection in the fetus before delivery. Intrapartum fever—often a symptom of chorioamnionitis—has been identified as risk factor for failure of IAP to prevent GBS disease in the newborn.[60,70] Given the association between epidural labor analgesia and fever, however, there is concern that chorioamnionitis may be overdiagnosed, resulting in unnecessary diagnostic evaluations of neonates.[71] Unpublished data from CDC surveillance sites across the United States in 2003 and 2004 demonstrated that while 67% of parturients received epidural labor analgesia, only 4% of those had fever, and the proportion of women diagnosed with chorioamnionitis (3%) was the same among the women with and without epidural labor analgesia. Thus, clinical chorioamnionitis is relatively uncommon—even among women with epidural labor analgesia—but warrants particular concern for clinicians caring for newborns.

Diagnostic Evaluations Among Infants Exposed to IAP

The 1996 and 2002 GBS prevention guidelines recommended a limited evaluation (complete blood cell [CBC] count with differential and blood culture) for infants exposed to IAP who are either less than 35 weeks gestational age or whose mother received less than 4 hours of IAP before delivery. The rationale behind the gestational age limit was that in the setting of IAP, it may be difficult to properly ascertain signs of sepsis in very preterm infants, and that CBC count and blood culture may aid in making the diagnosis. The recommendation regarding duration of IAP stems from evidence that IAP given for less than 4 hours is less effective at preventing colonization and early onset GBS disease compared with antibiotics given for longer durations[60,72](S. Schrag, PhD, unpublished data, 2009). Therefore, IAP given for less than 4 hours might be insufficient to decrease the risk of disease, but may impact the clinical presentation in a manner that would make it more difficult to diagnose sepsis.

Limited data available on the performance of CBC count as a screening test, however, suggest that while the test has a relatively high negative predictive value, the positive predictive value is quite limited, particularly among infants with no sings of sepsis.[73–75] A large study of neonatal sepsis evaluations among infants weighing at least 2000 g at birth conducted in 1995 and 1996 demonstrated that the presence of clinical signs of sepsis is a highly sensitive indicator of sepsis of all etiologies.[63] All infants with early onset GBS sepsis had clinical signs of infection within 8–12 hours of birth, regardless of whether their mother had received intrapartum antibiotics. The findings suggest that for many infants, careful clinicial observation performs well as a screen for early onset GBS sepsis.

False-Negative Cases of Early Onset GBS Disease

Studies reporting on patterns of early onset GBS disease in the era of widespread use of IAP have found approximately 60% to 80% of cases occur among infants born to women with a negative antenatal GBS screen.[21,49,64] False-negative cases are bound to occur; GBS culture at 35 to 37 weeks has a 95% to 97% negative predictive value for absence of colonization at the time of delivery. Therefore, a small proportion of women will not be colonized at the time of their screening and acquire GBS colonization between the time of the culture and the onset of labor.[76] Indeed, if the implementation of the guidelines were optimized (all pregnant women screened, and all women with indications for IAP receiving IAP), then those cases that continue to occur would highly likely be born to mothers who had screened negative, reflecting the inherent limitations of the prevention strategy. Clinicians should understand that a negative maternal GBS screen indicates that an infant is at low–but not zero—risk of GBS disease. GBS sepsis should be suspected in any infant with signs of sepsis, regardless of maternal screening results.

POTENTIAL UNINTENDED CONSEQUENCES OF GBS PREVENTION
Non-GBS Sepsis

Although GBS prevention efforts have very effectively decreased early onset GBS infections in the United States, there has been concern about the overall impact of widespread IAP on early onset neonatal sepsis. One question raised is whether the decrease in GBS infections is a true reduction in disease, or whether antibiotics are simply resulting in negative cultures while GBS continues to cause clinical sepsis. Nationally representative hospital discharge data, however, demonstrated a steady decrease in clinical sepsis rates from 1990 to 2002, with a marked decline in clinical sepsis among term infants during the 2 years following the issuance of the 1996 GBS prevention guidelines.[77]

Another concern is whether the decrease in GBS disease has been accompanied by an increase in other potentially more lethal neonatal pathogens. The predominant etiologies of neonatal sepsis have tended to change over time, and the leading causes of neonatal sepsis before the emergence of GBS in the 1970s were gram-negative pathogens, including E coli.[78,79] As the incidence of early onset GBS disease has declined over the past 15 years, the relative contribution of E coli and other non-GBS pathogens has increased. Yet, in terms of disease incidence, most studies have found overall stable[80–87] or decreasing[88,89] rates of sepsis caused by non-GBS pathogens during time periods in which the use of IAP has increased. An increased rate of E coli infections has been noted among preterm and low birth weight or very low birth weight infants,[90–94] although it is unclear whether GBS prevention efforts have contributed to the observed rise in E coli infections among preterm infants. Of note, a large, multicenter study of sepsis in preterm infants that reported an increase in E coli incidence between 1991 to 1993 and 1998 to 2000, found no significant change between 1998 to 2000 and 2002 to 2003.[95] The results of this study and one other also suggest that early onset sepsis caused by coagulase-negative staphylococci may be on the rise among preterm or very low birth weight infants.[87,95] Continued monitoring of trends in non-GBS pathogens among preterm and low birth weight infants is needed. Available evidence to date does not suggest any rise in non-GBS sepsis among term infants.

Another worry about widespread use of IAP is that it may select for ampicillin-resistant non GBS-pathogens, resulting in sepsis that is more difficult to treat. Some studies have found an increasing proportion of ampicillin-resistant isolates among preterm or very low birth weight infants with *E coli* sepsis over time.[85,93,96] A large multicenter study, however, found no significant change in the proportion of ampicillin-resistant *E coli* causing sepsis among very low birth weight infants between 1998 to 2000 and 2002 to 2003[95] In addition, ampicillin-resistant *E coli* is increasing in settings beyond the newborn nursery.[97] Therefore it is unclear to what extent IAP may be contributing to changes in resistance patterns.

Other studies have reported an association between IAP exposure and infection with ampicillin-resistant *E coli* and other gram-negative pathogens among infants of all gestational ages[45,90,98–100] and among preterm infants[93,94] These studies, however, have used infants infected with nonresistant pathogens as a control group; such a design does not account for the ampicillin-susceptible infections that are prevented by IAP and therefore tends to overestimate an association between antibiotic exposure and antibiotic resistance.[101] A large, case–control study that enrolled early onset *E coli* cases and uninfected infants born at the same hospitals found no association between IAP exposure and infection with ampicillin-resistant *E coli*.[102]

GBS Antibiotic Resistance

Another issue often raised regarding IAP is whether the extensive use of antibiotics in GBS-colonized women may exert selective pressure on the organism resulting in antibiotic resistance. Fortunately, GBS remains susceptible to penicillin and ampicillin, as well as most cephalosporins. In recent years there have been reports of isolates with increasing minimum inhibitory concentrations (MICs) to beta-lactam antibiotics, including 14 noninvasive isolates from adults in Japan,[103] and 22 invasive isolates recovered from patients of varying ages in the United States.[104] The isolates were not clustered geographically or temporally (collected from 1995 to 2005 in Japan and 1999 to 2005 in the United States). Alterations in a penicillin-binding protein, which may explain the elevated MICs, were found in all of the isolates from Japan and four of those from the United States. The measured MICs are just at the susceptibility threshold, and their clinical significance is as yet unclear. Although clinicians can confidently continue to use beta-lactam antibiotics for the prevention and treatment of GBS infections, continued surveillance of susceptibility patterns is warranted.

GBS resistance to macrolides, on the other hand, is clearly on the rise. Various studies in the United States have found the proportion of colonizing and invasive GBS isolates resistant to clindamycin to be in the range of 10% to 20%,[61,105–108] and rates of resistance as high as 41% have been reported.[109] Most studies have also reported increases in erythromycin resistance over time. The decreasing susceptibility of GBS to clindamycin and erythromycin underscores the importance of careful choice of IAP agent for penicillin-allergic GBS-colonized women at high risk for anaphylaxis.

2010 GBS GUIDELINES REVISION

The GBS prevention guidelines are currently under revision, and updated recommendations are expected by the end of 2010. A working group involving representatives from CDC, the Committee on Infectious Disease and Committee on the Fetus and Newborn of the AAP, the American College of Obstetricians and Gynecologists, the American College of Nurse Midwives, microbiologists, pharmacologists and other key stakeholders has been reviewing available data on the implementation and impact of the 2002 guidelines, as well as advances in laboratory methods for GBS detection. The revised guidelines will aim to strengthen and clarify recommendations where available data suggest that implementation has been suboptimal, such as preterm deliveries and the management of penicillin-allergic women. Recommendations regarding newer laboratory procedures, such as pigmented growth media and molecular methods for GBS detection will be included.

Efforts are underway to clarify and expand the scope of the algorithm and recommendations for the clinical care of infants as it pertains to GBS prevention, as reflected in the proposed revised algorithm in **Fig. 4**. Recognizing that an increasing proportion of cases of early onset GBS disease occur among infants born to women with negative

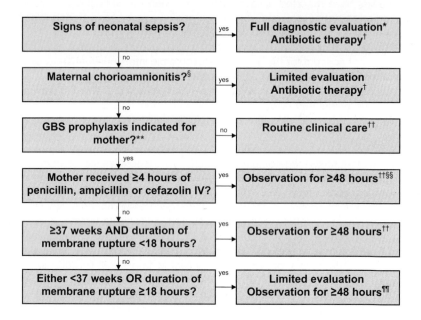

* Includes CBC with differential, platelets, blood culture, chest radiograph (if respiratory abnormalities are present), and LP (if patient stable enough to tolerate procedure and sepsis is suspected).

† Antibiotic therapy should be directed towards the most common causes of neonatal sepsis including GBS and other organisms (including gram negative pathgoens), and should take into account local antibiotic resistance patterns.

§ Consultation with obstetric providers is important to determine the level of clinical suspicion for chorioamnionitis. Chorioamnionitis is diagnosed clinically and some of the signs are non-specific.

¶ Includes blood culture (at birth), and CBC with differential and platelets. Some experts recommend a CBC with differential and platelets at 6-12 hours of age.

** GBS prophylaxis indicated if one or more of the following: (1) mother GBS positive at 35-37 weeks' gestation, (2) GBS status unknown with one or more intrapartum risk factors including <37 weeks' gestation, ROM ≥18 hours or T ≥100.4°F (38.0°C), (3) GBS bacteriuria during current pregnancy, (4) history of a previous infant with GBS disease.

†† If signs of sepsis develop, a full diagnostic evaluation should be done and antibiotic therapy initiated.

§§ If ≥37 weeks' gestation, observation may occur at home after 24 hours if there is a knowledgeable observer and ready access to medical care.

¶¶ Some experts recommend a CBC with differential and platelets at 6-12 hours of age.

Fig. 4. Algorithm for recommended management of newborns at risk for group B streptococcal disease.

GBS screens, the proposed revised algorithm will apply to all infants, regardless of maternal GBS status or exposure to IAP. Any infant with signs of sepsis should undergo a full diagnostic evaluation (including CBC count with differential and platelets, a blood culture, a chest radiograph if respiratory symptoms are present, and a lumbar puncture if the patient is stable enough to tolerate the procedure) and receive antibiotic treatment. Similarly, any infant whose mother had chorioamnionitis should have a diagnostic evaluation and receive antibiotic therapy. In the case of a well-appearing infant whose mother had chorioamnionitis, the evaluation need not include a chest radiograph or a lumbar puncture. Chorioamnionitis is diagnosed clinically and may be overdiagnosed in the setting of fevers resulting from epidural labor analgesia. Thus, clinicians caring for infants born to women with suspected chorioamnionitis may wish to confer with obstetric providers regarding the likelihood of true chorioamnionitis in the mother to avoid unnecessary evaluations and antibiotics in the neonate.

For well-appearing infants with no exposure to maternal chorioamnionitis, recommended management will depend on whether IAP was indicated for the mother. If IAP was not indicated and an infant is well appearing, then routine care is recommended. If IAP was indicated, then neonatal management will be guided by the adequacy of IAP and the presence of certain risk factors for early onset disease. If the mother received penicillin, ampicillin, or cefazolin for at least 4 hours, then the infant should be observed for at least 48 hours. If the IAP was less than 4 hours in duration, or another agent such as clindamycin or vancomycin (for which there are very limited data on effectiveness for preventing vertical GBS transmission), then the IAP is considered to be inadequate. However, in the absence of other risk factors, including gestational age less than 37 weeks or rupture of membranes greater than 18 hours, infants exposed to inadequate IAP may be managed through careful clinical observation for at least 48 hours; this is in contrast to the 2002 recommendation that all such infants have a screening CBC and blood culture. If the IAP was inadequate and the delivery was either preterm or complicated by prolonged rupture of membranes, then the infant should have a limited diagnostic evaluation; antibiotics are not warranted unless the laboratory or clinical findings are suggestive of sepsis. Adherence to the revised neonatal recommendations would be expected to result in fewer unnecessary diagnostic evaluations in well-appearing newborns. The recommendations and algorithm presented here are proposed changes to the 2002 guidelines and may undergo further revision before dissemination.

FUTURE OF GBS PREVENTION: VACCINES

Maternal immunization against GBS is an appealing approach to preventing perinatal GBS disease. A vaccine that effectively prevents or diminishes colonization in parturient women and results in transplacental transfer of antibody to infants could obviate the need for antenatal GBS screening and use of IAP. Additionally, a GBS vaccine might help prevent stillbirth caused by GBS, late-onset GBS disease, and invasive GBS infections in mothers. An effective vaccine also may help diminish the persistent racial disparities in neonatal GBS disease.

The protective effect of maternal antibodies against neonatal GBS disease has been demonstrated in several studies.[48,110,111] Several candidate vaccines targeting GBS surface proteins have been developed, and phase 1 and 2 human studies of capsular polysaccharide-protein conjugate vaccines have found the vaccines to be safe and immunogenic.[112-114] A recent double-blind randomized trial of a conjugate GBS (serotype 3) vaccine among nonpregnant women of reproductive age resulted in a significant delay in acquisition of the serotype contained in the vaccine among vaccine recipients compared with those who did not receive the vaccine.[115] Although GBS vaccines have shown promise, there remain hurdles to overcome. Clinical trials among pregnant women are complicated by ethical and medicolegal concerns. Furthermore, the primary outcome of interest—early onset GBS sepsis—has become a relatively rare endpoint as a result of antenatal screening and IAP. Trials using immunologic responses or maternal colonization may be more realistic approaches to obtaining vaccine licensure.[114]

SUMMARY

Much progress has been made toward decreasing the burden of early onset GBS disease in the United States. The incidence has declined by more than 80% since the preprevention era. Maternal GBS colonization, however, remains as common as during the preprevention era, and the risk for GBS infection in an infant born to a colonized mother who failed to receive IAP or received inadequate IAP is as high as it was in the early 1970s. Prevention efforts must be ongoing to maintain and further reduce the incidence of early onset disease. Further research is needed to identify effective means to reduce racial disparities for GBS disease and to decrease the burden of late-onset GBS disease, including vaccine trials.

The currently available GBS prevention strategies are highly effective at preventing early onset disease, but imperfect. Even with ideal implementation of universal screening and IAP, some cases will continue to occur among infants born to women who became colonized after their antenatal GBS screen, or who had a precipitous delivery that did not allow sufficient time for effective IAP. Clinicians must understand the risk factors for early onset GBS disease and the limitations of the prevention strategies to rapidly detect and treat cases that continue to occur in the era of GBS prevention through IAP. Revised GBS prevention guidelines will provide updated recommendations regarding the care of newborns in relation to GBS prevention.

REFERENCES

1. Baker CJ, Barrett FF, Gordon RC, et al. Suppurative meningitis due to streptococci of Lancefield group B: a study of 33 infants. J Pediatr 1973;82(4):724–9.
2. Barton LL, Feigin RD, Lins R. Group B beta hemolytic streptococcal meningitis in infants. J Pediatr 1973;82(4):719–23.
3. Franciosi RA, Knostman JD, Zimmerman RA. Group B streptococcal neonatal and infant infections. J Pediatr 1973;82(4):707–18.
4. Schuchat A. Epidemiology of group B streptococcal disease in the United States: shifting paradigms. Clin Microbiol Rev 1998;11(3):497–513.
5. CDC. Trends in perinatal group B streptococcal disease—United States, 2000–2006. MMWR Morb Mortal Wkly Rep 2009;58(5):109–12.
6. Jordan HT, Farley MM, Craig A, et al. Revisiting the need for vaccine prevention of late-onset neonatal group B streptococcal disease: a multistate, population-based analysis. Pediatr Infect Dis J 2008;27(12):1057–64.
7. Baker CJ, Barrett FF. Transmission of group B streptococci among parturient women and their neonates. J Pediatr 1973;83(6):919–25.
8. Desa DJ, Trevenen CL. Intrauterine infections with group B beta-haemolytic streptococci. Br J Obstet Gynaecol 1984;91(3):237–9.
9. Katz V, Bowes WA Jr. Perinatal group B streptococcal infections across intact amniotic membranes. J Reprod Med 1988;33(5):445–9.
10. Dillon HC Jr, Khare S, Gray BM. Group B streptococcal carriage and disease: a 6-year prospective study. J Pediatr 1987;110(1):31–6.

11. Easmon CS, Hastings MJ, Clare AJ, et al. Nosocomial transmission of group B streptococci. Br Med J 1981;283(6289):459–61.
12. Anthony BF, Okada DM, Hobel CJ. Epidemiology of the group B streptococcus: maternal and nosocomial sources for infant acquisitions. J Pediatr 1979;95(3): 431–6.
13. Olver WJ, Bond DW, Boswell TC, et al. Neonatal group B streptococcal disease associated with infected breast milk. Arch Dis Child 2000;83(1):F48–9.
14. Dinger J, Muller D, Pargac N, et al. Breast milk transmission of group B streptococcal infection. Pediatr Infect Dis J 2002;21(6):567–8.
15. Godambe S, Shah PS, Shah V. Breast milk as a source of late onset neonatal sepsis. Pediatr Infect Dis J 2005;24(4):381–2.
16. Wang LY, Chen CT, Liu WH, et al. Recurrent neonatal group B streptococcal disease associated with infected breast milk. Clin Pediatr (Phila) 2007;46(6): 547–9.
17. NIH. Summary of the workshop on perinatal infections due to group B *Streptococcus*. J Infect Dis 1977;136(1):137–52.
18. Phares CR, Lynfield R, Farley MM, et al. Epidemiology of invasive group B streptococcal disease in the United States, 1999–2005. JAMA 2008;299(17): 2056–65.
19. Baker CJ, Barrett FF. Group B streptococcal infections in infants. The importance of the various serotypes. JAMA 1974;230(8):1158–60.
20. Schrag SJ, Zywicki S, Farley MM, et al. Group B streptococcal disease in the era of intrapartum antibiotic prophylaxis. N Engl J Med 2000;342(1):15–20.
21. Puopolo KM, Madoff LC, Eichenwald EC. Early-onset group B streptococcal disease in the era of maternal screening. Pediatrics 2005;115(5):1240–6.
22. Edwards MS, Rench MA, Haffar AA, et al. Long-term sequelae of group B streptococcal meningitis in infants. J Pediatr 1985;106(5):717–22.
23. Lewin EB, Amstey MS. Natural history of group B streptococcus colonization and its therapy during pregnancy. Am J Obstet Gynecol 1981;139(5):512–5.
24. Hoogkamp-Korstanje JA, Gerards LJ, Cats BP. Maternal carriage and neonatal acquisition of group B streptococci. J Infect Dis 1982;145(6):800–3.
25. Hansen SM, Uldbjerg N, Kilian M, et al. Dynamics of *Streptococcus agalactiae* colonization in women during and after pregnancy and in their infants. J Clin Microbiol 2004;42(1):83–9.
26. Badri MS, Zawaneh S, Cruz AC, et al. Rectal colonization with group B *Streptococcus*: relation to vaginal colonization of pregnant women. J Infect Dis 1977; 135(2):308–12.
27. Meyn LA, Krohn MA, Hillier SL. Rectal colonization by group B *Streptococcus* as a predictor of vaginal colonization. Am J Obstet Gynecol 2009;201(1):76, e1–e7.
28. Schrag S, Gorwitz R, Fultz-Butts K, et al. Prevention of perinatal group B streptococcal disease. Revised guidelines from CDC. MMWR Recomm Rep 2002; 51(RR-11):1–22.
29. Campbell JR, Hillier SL, Krohn MA, et al. Group B streptococcal colonization and serotype-specific immunity in pregnant women at delivery. Obstet Gynecol 2000;96(4):498–503.
30. Newton ER, Butler MC, Shain RN. Sexual behavior and vaginal colonization by group B *Streptococcus* among minority women. Obstet Gynecol 1996;88: 577–82.
31. Stapleton RD, Kahn JM, Evans LE, et al. Risk factors for group B streptococcal genitourinary tract colonization in pregnant women. Obstet Gynecol 2005; 106(6):1246–52.

32. Katz VL, Moos MK, Cefalo RC, et al. Group B streptococci: results of a protocol of antepartum screening and intrapartum treatment. Am J Obstet Gynecol 1994; 170(2):521–6.
33. El Beitune P, Duarte G, Maffei CM, et al. Group B *Streptococcus* carriers among HIV-1 infected pregnant women: prevalence and risk factors. Eur J Obstet Gynecol Reprod Biol 2006;128(1–2):54–8.
34. Yancey MK, Duff P, Kubilis P, et al. Risk factors for neonatal sepsis. Obstet Gynecol 1996;87(2):188–94.
35. Regan JA, Klebanoff MA, Nugent RP, et al. Colonization with group B streptococci in pregnancy and adverse outcome. VIP Study Group. Am J Obstet Gynecol 1996;174(4):1354–60.
36. Liston TE, Harris RE, Foshee S, et al. Relationship of neonatal pneumonia to maternal urinary and neonatal isolates of group B streptococci. South Med J 1979;72(11):1410–2.
37. Wood EG, Dillon HC Jr. A prospective study of group B streptococcal bacteriuria in pregnancy. Am J Obstet Gynecol 1981;140(5):515–20.
38. Persson K, Christensen KK, Christensen P, et al. Asymptomatic bacteriuria during pregnancy with special reference to group B streptococci. Scand J Infect Dis 1985;17(2):195–9.
39. Boyer KM, Gotoff SP. Strategies for chemoprophylaxis of GBS early onset infections. Antibiot Chemother 1985;35:267–80.
40. CDC. Prevention of perinatal group B streptococcal disease: a public health perspective. Centers for Disease Control and Prevention. MMWR Recomm Rep 1996;45(RR-7):1–24.
41. Adams WG, Kinney JS, Schuchat A, et al. Outbreak of early onset group B streptococcal sepsis. Pediatr Infect Dis J 1993;12(7):565–70.
42. Boyer KM, Gadzala CA, Burd LI, et al. Selective intrapartum chemoprophylaxis of neonatal group B streptococcal early onset disease. I. Epidemiologic rationale. J Infect Dis 1983;148(5):795–801.
43. Schuchat A, Deaver-Robinson K, Plikaytis BD, et al. Multistate case–control study of maternal risk factors for neonatal group B streptococcal disease. The Active Surveillance Study Group. Pediatr Infect Dis J 1994;13(7):623–9.
44. Adair CE, Kowalsky L, Quon H, et al. Risk factors for early-onset group B streptococcal disease in neonates: a population-based case–control study. CMAJ 2003;169(3):198–203.
45. Schuchat A, Zywicki SS, Dinsmoor MJ, et al. Risk factors and opportunities for prevention of early-onset neonatal sepsis: a multicenter case–control study. Pediatrics 2000;105:21–6.
46. Schuchat A, Oxtoby M, Cochi S, et al. Population-based risk factors for neonatal group B streptococcal disease: results of a cohort study in metropolitan Atlanta. J Infect Dis 1990;162(3):672–7.
47. Oddie S, Embleton ND. Risk factors for early onset neonatal group B streptococcal sepsis: case–control study. BMJ 2002;325(7359):308.
48. Baker CJ, Kasper DL. Correlation of maternal antibody deficiency with susceptibility to neonatal group B streptococcal infection. N Engl J Med 1976;294(14):753–6.
49. Van Dyke MK, Phares CR, Lynfield R, et al. Evaluation of universal antenatal screening for group B *Streptococcus*. N Engl J Med 2009;360(25):2626–36.
50. Baker CJ, Edwards MS, Kasper DL. Role of antibody to native type III polysaccharide of group B *Streptococcus* in infant infection. Pediatrics 1981;68(4):544–9.

51. Vogel LC, Boyer KM, Gadzala CA, et al. Prevalence of type-specific group B streptococcal antibody in pregnant women. J Pediatr 1980;96(6):1047–51.
52. Christensen KK, Christensen P, Dahlander K, et al. Quantitation of serum antibodies to surface antigens of group B streptococci types Ia, Ib, and III: low antibody levels in mothers of neonatally infected infants. Scand J Infect Dis 1980;12(2):105–10.
53. Christensen KK, Dahlander K, Linden V, et al. Obstetrical care in future pregnancies after fetal loss in group B streptococcal septicemia. A prevention program based on bacteriological and immunological follow-up. Eur J Obstet Gynecol Reprod Biol 1981;12(3):143–50.
54. Faxelius G, Bremme K, Kvist-Christensen K, et al. Neonatal septicemia due to group B streptococci–perinatal risk factors and outcome of subsequent pregnancies. J Perinat Med 1988;16(5-6):423–30.
55. Carstensen H, Christensen KK, Grennert L, et al. Early-onset neonatal group B streptococcal septicaemia in siblings. J Infect 1988;17(3):201–4.
56. Lin FY, Weisman LE, Troendle J, et al. Prematurity is the major risk factor for late-onset group B Streptococcus disease. J Infect Dis 2003;188(2):267–71.
57. Boyer KM, Gotoff SP. Prevention of early-onset neonatal group B streptococcal disease with selective intrapartum chemoprophylaxis. New Engl J Med 1986; 314(26):1665–9.
58. Garland SM, Fliegner JR. Group B Streptococcus (GBS) and neonatal infections: the case for intrapartum chemoprophylaxis. Aust N Z J Obstet Gynaecol 1991;31(2):119–22.
59. Schrag SJ, Zell ER, Lynfield R, et al. A population-based comparison of strategies to prevent early onset group B streptococcal disease in neonates. New Engl J Med 2002;347(4):233–9.
60. Lin FY, Brenner RA, Johnson YR, et al. The effectiveness of risk-based intrapartum chemoprophylaxis for the prevention of early onset neonatal group B streptococcal disease. Am J Obstet Gynecol 2001;184(6):1204–10.
61. Castor ML, Whitney CG, Como-Sabetti K, et al. Antibiotic resistance patterns in invasive group B streptococcal isolates. Infect Dis Obstet Gynecol 2008;2008: 727505.
62. Bromberger P, Lawrence JM, Braun D, et al. The influence of intrapartum antibiotics on the clinical spectrum of early onset group B streptococcal infection in term infants. Pediatrics 2000;106:244–50.
63. Escobar GJ, Li DK, Armstrong MA, et al. Neonatal sepsis workups in infants ≥2000 grams at birth: a population-based study. Pediatrics 2000;106:256–63.
64. Pulver LS, Hopfenbeck MM, Young PC, et al. Continued early onset group B streptococcal infections in the era of intrapartum prophylaxis. J Perinatol 2009;29(1):20–5.
65. Pinto NM, Soskolne EI, Pearlman MD, et al. Neonatal early onset group B streptococcal disease in the era of intrapartum chemoprophylaxis: residual problems. J Perinatol 2003;23(4):265–71.
66. Mercer BM, Ramsey RD, Sibai BM. Prenatal screening for group B Streptococcus. II. Impact of antepartum screening and prophylaxis on neonatal care. Am J Obstet Gynecol 1995;173:842–6.
67. Peralta-Carcelen M, Fargason CA Jr, Cliver SP, et al. Impact of maternal group B streptococcal screening on pediatric management in full-term newborns. Arch Pediatr Adolesc Med 1996;150(8):802–8.
68. Balter S, Zell ER, O'Brien KL, et al. Impact of intrapartum antibiotics on the care and evaluation of the neonate. Pediatr Infect Dis J 2003;22(10):853–7.

69. Glasgow TS, Speakman M, Firth S, et al. Clinical and economic outcomes for term infants associated with increasing administration of antibiotics to their mothers. Paediatr perinat epidemiol 2007;21(4):338–46.
70. Ascher DP, Becker JA, Yoder BA, et al. Failure of intrapartum antibiotics to prevent culture-proved neonatal group B streptococcal sepsis. J Perinatol 1993;13(3):212–6.
71. Lieberman E, Lang JM, Frigoletto F Jr, et al. Epidural analgesia, intrapartum fever, and neonatal sepsis evaluation. Pediatrics 1997;99(3):415–9.
72. de Cueto M, Sanchez MJ, Sampedro A, et al. Timing of intrapartum ampicillin and prevention of vertical transmission of group B streptococcus. Obstet gynecol 1998;91(1):112–4.
73. Gerdes JS, Polin RA. Sepsis screen in neonates with evaluation of plasma fibronectin. Pediatr Infect Dis J 1987;6(5):443–6.
74. Greenberg DN, Yoder BA. Changes in the differential white blood cell count in screening for group B streptococcal sepsis. Pediatr Infect Dis J 1990;9(12):886–9.
75. Ottolini MC, Lundgren K, Mirkinson LJ, et al. Utility of complete blood count and blood culture screening to diagnose neonatal sepsis in the asymptomatic at risk newborn. Pediatr Infect Dis J 2003;22(5):430–4.
76. Yancey MK, Schuchat A, Brown LK, et al. The accuracy of late antenatal screening cultures in predicting genital group B streptococcal colonization at delivery. Obstet gynecol 1996;88(5):811–5.
77. Lukacs S, Schuchat A, Schoendorf K. National estimates of newborn sepsis: United States, 1990–2002. Presented at the annual meeting of Society for Pediatric and Perinatal Epidemiologic Research. June 14–15, 2004, Salt Lake City (Utah).
78. McCracken GH Jr. Group B streptococci: the new challenge in neonatal infections. J Pediatr 1973;82(4):703–6.
79. Freedman RM, Ingram DL, Gross I, et al. A half century of neonatal sepsis at Yale: 1928 to 1978. Am J Dis Child 1981;135(2):140–4.
80. Main EK, Slagle T. Prevention of early onset invasive neonatal group B streptococcal disease in a private hospital setting: the superiority of culture-based protocols. Am J Obstet Gynecol 2000;182(6):1344–54.
81. Baltimore RS, Huie SM, Meek JI, et al. Early onset neonatal sepsis in the era of group B streptococcal prevention. Pediatrics 2001;108(5):1094–8.
82. Cordero L, Sananes M, Ayers LW. Bloodstream infections in a neonatal intensive care unit: 12 years' experience with an antibiotic control program. Infect Control Hosp Epidemiol 1999;20(4):242–6.
83. Angstetra D, Ferguson J, Giles WB. Institution of universal screening for group B *Streptococcus* (GBS) from a risk management protocol results in reduction of early-onset GBS disease in a tertiary obstetric unit. Aust N Z J Obstet Gynaecol 2007;47(5):378–82.
84. Sutkin G, Krohn MA, Heine RP, et al. Antibiotic prophylaxis and nongroup B streptococcal neonatal sepsis. Obstet Gynecol 2005;105(3):581–6.
85. Alarcon A, Pena P, Salas S, et al. Neonatal early onset *Escherichia coli* sepsis: trends in incidence and antimicrobial resistance in the era of intrapartum antimicrobial prophylaxis. Pediatr Infect Dis J 2004;23(4):295–9.
86. Rentz AC, Samore MH, Stoddard GJ, et al. Risk factors associated with ampicillin-resistant infection in newborns in the era of group B streptococcal prophylaxis. Arch Pediatr Adolesc Med 2004;158(6):556–60.
87. Edwards RK, Jamie WE, Sterner D, et al. Intrapartum antibiotic prophylaxis and early onset neonatal sepsis patterns. Infect Dis Obstet Gynecol 2003;11(4):221–6.

88. Isaacs D, Royle JA. Intrapartum antibiotics and early onset neonatal sepsis caused by group B Streptococcus and by other organisms in Australia. Australasian Study Group for Neonatal Infections. Pediatr Infect Dis J 1999;18(6): 524–8.
89. Daley AJ, Isaacs D. Ten-year study on the effect of intrapartum antibiotic prophylaxis on early onset group B streptococcal and *Escherichia coli* neonatal sepsis in Australasia. Pediatr Infect Dis J 2004;23(7):630–4.
90. Joseph TA, Pyati SP, Jacobs N. Neonatal early onset *Escherichia coli* disease. The effect of intrapartum ampicillin. Arch Pediatr Adolesc Med 1998;152(1):35–40.
91. Towers CV, Carr MH, Padilla G, et al. Potential consequences of widespread antepartal use of ampicillin. Am J Obstet Gynecol 1998;179(4):879–83.
92. Levine EM, Ghai V, Barton JJ, et al. Intrapartum antibiotic prophylaxis increases the incidence of gram-negative neonatal sepsis. Infect Dis Obstet Gynecol 1999;7(4):210–3.
93. Bizzarro MJ, Dembry LM, Baltimore RS, et al. Changing patterns in neonatal *Escherichia coli* sepsis and ampicillin resistance in the era of intrapartum antibiotic prophylaxis. Pediatrics 2008;121(4):689–96.
94. Stoll BJ, Hansen N, Fanaroff AA, et al. Changes in pathogens causing early onset sepsis in very low birth weight infants. N Engl J Med 2002;347(4):240–7.
95. Stoll BJ, Hansen NI, Higgins RD, et al. Very low birth weight preterm infants with early onset neonatal sepsis: the predominance of gram-negative infections continues in the National Institute of Child Health and Human Development Neonatal Research Network, 2002–2003. Pediatr Infect Dis J 2005;24(7):635–9.
96. Hyde TB, Hilger TM, Reingold A, et al. Trends in incidence and antimicrobial resistance of early onset sepsis: population-based surveillance in San Francisco and Atlanta. Pediatrics 2002;110(4):690–5.
97. Al-Hasan MN, Lahr BD, Eckel-Passow JE, et al. Antimicrobial resistance trends of *Escherichia coli* bloodstream isolates: a population-based study, 1998-2007. J Antimicrob Chemother 2009;64(1):169–74.
98. Mercer BM, Carr TL, Beazley DD, et al. Antibiotic use in pregnancy and drug-resistant infant sepsis. Am J Obstet Gynecol 1999;181(4):816–21.
99. Terrone DA, Rinehart BK, Einstein MH, et al. Neonatal sepsis and death caused by resistant *Escherichia coli:* possible consequences of extended maternal ampicillin administration. Am J Obstet Gynecol 1999;180:1345–8.
100. Towers CV, Briggs GG. Antepartum use of antibiotics and early onset neonatal sepsis: the next 4 years. Am J Obstet Gynecol 2002;187(2):495–500.
101. Moore MR, Schrag SJ, Schuchat A. Effects of intrapartum antimicrobial prophylaxis for prevention of group B streptococcal disease on the incidence and ecology of early onset neonatal sepsis. Lancet Infect Dis 2003;3(4):201–13.
102. Schrag SJ, Hadler JL, Arnold KE, et al. Risk factors for invasive, early onset *Escherichia coli* infections in the era of widespread intrapartum antibiotic use. Pediatrics 2006;118(2):570–6.
103. Kimura K, Suzuki S, Wachino J, et al. First molecular characterization of group B streptococci with reduced penicillin susceptibility. Antimicrob Agents Chemother 2008;52(8):2890–7.
104. Dahesh S, Hensler ME, Van Sorge NM, et al. Point mutation in the group B streptococcal pbp2x gene conferring decreased susceptibility to beta-lactam antibiotics. Antimicrob Agents Chemother 2008;52(8):2915–8.
105. Manning SD, Foxman B, Pierson CL, et al. Correlates of antibiotic-resistant group B streptococcus isolated from pregnant women. Obstet Gynecol 2003; 101(1):74–9.

106. Varman M, Romero JR, Cornish NE, et al. Characterization and mechanisms of resistance of group B streptococcal isolates obtained at a community hospital. Eur J Clin Microbiol Infect Dis 2005;24(6):431–3.

107. Chohan L, Hollier LM, Bishop K, et al. Patterns of antibiotic resistance among group B streptococcus isolates: 2001–2004. Infect Dis Obstet Gynecol 2006; 2006:57492.

108. Panda B, Iruretagoyena I, Stiller R, et al. Antibiotic resistance and penicillin tolerance in ano-vaginal group B streptococci. J Matern Fetal Neonatal Med 2009; 22(2):111–4.

109. Borchardt SM, DeBusscher JH, Tallman PA, et al. Frequency of antimicrobial resistance among invasive and colonizing group B streptococcal isolates. BMC Infect Dis. 2006;6:57.

110. Lin FY, Philips JB 3rd, Azimi PH, et al. Level of maternal antibody required to protect neonates against early-onset disease caused by group B *Streptococcus* type Ia: a multicenter, seroepidemiology study. J Infect Dis 2001; 184(8):1022–8.

111. Lin FY, Weisman LE, Azimi PH, et al. Level of maternal IgG anti-group B *Streptococcus* type III antibody correlated with protection of neonates against early-onset disease caused by this pathogen. J Infect Dis 2004;190(5):928–34.

112. Baker CJ, Edwards MS. Group B streptococcal conjugate vaccines. Arch Dis Child 2003;88(5):375–8.

113. Heath PT, Feldman RG. Vaccination against group B *Streptococcus*. Expert Rev Vaccines 2005;4(2):207–18.

114. Edwards MS. Group B streptococcal conjugate vaccine: a timely concept for which the time has come. Hum Vaccin 2008;4(6):444–8.

115. Hillier S, Ferris D, Fine D, et al. Women receiving group B Streptococcus serotype III tetanus toxoid (GBS III-TT) vaccine have reduced vaginal and rectal acquisition of GBS type III. Presented at Infectious Diseases Society of America Annual Meeting. Philadelphia, October 29 to November 1, 2009.

Ureaplasma Species: Role in Diseases of Prematurity

Rose M. Viscardi, MD

KEYWORDS

- *Ureaplasma urealyticum* • *Ureaplasma parvum*
- Intrauterine infection • Prematurity
- Bronchopulmonary dysplasia • Intraventricular hemorrhage

Ureaplasma parvum (serotypes 1, 3, 6, and 14) and *U urealyticum* (serotypes 2, 4, 5, 7–13) are closely related species of the Mollicutes class, which are among the smallest free-living, self-replicating cells.[1–3] All serovars lack cell walls, exhibit limited biosynthetic abilities, hydrolyze urea to generate adenosine triphosphate (ATP), and adhere to human mucosal surfaces.[3] *U parvum* is the most common species isolated from clinical specimens.[3,4] Although *Ureaplasma* spp are not typically considered pathogens in early onset neonatal sepsis, they have been implicated in complications of human pregnancy and neonatal outcomes. As observed by Volgmann and colleagues[5] in the title of a recent review, *Ureaplasma* is a "harmless commensal or underestimated enemy of human reproduction." This article addresses this controversy and reviews evidence that the timing, duration, and intensity of the inflammatory response to *Ureaplasma* infection are major determinants of pregnancy and neonatal outcomes.

EPIDEMIOLOGY

Ureaplasma spp are the most common bacteria implicated in human urogenital infections, including nongonococcal urethritis in men and complications of pregnancy in women.[5] *Ureaplasma* spp can be detected in vaginal flora in 40% of sexually inactive and 67% of sexually active women of reproductive age, and 25% of postmenopausal women.[6] Despite the detection of viable *Ureaplasma* on toilets for up to 2 hours,[7] infection from exposure to contaminated surfaces is unlikely. Known transmission routes involve sexual contact or maternal-infant transfer.

EFFECT OF *UREAPLASMA* UROGENITAL TRACT COLONIZATION ON REPRODUCTION

Because *Ureaplasma* is a commensal in the adult female genital tract, it has been considered of low virulence. However, *Ureaplasma* urogenital tract colonization has

Funding support: This work was funded by NIH grants HL071113 and HL087166.
Department of Pediatrics, University of Maryland School of Medicine, 29 South Greene Street, Rm GS110, Baltimore, MD 21201, USA
E-mail address: rviscard@umaryland.edu

been causally linked to infertility,[8,9] early pregnancy loss,[10] stillbirth,[11,12] and preterm birth.[13–17] The relationship with these outcomes remains controversial because a causal relationship has been difficult to prove for each condition because of (1) accuracy of differentiating the presence of bacteria as specimen contaminants versus pathogens, (2) the polymicrobial nature of vaginal flora, (3) difficulty in detecting *Ureaplasma* and other fastidious microbes,[18] and (4) the contribution of other factors to the pathophysiology of these complex disorders. In vitro and in vivo experimental models have provided additional evidence in support of a role for *Ureaplasma* in these obstetric disorders.

Ureaplasma Intrauterine Infection/Chorioamnionitis

Intrauterine infection has been implicated as a major cause of preterm birth, especially in gestations of less than 30 weeks.[19] *Ureaplasma* spp are the most common organisms isolated from amniotic fluid obtained from women who present with premature onset of labor (POL) with intact membranes,[20,21] preterm premature rupture of membranes (pPROM),[22] and short cervix associated with microbial invasion of the amniotic cavity,[23] and from infected placentas.[22] The prevalence of infected amniotic fluid with cultivated *Ureaplasma* as the only microbe ranges from between 6% and 9% for pregnancies complicated by POL with intact membranes[21,24] to 22% for a cohort of women with POL or pPROM.[25] Detection of cultivated *Ureaplasma* in placental chorion in pregnancies producing very low birth weight (VLBW) infants ranges from between 6% and 10% in homogenized frozen tissue[26,27] to 28% in fresh tissue, and is inversely related to gestational age.[13] Recovery of *Ureaplasma* from the chorion increased with duration of rupture membranes, suggesting an ascending route of infection.[13] However, *Ureaplasma* has also been detected in 22% of placentas with duration of ROM less than 1 hour, suggesting the possibility of a preexisting infection. Indeed, *Ureaplasma* species have been detected in amniotic fluid as early as the time of genetic amniocentesis (16–20 weeks) in up to 13% of asymptomatic women.[16,28–30] Placentas with the lowest rate of *Ureaplasma* recovery were from women delivered for preeclampsia or intrauterine growth restriction.[13] Recent analysis of amniotic fluid from women with POL and intact membranes using advanced molecular techniques has demonstrated a greater prevalence (15%) and diversity of microbes including those uncultivated and uncharacterized compared with culture or species-specific polymerase chain reaction (PCR) studies.[18] In this study, only half of *Ureaplasma*-positive amniotic fluid samples were identified by culture with increased detection by combined culture and PCR.

The presence of *Ureaplasma* as the only identified microbial isolate in the upper genital tract is significantly associated with adverse pregnancy outcomes, including premature delivery, neonatal morbidity, and perinatal death.[13,21,22,25] Experimental models of intrauterine *Ureaplasma* infection in mice,[31] sheep,[32,33] and nonhuman primates[34] have been described. Intra-amniotic inoculation of *U parvum* did not stimulate POL in mice or sheep, but did stimulate progressive uterine contractions and preterm delivery in rhesus macaques inoculated at 136 days gestation (80% term),[34] suggesting species differences in the host response or serovar differences in virulence. The rhesus macaque model is the first experimental model to definitely show a causal link between *Ureaplasma* intrauterine infection and POL.

Ureaplasma-mediated Inflammation and POL

There is accumulating evidence that intrauterine infection–induced POL is the result of an inflammatory cascade initiated by bacterial interaction with host pattern recognition receptors (PRR) such as the toll-like receptors.[35] Following engagement with PRRs, there is a sequential increase in inflammatory cytokines such as interleukin

(IL)-1β, tumor necrosis factor (TNF)-α, IL-6, and IL-8 followed by leukocyte recruitment, increases in prostaglandins such as PGE2 and PGF2-α and matrix metalloproteinases (MMPs). These mediators contribute to uterine contractions, cervical dilatation and effacement, and membrane rupture.[35]

In the presence of pPROM, cultivated *Ureaplasma* as the sole microbe was associated with increased leukocytes and proinflammatory cytokines (IL-6, IL-1β, and TNF-α) in amniotic fluid and increased cord blood IL-6 concentrations, indicating a robust inflammatory response to this infection. Although most women in whom subclinical *Ureaplasma* amniotic cavity infection is detected midtrimester deliver at term,[16] those with elevated amniotic fluid IL-6 levels have increased risk for adverse pregnancy outcome including fetal loss and preterm delivery.[36] In the rhesus *U parvum* intrauterine infection model, uterine activity was preceded by an increase in amniotic fluid leukocytes, inflammatory cytokines, prostaglandins PGE2 and PGF2α, and MMP-9, demonstrating that *Ureaplasma* alone stimulates the mediators of POL.[34] In contrast, heat-killed *U parvum* serotype 1 failed to stimulate a significant increase in cytokine and PGE2 response in fetal membrane explants derived from term placentas. High inoculum (10^6 color changing units [CCU]/ml), but not low inoculum (10^2–10^4 CCU/mL) heat-killed *U urealyticum* serotype 8 stimulated TNF-α, IL-10 and PGE2 production by choriodecidual explants in vitro. The apparent low virulence of *Ureaplasma* serotypes in these in vitro studies may be due, in part, to the use of laboratory reference strains from the American Tissue Culture Collection (ATCC, Manassas, VA) rather than more virulent clinical isolates, or killed rather than live organisms. Alternatively, a decreased capacity to stimulate an inflammatory response in the intrauterine compartment may allow *Ureaplasma* infections to persist for long periods of time. **Fig. 1** summarizes the inflammatory pathways initiated by *Ureaplasma* infection that may contribute to POL.

ASSOCIATION OF *UREAPLASMA* SPP AND NEONATAL OUTCOMES

The timing and duration of fetal exposure to *Ureaplasma* and the intensity of the maternal and fetal inflammatory responses may be variable, but these factors likely contribute to the effect of *Ureaplasma* on neonatal outcomes. The rate of *Ureaplasma* respiratory tract colonization increases with duration of ROM,[37,38] indicating that, for most cases, *Ureaplasma* is likely vertically transmitted from mothers to their infants just before or at the time of preterm birth as the result of an ascending infection from the lower genital tract. However, in a prospective cohort from our institution, we observed that 23% of preterm infants with *Ureaplasma* respiratory colonization (unpublished observations), and 28% of infants with invasive *Ureaplasma* detected in blood or cerebrospinal fluid (CSF) by PCR[39] experienced ROM less than 1 hour, suggesting that colonization/infection in these infants was the result of preexisting (intrauterine) infection.[40,41] This is in agreement with Dammann and colleagues[40] who noted that ROM was less than 1 hour in 31% of pregnancies with *Ureaplasma* culture–positive placentas. In our cohort, 78% of placentas of infants with *Ureaplasma* respiratory tract colonization and duration of rupture of membranes (ROM) less than 1 hour showed evidence of histologic chorioamnionitis, in contrast to 36% of culture-negative infants with duration of ROM less than 1 hour. The placentas of *Ureaplasma*-positive infants in this group were more likely to have advanced maternal and fetal stages, indicating a more long-standing infection.[42]

These data suggest that fetal exposure to *Ureaplasma* spp may occur early in pregnancy and may be sustained during critical periods of development. We propose that *Ureaplasma*-induced injury to the preterm lung and brain occurs during a common

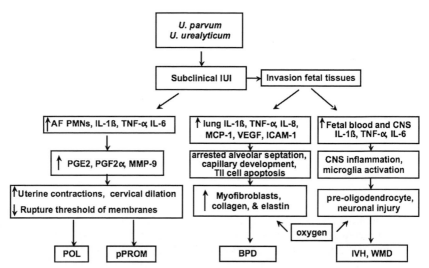

Fig. 1. Overview of potential inflammatory pathways involved in *Ureaplasma*-mediated POL, and common neonatal morbidities. Intrauterine *Ureaplasma* infections may develop by ascending infection or transplacental route. Engagement with host pathogen recognition receptors initiates a maternal and fetal inflammatory cascade. In the amniotic cavity, there is sequential upregulation of inflammatory cytokines, recruitment of leukocytes, release of prostaglandins and metalloproteinases leading to uterine contractions, cervical dilatation and effacement, and membrane rupture.[34,35] In the fetal lung, prolonged exposure to inflammatory cytokines inhibits alveolar development.[110] Systemic invasion via the umbilical cord stimulates a cytokinemia in blood and/or CNS resulting in microglia activation and preoligodendrocyte and neuronal injury.[31]

developmental-dependent window of vulnerability and is mediated by the inflammatory response in placental, blood, lung, and central nervous system (CNS) compartments.[43] During the period from 23 to 32 weeks' gestation, the lung and brain share a vulnerability to injury mediated by infection/inflammation.[44–46] During this period of saccular lung development[45,46] and predominance of the oxidative stress–sensitive preoligodendrocyte in the fetal brain,[47–49] exposure of the fetus to intrauterine *Ureaplasma* infection–mediated inflammation and postnatal interactions with other inflammatory stimuli may alter developmental signaling. The evidence supporting this hypothesis and potential mechanisms are reviewed in the following sections.

Ureaplasma spp and Neonatal Lung Injury

The rate of respiratory tract colonization with *Ureaplasma* in infants less than 1500 g birth weight ranges from 20% to 45%, depending on study entry criteria, frequency of sampling, and detection methods.[50,51] In a recent cohort of infants less than 33 weeks' gestation, *Ureaplasma* spp were detected during the first week of life in tracheal aspirates or nasopharyngeal specimens in 35% of infants.[39] *Ureaplasma* respiratory tract colonization is associated with a peripheral blood leukocytosis[52] and early radiographic emphysematous changes of bronchopulmonary dysplasia (BPD).[53,54] These findings may be explained, in part, by an in utero onset of the inflammatory response and lung injury.

The contribution of *Ureaplasma* respiratory tract colonization to the development of BPD has been debated; however, a meta-analysis of 17 clinical studies published before 1995 supported a significant association between *Ureaplasma* respiratory tract colonization and development of BPD defined as oxygen dependence at 28 to 30 days postnatal age.[50] In a meta-analysis of 36 published studies involving approximately 3000 preterm infants, Schelonka and colleagues[51] observed a significant association between *Ureaplasma* respiratory colonization and development of BPD whether defined as oxygen dependence at 28 days or at 36 weeks postmenstrual age (PMA). Studies published since the last meta-analysis support the *Ureaplasma* respiratory colonization-BPD association,[55,56] particularly for the subset of *Ureaplasma*-colonized infants exposed to chorioamnionitis and leukocytosis at birth.[56]

Evidence from studies of human preterm infants,[57–59] and intrauterine infection models in mice,[31] sheep,[32,33] and nonhuman primates[34,60] supports that *Ureaplasma* infection is proinflammatory and profibrotic and results in a BPD phenotype. In a review of lung pathology of archived autopsy specimens from *Ureaplasma*-infected preterm infants, the most striking findings were (1) the presence of moderate to severe fibrosis, (2) increased myofibroblasts, (3) disordered elastin accumulation, and (4) increased numbers of TNF-α and transforming growth factor β_1 (TGF β_1) immunoreactive cells in all *Ureaplasma*-infected infants compared with gestational controls and infants who died with pneumonia from other causes.[58,59] Experimental murine intrauterine *U parvum* exposure stimulated fetal lung cytokine expression and augmented hyperoxia-induced lung injury.[31] In the 125-day immature baboon model, we observed extensive fibrosis (**Fig. 2**), an increase in the myofibroblast phenotype, and increased

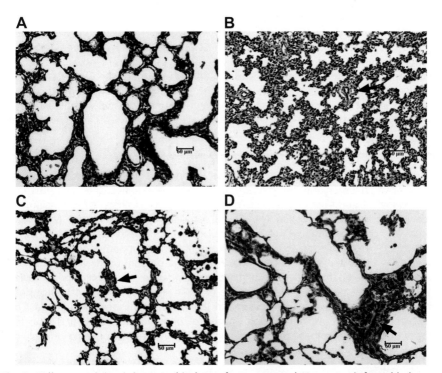

Fig. 2. Collagen staining is increased in lungs from antenatal *U parvum*–infected baboons. Lung specimens from 125-day gestation baboon newborns ventilated for 14 days that were infected antenatally with *U parvum* serovar 1 (*D*) or noninfected (*C*) were stained with trichome for collagen and compared with stained lung sections from 125-day (*A*) and 140-day (*B*) gestational controls. The most marked fibrosis occurred in the *U parvum*–infected lungs (*arrows*). Magnification ×200.

expression of proinflammatory (TNF-α, IL-1β) and profibrotic cytokines (TGFβ_1; oncostatin M) in lungs of antenatal *Ureaplasma*-infected animals compared with gestational controls or noninfected ventilated animals.[60] In a study of rhesus macaques, histologic changes in the fetus' lungs depended on the duration of intrauterine exposure to *U parvum*.[34] Infection exposure duration less than 136 hours resulted in neutrophil infiltration without epithelial injury. With progressive duration of exposure there was an influx of neutrophils and macrophages, epithelial necrosis, and type II cell proliferation. For exposure duration longer than 10 days, increased collagen and thickened alveolar walls were evident. These data confirm that *Ureaplasma* infection contributes to chronic inflammation and fibrosis in the preterm lung. Moreover, these data suggest that *Ureaplasma* acts as a coinflammatory stimulus by causing an augmented, dysregulated inflammatory response to subsequent inflammatory insults such as hyperoxia and volutrauma.

Insights into how *Ureaplasma* infection–mediated inflammation produces the BPD phenotype are provided by studies of transgenic mice overexpressing proinflammatory cytokines. In transgenic mice, overexpression of TNF-α, IL-6, and IL-11 each inhibited alveolarization, indicating that prolonged exposure of the preterm lung to a proinflammatory environment may contribute to abnormal alveolar septation, the hallmark of the new BPD.[61] In a recently developed bitransgenic CCSP-rtTA-(tetO)-CMV-IL-1β mouse, IL-1β was expressed under conditional control in airway epithelial cells in the fetal and neonatal lung.[62] IL-1β expression increased on E14.5 and was maximal by E16.5 (pseudoglandular period) and decreased postnatally. In this model, postnatal growth was impaired and mortality was higher in the newborn mice expressing IL-1β. The lungs of these newborn mice demonstrated many features of the BPD phenotype, including disrupted alveolar septation and capillary development, and disordered α-smooth muscle actin and elastin deposition in alveolar septa of distal airspaces.[62] These observations suggest that an early and prolonged exposure to *Ureaplasma*-mediated inflammation may be necessary to adversely affect lung development (see **Fig. 1**).

Ureaplasma spp and Other Neonatal Lung Disorders

There have been case[63,64] and small series reports of culture-confirmed congenital *Ureaplasma* pneumonia in late preterm infants.[65] In one series, 3 infants presented with clinical features of pneumonia and persistent pulmonary hypertension.[65] In each infant, tracheal aspirates and blood samples were positive for *Ureaplasma* culture and postmortem lung cultures were positive for *Ureaplasma* in 2 infants who died. In a 5-year series of 159 perinatal autopsies, postmortem lung cultures were positive for *Ureaplasma* in 9% of cases. Forty-three percent of the autopsied cases were intrauterine deaths and 45% had histologic evidence of congenital pneumonia.[66] This was in agreement with a larger series of 430 stillborn and neonatal autopsies in which 8% were positive for *Ureaplasma* in the lungs.[67] These studies suggest that *Ureaplasma* species are uncommon causes of pneumonia in term and near-term infants, but cultures for these organisms should be considered in cases of unexplained congenital pneumonia or fetal demise.

UREAPLASMAL INVASIVE DISEASE

Although *Ureaplasma* spp are most commonly isolated from respiratory secretions, the organisms have also been isolated from gastric aspirates,[68] blood,[69,70] CSF,[71,72] lung,[65] and brain[73,74] tissue. Isolation of *Ureaplasma* from cord blood was first described in 1969[75] and isolation from cord or venous blood in association with pneumonia was documented in several other studies.[65,69,76] In 2 recent large prospective cohorts, *Ureaplasma* was detected in 17% of cord blood cultures[70] and 23.6% of serum or CSF PCR samples,[39] but invasive disease was not associated with BPD at 36 weeks PMA in either cohort. *U parvum* was the predominant species detected in serum and CSF. In infants for whom *Ureaplasma* respiratory status was known, 19% of serum and 11% of CSF samples from infants with *Ureaplasma* respiratory colonization and 15% of serum and 19% of CSF samples from infants without *Ureaplasma* respiratory colonization were PCR positive. In all cases, the *Ureaplasma* detected in respiratory samples was the same species as the one detected in serum or CSF from the same subject.[39]

Ureaplasma-mediated Inflammation and Neonatal Brain Injury

Although considerable evidence has been published linking *Ureaplasma* respiratory colonization with neonatal lung morbidity, less is known about possible links between intrauterine *Ureaplasma* exposure, invasive disease, and neurologic morbidities such as intraventricular hemorrhage (IVH) and white matter injury. In a prospective series of infants with suspected sepsis/meningitis or hydrocephalus, *M hominis*, a related genital mycoplasma, was isolated in 5 and *Ureaplasma* spp in 8 CSF samples.[71] Six infants with *Ureaplasma*-positive CSF had severe IVH complicated by posthemorrhagic hydrocephalus in 3. There are additional case reports of IVH complicated by hydrocephalus or death in association with *Ureaplasma*-positive CSF.[73,77] In our study of invasive *Ureaplasma*,[39] the risk of severe IVH ($\geq$grade 3) was 2.5-fold higher in serum PCR-positive than PCR-negative infants after adjustment for gestational age, but there was no association of cranial ultrasound abnormalities with detection of *Ureaplasma* in CSF. This result may have been due to selection bias of lumbar punctures more likely being performed in more stable infants. *U parvum* was the species detected in all PCR-positive infants with severe IVH. There was a fivefold increased risk for severe IVH in the presence of *Ureaplasma* PCR-positive serum combined with elevated serum IL-1β,[39] suggesting a possible link between invasive *Ureaplasma*, cytokinemia, and neonatal brain injury (see **Fig. 1**).

A role for *Ureaplasma* in neonatal brain injury is supported by recent studies in experimental animal models. In the murine intrauterine *U parvum* infection model, the brains of fetal and newborn mice showed evidence of microglial activation, delayed myelination, and disturbed neuronal development.[31] In antenatal *U parvum*–exposed immature rhesus macaques, CSF and brain tissue were culture-positive in 20%.[34] Although there was no evidence of hemorrhage on gross and microscopic examinations of the brains of these animals, specific immunohistochemical analyses were not performed. Future studies in these models will provide additional insights into the mechanisms of *Ureaplasma*-mediated brain injury and could evaluate potential therapeutic interventions.

The effect of intrauterine *Ureaplasma* infection on neurodevelopmental outcome is unknown. A recent study comparing outcomes of infants born at less than 33 weeks' gestation with and without amniotic cavity infection with *Ureaplasma* or other microbes at time of delivery reported lower psychomotor developmental index scores on the Bayley Scales of Infant Development and a higher rate of cerebral palsy at 2 years adjusted age in infants exposed to intrauterine infection compared with nonexposed infants.[78] Infants exposed to intrauterine *Ureaplasma* were more severely affected than those exposed to other bacteria. Additional studies are needed to assess the contribution of *Ureaplasma* to adverse neurodevelopment.

Ureaplasma spp and Neonatal Meningitis

The prevalence, clinical risk factors, and CSF parameters in Ureaplasma CNS infections have not been fully elucidated. Most series have focused on the preterm population, but there have been case reports of Ureaplasma isolation in CSF of term infants.[69,79] The rate of Ureaplasma culture–positive CSF in prospective series in preterm infants varied from 0.2% to 9%.[71,72,80–82] The prevalence for Ureaplasma is higher than for other causes of bacterial meningitis (1%–2%)[83,84] Although CSF pleocytosis has been described, it is absent in most cases.[69,82] The usefulness of CSF parameters in the diagnosis of bacterial meningitis in preterm infants is debated.[84] In our prospective series,[39] the CSF white blood cell count, percent neutrophils, and glucose and protein concentrations did not differ between Ureaplasma-positive and -negative samples on PCR (**Table 1**). Only 25% of Ureaplasma-positive CSF samples had a white blood cell count greater than 20 cells/mm^3 compared with 16% of Ureaplasma-negative samples. No other bacteria were detected in these samples. These observations suggest that Ureaplasma infections may be the most common cause of CNS infections in neonates, but most infections are asymptomatic. Because most infections seem to resolve without therapy, it is unclear whether culture for these organisms should be included in the routine evaluation of sepsis in the newborn. Additional studies focused on long-term outcomes of Ureaplasma CNS infections are warranted before specific recommendations can be made for clinical management.

UREAPLASMA INFECTIONS IN INFANTS AND CHILDREN

The duration of Ureaplasma respiratory tract colonization is unknown. In a study conducted in 1969, 12 of 21 Ureaplasma-colonized newborns remained culture-positive for up to 10 months. In addition, 7 of 52 initially culture-negative infants converted to culture-positive during the same time period, confirming the importance of multiple cultures for definitive diagnosis, and suggesting the possibility of horizontal transmission. Over a 10-year period, 31% of more than 45,000 cultures at a national reference laboratory for mycoplasma cultures were positive for Mycoplasma spp not including M pneumoniae.[4] In children, most Ureaplasma-positive respiratory cultures were from children less than 12 months old (92%), but 4% were from children 1 to 7 years of age. In agreement, Matlow and colleagues[85] reported that only 1.8% of nonneonatal respiratory samples submitted to a single institution laboratory were positive for Ureaplasma.

Table 1		
CSF characteristics in infants with invasive Ureaplasma		
CSF Parameter	**CSF PCR (+) N = 36**	**CSF PCR (−) N = 153**
WBC/mm^{3,a}	4 (0–172)	3 (0–193)
% neutrophils	31 (0–92)	17 (0–87)
% lymphocytes	14 (0–100)	16 (0–100)
% monocytes	23 (0–100)	42 (0–100)
Glucose (mg/dL)	47 (26–105)	52 (0–171)
Protein (mg/dL)	154 (64–527)	152 (47–558)

[a] CSF white blood cell counts were corrected for red blood cells. Data are expressed as median with range in parentheses.

Ureaplasma respiratory tract colonization has also been proposed as a causative factor in reactive airway disease in young infants. Wheezing in infants and children less than 3 years of age has been associated with isolation of *Ureaplasma* from the upper respiratory tract.[86] In a large study of almost 3000 women and their offspring in Sweden, maternal vaginal colonization with *Ureaplasma* during pregnancy was associated with a twofold increased risk for infant wheezing defined as 1 or more hospitalizations for asthma during the first 3 years of life.[87] The investigators proposed that acquisition of microorganisms such as *Ureaplasma* spp at birth affects the establishment of infant microflora and subsequent development of allergy and wheezing.

Ureaplasma as a significant cause of sepsis or meningitis beyond the newborn period seems unlikely. In a series of infants less than 3 months of age evaluated for sepsis, *Ureaplasma* was not detected in any blood or CSF sample, but it was isolated from 6% of urine cultures.[88] Other diseases associated with *Ureaplasma* include pediatric joint disorders.[86]

UREAPLASMA DIAGNOSTIC METHODS

Ureaplasma spp may be isolated from blood, amniotic fluid, CSF, sputum, bronchoalveolar lavage, pleural fluid, and semen. Because these organisms are susceptible to desiccation and are sensitive to temperature changes, attention to sample collection and processing are of utmost importance. Samples should be directly inoculated into 10B broth for transport on ice to the laboratory. The specimen should be inoculated in 10B broth with serial 1:10 dilutions and incubated under atmospheric conditions and on A8 agar and incubated in 5% CO_2 at 37°C. Cultures are observed for up to 7 days for broth color change from yellow to pink, indicating pH change due to urease activity in the absence of turbidity. Any broth with color change should be subcultured on A8 agar. Colonies of *Ureaplasma* spp are identified presumptively by their characteristic brown appearance on A8 agar in the presence of the $CaCl_2$ indicator. *Ureaplasma* can be differentiated from *M hominis* by the larger size, lack of precipitate, and fried-egg appearance of *M hominis*. Cultures usually grow within 24 to 48 hours. Because most clinical laboratories lack the expertise for culture of these organisms, cultures may need to be shipped for processing to a reference laboratory such as the University of Alabama Mycoplasma Diagnostic Laboratory.

PCR protocols for detection of the common *Ureaplasma* spp mba or urease genes,[89–91] and species- and serovar-specific primers are available.[89,92,93] These methods have the advantage of more rapid results and potentially increased sensitivity compared with traditional culture.

THERAPEUTIC CONSIDERATIONS
Interventions During Pregnancy

Antibiotic therapy is now standard of care for management of pPROM.[94] However, usual regimens failed to eradicate organisms including *Ureaplasma* or diminish inflammation in the amniotic cavity in pregnancies complicated by pPROM.[95] In a small series of women with microbial invasion of the amniotic cavity with short cervix, parenteral azithromycin eradicated *Ureaplasma* in 3 of 4 cases and delivery occurred at term. Combination of antibiotics with antiinflammatory drugs may improve efficacy. In an experimental *Ureaplasma* intra-amniotic infection in rhesus macaques, azithromycin alone or in combination with dexamethasone and indocin prevented fetal lung damage (Novy, MJ and colleagues, Maternal azithromycin (AZI) therapy for *Ureaplasma* intra-amnioitc infection (IAI) prevents advanced fetal lung lesions in rhesus monkeys, 2008 SGI Annual Scientific Meeting, March 26–29, 2008, San Diego, CA,

Abstract 438, unpublished data). Whether this approach will be beneficial for CNS outcomes is unknown.

BPD Prevention

Despite in vitro susceptibility of *Ureaplasma* to erythromycin,[96] trials of erythromycin therapy in the first few weeks of life in *Ureaplasma*-colonized preterm infants have failed to demonstrate efficacy to prevent BPD[97,98] or eradicate respiratory tract colonization.[99] The failure to prevent BPD in these studies may have been due to the small sample size of each study, or to the initiation of erythromycin therapy too late to prevent the lung inflammation and injury that contribute to the pathogenesis of BPD. Demonstration of efficacy of antibiotic therapy to prevent BPD in *Ureaplasma*-colonized preterm infants will require carefully designed and adequately powered studies.

The new 14-member macrolides that are derivatives of erythromycin and the related 15-member azalides have immunomodulatory effects, including effects on neutrophil function (eg, chemotaxis, cell adhesion, oxidative burst, and phagocytosis) and inhibition of cytokine release (eg, IL-1β, IL-8, TNFα)[100] and nitric oxide production in vitro.[101] Macrolide antibiotics may exert immunomodulatory antiinflammatory effects in the setting of infection, and these may occur independently of a direct bactericidal effect.[102] In addition, azithromycin exhibits higher potency than erythromycin against clinical *Ureaplasma* isolates in vitro.[103] Pharmacokinetic studies in mice and humans have shown that azithromycin is preferentially concentrated in pulmonary epithelial lining fluid and alveolar macrophages.[104–106] Because neutrophil recruitment and activation has been implicated in BPD pathogenesis,[107,108] the experimental effects observed with azithromycin in vitro and in vivo indicate that this drug may be beneficial in the treatment of *Ureaplasma* infection and the prevention of BPD in preterm infants.

Because *Ureaplasma*-mediated lung injury may be initiated in utero and augmented postnatally by exposure to mechanical ventilation and hyperoxia, therapy to prevent BPD should be initiated as soon as possible after birth in infants at risk. Recently, Walls and colleagues[109] demonstrated that azithromycin, but not erythromycin, prophylaxis improved outcomes and reduced inflammation in a murine neonatal *Ureaplasma* infection model. This finding suggests that azithromycin may be effective if administered immediately after birth. However, until appropriate pharmacokinetics and efficacy trials are conducted, a dosing regimen for azithromycin in neonates cannot be recommended.

SUMMARY

Ureaplasma species may indeed be an "underestimated enemy of human reproduction." However, there are many questions yet to be answered before recommendations for changes in clinical practices can be recommended. More needs to be learned about the relative contribution of *Ureaplasma* virulence factors, host immune factors that affect susceptibility to these pathogens and the variability in the inflammatory response, and interactions with environmental factors such as oxygen exposure and mechanical ventilation. Routine antibiotic use should be limited to clinical trials until clear benefit can be established. However, culture or PCR for these organisms should be considered in cases of unexplained fetal demise, congenital pneumonia, or meningitis unresponsive to broad-spectrum antibiotics. Follow-up cultures should be obtained in any treated infant because effective clearance has proven difficult in erythromycin trials.

REFERENCES

1. Kong F, James G, Zhenfang M, et al. Phylogenetic analysis of *Ureaplasma urealyticum* – support for the establishment of a new species, *Ureaplasma parvum*. Int J Syst Bacteriol 1999;49:1879–89.
2. Glass JI, Lefkowitz EJ, Glass JS, et al. The complete sequence of the mucosal pathogen *Ureaplasma urealyticum*. Nature 2000;407(6805):757–62.
3. Waites KB, Katz B, Schelonka RL. Mycoplasmas and ureaplasmas as neonatal pathogens. Clin Microbiol Rev 2005;18(4):757–89.
4. She RC, Simmon KE, Bender JM, et al. Mollicute infections in neonates. Pediatr Infect Dis J 2009;28(3):248–50.
5. Volgmann T, Ohlinger R, Panzig B. *Ureaplasma urealyticum*-harmless commensal or underestimated enemy of human reproduction? A review. Arch Gynecol Obstet 2005;273(3):133–9.
6. Iwasaka T, Wada T, Kidera Y, et al. Hormonal status and mycoplasma colonization in the female genital tract. Obstet Gynecol 1986;68(2):263–6.
7. Potasman I, Oren A, Srugo I. Isolation of *Ureaplasma urealyticum* and *Mycoplasma hominis* from public toilet bowls. Infect Control Hosp Epidemiol 1999;20(1):66–8.
8. Zeighami H, Peerayeh SN, Yazdi RS, et al. Prevalence of *Ureaplasma urealyticum* and *Ureaplasma parvum* in semen of infertile and healthy men. Int J STD AIDS 2009;20(6):387–90.
9. Gupta A, Gupta S, Mittal A, et al. Correlation of mycoplasma with unexplained infertility. Arch Gynecol Obstet 2009;280(6):981–5.
10. Joste NE, Kundsin RB, Genest DR. Histology and *Ureaplasma urealyticum* culture in 63 cases of first trimester abortion. Am J Clin Pathol 1994;102(6):729–32.
11. Tafari N, Ross S, Naeye RL, et al. Mycoplasma T strains and perinatal death. Lancet 1976;1(7951):108–9.
12. Gibbs RS. The origins of stillbirth: infectious diseases. Semin Perinatol 2002;26(1):75–8.
13. Kundsin RB, Leviton A, Allred EN, et al. *Ureaplasma urealyticum* infection of the placenta in pregnancies that ended prematurely. Obstet Gynecol 1996;87:122–7.
14. Yoon BH, Romero R, Chang JW, et al. Microbial invasion of the amniotic cavity with *Ureaplasma urealyticum* is associated with a robust host response in fetal, amniotic, and maternal compartments. Am J Obstet Gynecol 1998;179:1254–60.
15. Gerber S, Vial Y, Hohlfeld P, et al. Detection of *Ureaplasma urealyticum* in second-trimester amniotic fluid by polymerase chain reaction correlates with subsequent preterm labor and delivery. J Infect Dis 2003;187(3):518–21.
16. Perni SC, Vardhana S, Korneeva I, et al. *Mycoplasma hominis* and *Ureaplasma urealyticum* in midtrimester amniotic fluid: association with amniotic fluid cytokine levels and pregnancy outcome. Am J Obstet Gynecol 2004;191(4):1382–6.
17. Witt A, Berger A, Gruber CJ, et al. Increased intrauterine frequency of *Ureaplasma urealyticum* in women with preterm labor and preterm premature rupture of the membranes and subsequent cesarean delivery. Am J Obstet Gynecol 2005;193(5):1663–9.
18. DiGiulio DB, Romero R, Amogan HP, et al. Microbial prevalence, diversity and abundance in amniotic fluid during preterm labor: a molecular and culture-based investigation. PLoS One 2008;3(8):e3056.

19. Goldenberg RL, Hauth JC, Andrews WW. Intrauterine infection and preterm delivery. N Engl J Med 2000;342(20):1500–7.
20. Gomez R, Ghezzi F, Romero R, et al. Premature labor and intra-amniotic infection. Clin Perinatol 1995;22:281–342.
21. Yoon BH, Chang JW, Romero R. Isolation of *Ureaplasma urealyticum* from the amniotic cavity and adverse outcome in preterm labor. Obstet Gynecol 1998; 92:77–82.
22. Romero R, Yoon BH, Mazor M, et al. A comparative study of the diagnostic performance of amniotic fluid glucose, white blood cell count, interleukin-6, and Gram stain in the detection of microbial invasion in patients with preterm premature rupture of membranes. Am J Obstet Gynecol 1993;169:839–51.
23. Hassan S, Romero R, Hendler I, et al. A sonographic short cervix as the only clinical manifestation of intra-amniotic infection. J Perinat Med 2006;34(1):13–9.
24. Yoon BH, Romero R, Lim JH, et al. The clinical significance of detecting *Ureaplasma urealyticum* by the polymerase chain reaction in the amniotic fluid of patients with preterm labor. Am J Obstet Gynecol 2003;189:919–24.
25. Kirchner L, Helmer H, Heinze G, et al. Amnionitis with *Ureaplasma urealyticum* or other microbes leads to increased morbidity and prolonged hospitalization in very low birth weight infants. Eur J Obstet Gynecol Reprod Biol 2007;134(1):44–50.
26. Onderdonk AB, Delaney ML, DuBois AM, et al. Detection of bacteria in placental tissues obtained from extremely low gestational age neonates. Am J Obstet Gynecol 2008;198(1)(110):e111–7.
27. Olomu IN, Hecht JL, Onderdonk AO, et al. Perinatal correlates of *Ureaplasma urealyticum* in placenta parenchyma of singleton pregnancies that end before 28 weeks of gestation. Pediatrics 2009;123(5):1329–36.
28. Gray DJ, Robinson HB, Malone J, et al. Adverse outcome in pregnancy following amniotic fluid isolation of *Ureaplasma urealyticum*. Prenat Diagn 1992;12(2):111–7.
29. Horowitz S, Mazor M, Romero R, et al. Infection of the amniotic cavity with *Ureaplasma urealyticum* in the midtrimester of pregnancy. J Reprod Med 1995; 40(5):375–9.
30. Berg TG, Philpot KL, Welsh MS, et al. *Ureaplasma/Mycoplasma*-infected amniotic fluid: pregnancy outcome in treated and nontreated patients. J Perinatol 1999;19(4):275–7.
31. Normann E, Lacaze-Masmonteil T, Eaton F, et al. A novel mouse model of *Ureaplasma*-induced perinatal inflammation: effects on lung and brain injury. Pediatr Res 2009;65(4):430–6.
32. Moss TJ, Nitsos I, Ikegami M, et al. Experimental intrauterine *Ureaplasma* infection in sheep. Am J Obstet Gynecol 2005;192(4):1179–86.
33. Moss TJ, Knox CL, Kallapur SG, et al. Experimental amniotic fluid infection in sheep: effects of *Ureaplasma parvum* serovars 3 and 6 on preterm or term fetal sheep. Am J Obstet Gynecol 2008;198(1):122, e1–8.
34. Novy MJ, Duffy L, Axthelm MK, et al. *Ureaplasma parvum* or *Mycoplasma hominis* as sole pathogens cause chorioamnionitis, preterm delivery, and fetal pneumonia in rhesus macaques. Reprod Sci 2009;16(1):56–70.
35. Peltier MR. Immunology of term and preterm labor. Reprod Biol Endocrinol 2003;1:122.
36. Bashiri A, Horowitz S, Huleihel M, et al. Elevated concentrations of interleukin-6 in intra-amniotic infection with *Ureaplasma urealyticum* in asymptomatic women during genetic amniocentesis. Acta Obstet Gynecol Scand 1999;78(5):379–82.

37. Grattard F, Soleihac B, De Barbeyrac B, et al. Epidemiologic and molecular investigations of genital mycoplasmas from women and neonates at delivery. Pediatr Infect Dis J 1995;14:853–8.

38. Kafetzis DA, Skevaki CL, Skouteri V, et al. Maternal genital colonization with *Ureaplasma urealyticum* promotes preterm delivery: association of the respiratory colonization of premature infants with chronic lung disease and increased mortality. Clin Infect Dis 2004;39(8):1113–22.

39. Viscardi RM, Hashmi N, Gross GW, et al. Incidence of invasive *Ureaplasma* in VLBW infants: relationship to severe intraventricular hemorrhage. J Perinatol 2008;28(11):759–65.

40. Dammann O, Allred EN, Genest DR, et al. Antenatal mycoplasma infection, the fetal inflammatory response and cerebral white matter damage in very-low-birth-weight infants. Paediatr Perinat Epidemiol 2003;17(1):49–57.

41. McElrath TF, Allred EN, Leviton A. Prolonged latency after preterm premature rupture of membranes: an evaluation of histologic condition and intracranial ultrasonic abnormality in the neonate born at <28 weeks of gestation. Am J Obstet Gynecol 2003;189(3):794–8.

42. Redline RW, Wilson-Costello D, Borawski E, et al. Placental lesions associated with neurologic impairment and cerebral palsy in very low-birth-weight infants. Arch Pathol Lab Med 1998;122:1091–8.

43. Viscardi RM, Muhumuza CK, Rodriguez A, et al. Inflammatory markers in intrauterine and fetal blood and cerebrospinal fluid compartments are associated with adverse pulmonary and neurologic outcomes in preterm infants. Pediatr Res 2004;55:1009–17.

44. Vigneswaran R. Infection and preterm birth: evidence of a common causal relationship with bronchopulmonary dysplasia and cerebral palsy. J Paediatr Child Health 2000;36:293–6.

45. Jobe AH, Ikegami M. Antenatal infection/inflammation and postnatal lung maturation and injury. Respir Res 2001;2:27–32.

46. Bose CL, Dammann CE, Laughon MM. Bronchopulmonary dysplasia and inflammatory biomarkers in the premature neonate. Arch Dis Child Fetal Neonatal Ed 2008;93(6):F455–61.

47. Back SA, Gan X, Li Y, et al. Maturation-dependent vulnerability of oligodentrocytes to oxidative stress-induced death caused by glutathione depletion. J Neurosci 1998;18:6241–53.

48. Back SA, Luo NL, Borenstein NS, et al. Late oligodendrocyte progenitors coincide with the developmental window of vulnerability for human perinatal white matter injury. J Neurosci 2001;21:1302–12.

49. Volpe JJ. Neurobiology of periventricular leukomalacia in the premature infant. Pediatr Res 2001;50:553–62.

50. Wang EL, Ohlsson A, Kellner JD. Association of *Ureaplasma urealyticum* colonization with chronic lung disease of prematurity: Results of a metaanalysis. J Pediatr 1995;127:640–4.

51. Schelonka RL, Katz B, Waites KB, et al. Critical appraisal of the role of *Ureaplasma* in the development of bronchopulmonary dysplasia with metaanalytic techniques. Pediatr Infect Dis J 2005;24(12):1033–9.

52. Panero A, Pacifico L, Roggini M, et al. *Ureaplasma urealyticum* as a cause of pneumonia in preterm infants: analysis of the white cell response. Arch Dis Child 1995;73:F37–40.

53. Crouse DT, Odrezin GT, Cutter GR, et al. Radiographic changes associated with tracheal isolation of *Ureaplasma urealyticum* from neonates. Clin Infect Dis 1993;17(Suppl 1):S122–30.

54. Pacifico L, Panero A, Roggini M, et al. *Ureaplasma urealyticum* and pulmonary outcome in a neonatal intensive care population. Pediatr Infect Dis 1997;16: 579–86.

55. Colaizy TT, Morris CD, Lapidus J, et al. Detection of ureaplasma DNA in endotracheal samples is associated with bronchopulmonary dysplasia after adjustment for multiple risk factors. Pediatr Res 2007;61(5 Pt 1):578–83.

56. Honma Y, Yada Y, Takahashi N, et al. Certain type of chronic lung disease of newborns is associated with *Ureaplasma urealyticum* infection in utero. Pediatr Int 2007;49(4):479–84.

57. Patterson AM, Taciak V, Lovchik J, et al. *Ureaplasma urealyticum* respiratory tract colonization is associated with an increase in IL-1ß and TNF-a relative to IL-6 in tracheal aspirates of preterm infants. Pediatr Infect Dis J 1998;17: 321–8.

58. Viscardi RM, Manimtim WM, Sun CCJ, et al. Lung pathology in premature infants with *Ureaplasma urealyticum* infection. Pediatr Dev Pathol 2002;5:141–50.

59. Viscardi R, Manimtim W, He JR, et al. Disordered pulmonary myofibroblast distribution and elastin expression in preterm infants with *Ureaplasma urealyticum* pneumonitis. Pediatr Dev Pathol 2006;9(2):143–51.

60. Viscardi RM, Atamas SP, Luzina IG, et al. Antenatal *Ureaplasma urealyticum* respiratory tract infection stimulates proinflammatory, profibrotic responses in the preterm baboon lung. Pediatr Res 2006;60(2):141–6.

61. Jobe AH, Bancalari E. Bronchopulmonary dysplasia. Am J Respir Crit Care Med 2001;163:1723–9.

62. Bry K, Whitsett JA, Lappalainen U. IL-1beta disrupts postnatal lung morphogenesis in the mouse. Am J Respir Cell Mol Biol 2007;36(1):32–42.

63. Quinn PA, Gillan JE, Markestad T, et al. Intrauterine infection with *Ureaplasma urealyticum* as a cause of fatal neonatal pneumonia. Pediatr Infect Dis 1985;4: 538–43.

64. Brus F, van Waarde WM, Schoots C, et al. Fatal ureaplasmal pneumonia and sepsis in a newborn infant. Eur J Pediatr 1991;150:782–3.

65. Waites KB, Crouse DT, Philips JB, et al. Ureaplasmal pneumonia and sepsis associated with persistent pulmonary hypertension of the newborn. Pediatrics 1989;83:79–85.

66. Madan E, Meyer MP, Amortequi A. Chorioamnionitis: a study of organisms isolated in perinatal autopsies. Ann Clin Lab Sci 1988;18(1):39–45.

67. Madan E, Meyer MP, Amortegui AJ. Isolation of genital mycoplasmas and *Chlamydia trachomatis* in stillborn and neonatal autopsy material. Arch Pathol Lab Med 1988;112(7):749–51.

68. Wang EE, Frayha H, Watts J, et al. Role of *Ureaplasma urealyticum* and other pathogens in the development of chronic lung disease of prematurity. Pediatr Infect Dis J 1988;7(8):547–51.

69. Waites KB, Crouse DT, Cassell GH. Systemic neonatal infection due to *Ureaplasma urealyticum*. Clin Infect Dis 1993;17(Suppl 1):S131–5.

70. Goldenberg RL, Andrews WW, Goepfert AR, et al. The Alabama Preterm Birth Study: umbilical cord blood *Ureaplasma urealyticum* and *Mycoplasma hominis* cultures in very preterm newborn infants. Am J Obstet Gynecol 2008;198(1):43 e41–5.

71. Waites KB, Crouse DT, Nelson KG, et al. Chronic *Ureaplasma urealyticum* and *Mycoplasma hominis* infections of central nervous system in preterm infants. Lancet 1988;2:17–21.

72. Waites KB, Duffy LB, Crouse DT, et al. Mycoplasmal infections of cerebrospinal fluid in newborn infants from a community hospital population. Pediatr Infect Dis J 1990;9(4):241–5.

73. Ollikainen J, Hiekkaniemi H, Korppi M, et al. *Ureaplasma urealyticum* cultured from brain tissue of preterm twins who died of intraventricular hemorrhage. Scand J Infect Dis 1993;25:529–31.

74. Rao RP, Ghanayem NS, Kaufman BA, et al. *Mycoplasma hominis* and *Ureaplasma* species brain abscess in a neonate. Pediatr Infect Dis J 2002; 21(11):1083–5.

75. Klein JO, Buckland D, Finland M. Colonization of newborn infants by mycoplasmas. N Engl J Med 1969;280(19):1025–30.

76. Cassell GH, Waites KB, Crouse DT, et al. Association of *Ureaplasma urealyticum* infection of the lower respiratory tract with chronic lung disease and death in very-low-birth-weight infants. Lancet 1988;2:240–4.

77. Hentschel J, Abele-Horn M, Peters J. *Ureaplasma urealyticum* in the cerebrospinal fluid of a premature infant. Acta Paediatr 1993;82(8):690–3.

78. Berger A, Witt A, Haiden N, et al. Intrauterine infection with *Ureaplasma* species is associated with adverse neuromotor outcome at 1 and 2 years adjusted age in preterm infants. J Perinat Med 2009;37(1):72–8.

79. Stahelin-Massik J, Levy F, Friderich P, et al. Meningitis caused by *Ureaplasma urealyticum* in a full term neonate. Pediatr Infect Dis J 1994; 13(5):419–21.

80. Zheng X, Watson HL, Waites KB, et al. Serotype diversity and antigen variation among invasive isolates of *Ureaplasma urealyticum* from neonates. Infect Immun 1992;60:3472–4.

81. Heggie AD, Jacobs MR, Butler VT, et al. Frequency and significance of isolation of *Ureaplasma urealyticum* and *Mycoplasma hominis* from cerebrospinal fluid and tracheal aspirate specimens from low birth weight infants. J Pediatr 1994; 124:956–61.

82. Sethi S, Sharma M, Narang A, et al. Isolation pattern and clinical outcome of genital mycoplasma in neonates from a tertiary care neonatal unit. J Trop Pediatr 1999;45(3):143–5.

83. Schwersenski J, McIntyre L, Bauer CR. Lumbar puncture frequency and cerebrospinal fluid analysis in the neonate. Am J Dis Child 1991;145:54–8.

84. Smith PB, Garges HP, Cotton CM, et al. Meningitis in preterm neonates: importance of cerebrospinal fluid parameters. Am J Perinatol 2008;25(7):421–6.

85. Matlow AG, Richardson SE, Quinn PA, et al. Isolation of *Ureaplasma urealyticum* from nonneonatal respiratory tract specimens in a pediatric institution. Pediatr Infect Dis J 1996;15(3):272–4.

86. Pinna GS, Skevaki CL, Kafetzis DA. The significance of *Ureaplasma urealyticum* as a pathogenic agent in the paediatric population. Curr Opin Infect Dis 2006; 19(3):283–9.

87. Benn CS, Thorsen P, Jensen JS, et al. Maternal vaginal microflora during pregnancy and the risk of asthma hospitalization and use of anti-asthma medication in early childhood. J Allergy Clin Immunol 2002;110(1):72–7.

88. Likitnukul S, Kusmiesz H, Nelson JD, et al. Role of genital mycoplasmas in young infants with suspected sepsis. J Pediatr 1986;109(6):971–4.

89. Kong F, Ma Z, James G, et al. Species identification and subtyping of *Ureaplasma parvum* and *Ureaplasma urealyticum* using PCR-based assays. J Clin Microbiol 2000;38(3):1175–9.

90. Scheurlen W, Frauendienst G, Schrod L, et al. Polymerase chain reaction-amplification of urease genes: rapid screening for ureaplasma infection in endotracheal aspirates of ventilated newborns. Eur J Pediatr 1992;151:740–2.

91. Blanchard A, Hentschel J, Duffy L, et al. Detection of *Ureaplasma urealyticum* by polymerase chain reaction in the urogenital tract of adults, in amniotic fluid, and in the respiratory tract of newborns. Clin Infect Dis 1993;17(Suppl 1): S148–53.

92. Stellrecht KA, Woron AM, Mishrik NG, et al. Comparison of multiplex PCR assay with culture for detection of genital mycoplasmas. J Clin Microbiol 2004;42(4): 1528–33.

93. Mallard K, Schopfer K, Bodmer T. Development of real-time PCR for the differential detection and quantification of *Ureaplasma urealyticum* and *Ureaplasma parvum*. J Microbiol Methods 2005;60(1):13–9.

94. Kirschbaum T. Antibiotics in the treatment of preterm labor. Am J Obstet Gynecol 1993;168(4):1239–46.

95. Gomez R, Romero R, Nien JK, et al. Antibiotic administration to patients with preterm premature rupture of membranes does not eradicate intra-amniotic infection. J Matern Fetal Neonatal Med 2007;20(2):167–73.

96. Renaudin H, Bebear C. Comparative in vitro activity of azithromycin, clarithromycin, erythromycin and lomefloxacin against *Mycoplasma pneumoniae*, *Mycoplasma hominis* and *Ureaplasma urealyticum*. Eur J Clin Microbiol Infect Dis 1990;9(11):838–41.

97. Bowman ED, Dharmalingam A, Fan WQ, et al. Impact of erythromycin on respiratory colonization of *Ureaplasma urealyticum* and the development of chronic lung disease in extremely low birth weight infants. Pediatr Infect Dis J 1998; 17:615–20.

98. Jonsson B, Rylander M, Faxelius G. *Ureaplasma urealyticum*, erythromycin and respiratory morbidity in high-risk preterm neonates. Acta Paediatr 1998;87: 1079–84.

99. Baier RJ, Loggins J, Kruger TE. Failure of erythromycin to eliminate airway colonization with *Ureaplasma urealyticum* in very low birth weight infants. BMC Pediatr 2003;3:10.

100. Rubin BK. Macrolides as biologic response modifiers. J Respir Dis 2002;23: S31–8.

101. Ianaro A, Ialenti A, Maffia P, et al. Anti-inflammatory activity of macrolide antibiotics. J Pharmacol Exp Ther 2000;292(1):156–63.

102. Tsai WC, Standiford TJ. Immunomodulatory effects of macrolides in the lung: lessons from *in-vitro* and *in-vivo* models. Curr Pharm 2004;10(25):3081–93.

103. Duffy LB, Crabb D, Searcey K, et al. Comparative potency of gemifloxacin, new quinolones, macrolides, tetracycline and clindamycin against *Mycoplasma* spp. J Antimicrob Chemother 2000;45(Suppl 1):29–33.

104. Girard AE, Cimochowski CR, Faiella JA. Correlation of increased azithromycin concentrations with phagocyte infiltration into sites of localized infection. J Antimicrob Chemother 1996;37(Suppl C):9–19.

105. Patel KB, Xuan D, Tessier PR, et al. Comparison of bronchopulmonary pharmacokinetics of clarithromycin and azithromycin. Antimicrobial Agents Chemother 1996;40(10):2375–9.

106. Capitano B, Mattoes HM, Shore E, et al. Steady-state intrapulmonary concentrations of moxifloxacin, levofloxacin, and azithromycin in older adults. Chest 2004; 125(3):965–73.
107. Auten RL, Ekekezie II. Blocking leukocyte influx and function to prevent chronic lung disease of prematurity. Pediatr Pulmonol 2003;35(5):335–41.
108. Liao L, Ning Q, Li Y, et al. CXCR2 blockade reduces radical formation in hyperoxia-exposed newborn rat lung. Pediatr Res 2006;60(3):299–303.
109. Walls SA, Kong L, Leeming HA, et al. Antibiotic prophylaxis improves *Ureaplasma*-associated lung disease in suckling mice. Pediatr Res 2009; 66(2):197–202.
110. Viscardi RM, Hasday JD. Role of *Ureaplasma* species in neonatal chronic lung disease: epidemiologic and experimental evidence. Pediatr Res 2009;65: 84R–90R.

Molecular Diagnosis of Neonatal Sepsis

Jeanne A. Jordan, PhD[a,b,*]

KEYWORDS

• Neonate • Bloodstream infection • Molecular testing

Bloodstream infections (BSI) in newborns are a significant cause of mortality and morbidity, including developmental delay and hearing loss, especially for the premature or low birth weight infant. Ten percent of infants born in the United States are admitted to a neonatal intensive care unit (NICU) annually. Roughly half of these admissions are infants with risk factors for BSI. Nearly 25% of all NICU days represent infant stays for evaluations to rule out sepsis. Current recommendations for treating early onset sepsis include broad-spectrum antimicrobial therapy covering gram-positive and gram-negative bacteria. Therefore, many institutions prescribe 1 of 2 antibiotic regimens: ampicillin and gentamicin, or ampicillin and a third-generation cephalosporin.

In the United States, Group B *Streptococcus* (*Streptococcus agalactiae*) is the most common cause of early onset sepsis in the near-term and term infant, whereas *Escherichia coli* is isolated most often in the preterm infant. Less frequent causes of early onset bacterial sepsis in the neonate include *Streptococcus* spp, *Staphylococcus* spp, *Haemophilus influenza*, and *Listeria monocytogenes*.[1]

In newborn infants with suspected sepsis, it is critically important to determine whether clinical symptoms are caused by the presence of bacteria in the bloodstream. The sooner an answer can be made available, the better the chances for survival and an improved outcome. Among the current, commonly used diagnostic laboratory methods, growth in culture using an automated instrument is considered the gold standard. However, even the automated blood-culturing systems have unacceptably low sensitivities.[2] Of the factors affecting the yield from blood culture, the most important is the volume of blood collected from the patient. The smaller the blood volume collected for culture, the lower the chances of recovering microorganisms.[3,4] To optimize bacterial recovery, it is recommended that a minimum of 0.5 mL of whole blood

[a] Department of Epidemiology and Biostatistics, School of Public Health and Health Services, The George Washington University, 231 Ross Hall, 2300 Eye Street, NW, Washington, DC 20037, USA
[b] GWU-APHL International Institute for Public Health Laboratory Management, 2300 Eye Street, NW, Washington, DC 20037, USA
* Department of Epidemiology and Biostatistics, School of Public Health and Health Services, The George Washington University, 231 Ross Hall, 2300 Eye Street, NW, Washington, DC 20037.
E-mail address: sphjaj@gwumc.edu

Clin Perinatol 37 (2010) 411–419
doi:10.1016/j.clp.2010.02.001
0095-5108/10/$ – see front matter © 2010 Elsevier Inc. All rights reserved.

be added to each blood culture bottle. Other factors affecting the ability of blood cultures to detect BSI include (1) the time of collection of the blood sample relative to the time of initiation of antibiotics (collecting blood after antibiotics are administered to the neonate or the mother lowers the yield), (2) intermittent bacteremia, (3) low colony count per milliliter of blood, (4) collecting only a single-bottle blood culture specimen, and (5) inoculating only an aerobic blood culture bottle.[5]

Currently, most blood culturing is performed using an automated instrument like the Bactec 9240 (Becton Dickinson Diagnostics Instrument Systems, Sparks, MD, USA), which detects viable culturable microorganisms within a pediatric blood culture bottle. Detecting growth usually requires 12 to 24 hours for gram-negative microorganisms, or 24 to 48 hours for gram-positive microorganisms. After that, 1 to 2 additional days are needed to obtain a pure culture for phenotypic identification and antimicrobial susceptibility testing. The delay in receiving laboratory results, beyond the initial Gram stain from the positive blood culture bottle, promotes the extended use of 2 or more broad-spectrum antibiotics, when 1 broad-spectrum or a narrow-spectrum antibiotic would usually suffice. Obtaining culture results sooner would reduce the use of unnecessary or inefficient antibiotics and thus reduce the emergence of antimicrobial resistance, avoid the suppression of beneficial commensal organisms, and potentially reduce the length of NICU or hospital stay. Recent studies from academic and industrial laboratories describe the use of rapid molecular approaches for diagnosing BSI. At present, however, there are no molecular systems that can replace culture-based methods, because with few exceptions, most antimicrobial susceptibility testing requires purified bacterial isolates.

This article describes the following molecular-based approaches to detecting BSI: (1) whole blood tested directly by target amplification, (2) preenrichment of whole blood before target amplification, (3) fluids from positive blood culture bottles tested by polymerase chain reaction (PCR), (4) nucleic acid sequence-based amplification (NASBA), (5) PCR in conjunction with sequencing or microarray analysis, and (6) non-amplification-based fluorescence in situ hybridization (FISH). Other promising new technologies have been described for diagnosing chorioamnionitis and sepsis, such as proteomics and mass spectrometry, and these methods are discussed elsewhere.[6,7]

Whole blood DNA extraction protocols must be improved for more efficient recovery of low numbers of bacteria in small blood volumes routinely collected from infants. When improving extraction protocols for the purpose of isolating the nucleic acid microorganisms, it is important to consider that microorganisms can be present in whole blood in various forms. These forms include (1) viable intact bacteria (the only form that blood cultures are designed to detect), (2) intracellular or phagocytized bacteria, (3) nonviable bacteria, and (4) free nucleic acid from lysed bacterial cells. Most commonly used nucleic acid extraction and purification methods do not enrich or specifically select for microbial nucleic acid, but purify all nucleic acid present in a specimen. In whole blood, most of the purified nucleic acid is human genomic DNA. The abundance of human genomic DNA from white blood cells (WBC) effectively outcompetes microbial DNA for binding sites. As a result, recovery of bacterial nucleic acid is sacrificed and assay sensitivity reduced, especially when the neonate's WBC count is elevated.

To circumvent these obstacles that limit pathogen DNA yield, alternative approaches are being developed and evaluated. One approach is selective lysis and degradation of DNA from eukaryotic cells before bacterial lysis and DNA purification.[8] This approach also degrades free bacterial DNA within a sample, which may reduce the number of discordant PCR-positive, blood culture-negative results.

However, because the significance of nonviable bacterial DNA in a patient's blood is not yet known, this approach may limit the sensitivity for detecting true septicemia.

BACTERIAL DNA AMPLIFICATION DIRECTLY FROM WHOLE BLOOD OF INFANTS

The most appealing approach to detect BSI would be to use whole blood directly as the specimen for sample extraction and target detection in a molecular-based system. This approach would allow faster turnaround time in getting results to clinicians making decisions about patient care. Using a simple platform that would detect, identify, and provide antibiotic susceptibility information about the microorganism around the clock is the end goal. Despite considerable efforts in academia and industry, this goal has been elusive to date.

A small number of studies in infants have been published in which whole blood was used directly for screening for bacterial nucleic acid by a target amplification assay. In a study of blood samples collected from 85 neonates, using a highly conserved universal 16S ribosomal DNA (rDNA) target present in nearly all bacteria but not in human cells, Jordan and Durso[9] demonstrated 94.1% (83 of 85) agreement between real-time PCR and culture results. This study included NICU patients being evaluated for either early or late onset sepsis. The volume of whole blood collected for extraction and PCR analysis ranged from 100 to 600 µL. The sensitivity and specificity of this real-time PCR assay was 96.2% and 100%, respectively, with a limit of detection for E coli and group B Streptococcus of 40 or 50 colony-forming units per milliliter of blood, respectively.

Reier-Nilsen and colleagues[10] enrolled 48 infants being evaluated for early onset sepsis. These investigators targeted several larger 16S rDNA targets using conventional PCR and gel-based detection methods. The volume of whole blood used in this study ranged between 1 and 2 mL. The sensitivity of their molecular approach was 66.7% and the specificity was 87.5% compared with culture.

Chan and colleagues[11] enrolled preterm infants with clinical features suggestive of late onset sepsis and tested the blood samples for bacteremia, using a quantitative PCR assay that differentiated gram-negative and gram-positive organisms. The study used 0.5 mL of whole blood for the molecular testing. The sensitivity and specificity for gram-negative bacteria were 86.4% and 99.0%, respectively, whereas they were slightly lower at 73.7% and 98.5%, respectively, for gram-positive bacteria.

In summary, using whole blood directly in a target amplification-based assay for detecting bacteria has the advantage of rapid diagnosis but the challenges of suboptimal sensitivity and specificity. In a significant subset of cases in the studies summarized earlier, bacteria were detected sooner when using PCR compared with culture. However, these varied molecular approaches failed to detect culture-positive samples in some cases. Areas for further research include improving sensitivity, increasing the number of informative sequences for primer and probe design, and identifying additional antimicrobial resistance gene targets.

IMPROVING SENSITIVITY OF PCR FOR DETECTING BACTEREMIA

Sensitivity of whole blood PCR for pathogen detection has been suboptimal to date, and several strategies are under investigation to improve this. An obvious approach, which is perhaps not feasible in many NICU patients, is to increase the volume of blood used in the extraction and amplification processes. Another option is improving sample extraction procedures to obtain greater recovery of bacterial nucleic acid over human genomic DNA. In an attempt to improve sensitivity for detecting small numbers of bacteria in small volumes of whole blood, some investigators have used a preenrichment step before target amplification.

Jordan and Durso[12] described an approach in which whole blood was incubated in tryptic soy broth (TSB) for up to 5 hours before nucleic acid extraction and PCR. A total of 548 paired blood samples from NICU patients with suspected early or late onset sepsis were screened by culture and by PCR for bacterial 16S ribosomal DNA after the preamplification step. The culture positivity rate in this study was 5%. PCR had an analytical sensitivity and specificity of 96% and 88.9%, respectively. These numbers are similar to those obtained in studies by the same group with no amplification step, possibly because smaller volumes of blood were tested, a single PCR target was amplified rather than 4 targets, and the universal 16S rDNA target is relatively less sensitive than the organism-specific PCR targets used in the later study.[9]

Another study by Jordan and colleagues[13] was undertaken using the same TSB enrichment protocol in conjunction with PCR and pyrosequencing. The advantage of sequencing is that it allows not only for microbial detection but also for identification of the bloodstream pathogen. In this study, 1233 term or near-term neonates evaluated for early onset sepsis were enrolled. The culture positivity rate in this study was less than 1.5%. The results of this study revealed a high level of overall agreement (96.8%), specificity (97.5%), and negative predictive value (99.2%), but also revealed the inability of PCR to detect several culture-proved cases of early onset sepsis in these infants. Other strategies are needed to improve sensitivity of PCR compared with blood culture for detecting bacteria in whole blood.

PCR-BASED PATHOGEN IDENTIFICATION FROM BLOOD CULTURE BOTTLE FLUIDS WITH DETECTABLE GROWTH

Several studies have described the use of fluids from positive blood culture bottles as specimens for target amplification assays. In these studies, as little as 0.1 mL of fluid was removed from positive blood culture bottles, and nucleic acid extraction and PCR or NASBA target amplification were performed. This strategy, if optimized, could provide clinicians with pathogen identification and antibiotic susceptibility information much more rapidly than current methods, resulting in more tailored empirical antibiotic therapy and promoting responsible antibiotic stewardship.

Eigner and colleagues[14] evaluated a commercially available assay for detection of 32 common bacterial pathogens in fluid from 279 positive blood culture bottles (35.5% gram-negative and 64.5% gram-positive bacteria). In this system, bacterial DNA is isolated from the specimen, amplified, detected, and identified via hybridization and an alkaline phosphatase reaction on a membrane strip. This assay correctly identified 148 of 152 (97.4%) gram-positive cocci and 89 of 91 (97.8%) gram-negative rods. The overall agreement between this assay and conventional blood culture processing was 87.1% (243 of 279).

Gebert and colleagues[8] assessed whether time could be saved by testing fluids from positive blood culture using PCR compared with automated blood culture systems. The study included adult and pediatric populations. DNA was extracted from blood culture bottle fluids and analyzed by PCR for bacteria and *Candida* targets. Of the 18 positive blood cultures, only 11 were positive by PCR, but of those that were detected by PCR there was an average net gain of 10.7 hours (range of 1.2–37.7 hours) in diagnosing BSI. The sensitivity of PCR in this study was much lower than that in other studies, may be as a result of differences in the DNA extraction kits used. This highlights the importance of optimizing the DNA extraction methodology, particularly when analyzing small sample volumes such as those available from neonates. In a much larger study of 482 positive blood culture bottles, Wellinghausen and colleagues[15] described a multiplex PCR-enzyme-linked immunosorbent assay with overall sensitivity of 100% and specificities ranging from 92.5% to 100%, depending on the bacterial type identified.

Jordan and colleagues[16] combined real-time PCR with pyrosequencing to detect and identify the microorganisms in 255 consecutive positive blood culture bottles containing 270 bacterial isolates. This study included blood culture bottles from neonates and adults. Four separate targets (2 16S rDNA and 2 23S rDNA) were analyzed. The investigators found 98.7% agreement between the phenotypic and genotypic results in this study. Agreement remained high even in the 5.1% of bottles with polymicrobial growth.

SPECIFICITY: ABILITY OF PCR TO RULE OUT BACTEREMIA

In addition to enhancing sensitivity of PCR for detecting BSI pathogens, another important challenge to address is specificity, or the significance of PCR-positive, culture-negative results. Because the current gold standard blood culture is less than perfect for detecting BSI, comparing new methods to culture may be misleading. Discordant results could represent false-positive PCR because of sample or reagent contamination or false-negative blood culture because of low sample volume or other factors. PCR has potential advantages over blood culture, such as detection of DNA from dead or intracellular bacteria, which is not detected by culture, but which may be clinically important. Another advantage of a molecular method that uses target amplification is identification of novel or emerging organisms associated with BSI that are uncultivable or fastidious in nature.[17,18]

One confounding problem when using blood culture bottles for nucleic acid amplification testing is detection of nonviable fragments of DNA presumably present within the culture medium that is added to the blood culture bottle during the manufacturing process. Several investigators have described finding *Bacillus* spp or *Streptococcus* spp within uninoculated blood culture bottles (Jordan, unpublished data, 2005).[19,20]

PCR FOR IDENTIFICATION OF FALSE-POSITIVE BLOOD CULTURES

False-positive blood cultures have been reported to occur at a rate of 1% to 10% and generate uncertainty about whether these results represent growth of fastidious organisms that cannot be subcultured or instrument false-positives. Molecular methods have been used to rapidly rule out bacteremia in cases of false-positive blood cultures flagged by automated blood culture instruments.[19,21] Karahan and colleagues[21] analyzed 169 subculture-negative aerobic blood culture bottles obtained from different patients using PCR and sequencing to determine whether a positive blood culture bottle represented a true-positive or a false-positive. Eubacterial PCR yielded a total of 10 positive results, whereas the remaining 159 instrument positive bottles were negative by PCR. Qian and colleagues[19] analyzed 76 instrument false-positive samples for 16S rDNA target. None of these specimens were PCR positive, but all were found to have significantly higher WBC counts than the 20 instrument true-negatives and the 45 instrument true-positive specimens. Rapid screening in these instances would provide important information to clinicians.

Newer Amplification-based Technologies for Blood Pathogen Detection

Several newer methods have been developed to enhance sensitivity, speed, or ease of pathogen detection, including NASBA and mass-tag PCR. Zhao and colleagues[22] were the first to describe an approach using NASBA in conjunction with 5 broad-range molecular beacons to screen blood culture bottles for fungal and bacterial pathogens. NASBA is an isothermal nucleic acid amplification assay that targets single-stranded templates so it preferentially amplifies RNA targets, and thus has an advantage over PCR in that ribosomal RNA (rRNA) genes are expressed at much higher levels at thousands of copies per cell. Five hundred and twenty randomly selected samples from positive blood culture bottles were evaluated in this study (362 gram-positive, 149 gram-negative and 10 *Candida* spp). The investigators found their approach to have an overall sensitivity and specificity for gram-positive and gram-negative bacteria of 96.1% and 98.6% and 100% and 95.9%, respectively, and found 100% sensitivity and specificity for *Candida*.

Nonamplification Methods for Blood Pathogen Detection

Bacterial detection platforms such as DNA microarray, FISH, and mass spectrometry that do not require target amplification have been developed, thus shortening the time to obtain results. For example, Cleven and colleagues[23] developed a DNA microarray that directly identified 3 common bloodstream pathogens (*Staphylococcus aureus*, *E coli*, and *Pseudomonas aeruginosa*) from positive blood culture bottles without prior nucleic acid target amplification. The array contained recombinant plasmid-based species-specific probes, 200 to 800 base pairs in length, that targeted housekeeping genes, virulence factors, and antibiotic resistance genes. This study included 13 positive blood culture bottles, along with clinical isolates and reference strains. A high level of correlation was found between the microarray analysis and conventional phenotypic identification for all 3 pathogens. Antibiotic susceptibility testing showed perfect correlation for *S aureus*, with slightly lower correlations for antibiotic resistance genes in *E coli* and *P aeruginosa*; more comprehensive gene targets were needed for *E coli*, and some nonspecific cross-hybridization was seen with *P aeruginosa* strains.

FISH has been used to rapidly identify microorganisms from positive blood culture fluids. Waar and colleagues[24] used FISH to detect and differentiate several *Enterococcus* spp present in 30 positive blood cultures containing gram-positive cocci in chains. Fifteen microliters of positive fluid were smeared onto a glass slide, and hybridization was performed using specific probes. Ten of 30 blood culture bottles yielded *Enterococcus faecalis*. Of these, all 10 were positive when hybridized to the *E faecalis*-specific probe. None of the remaining 20 bottles containing nonenterococcal gram-positive cocci reacted with any of the *Enterococcus* spp probes. In a much larger study, Gescher and colleagues[25] used FISH to accelerate identification of gram-positive cocci from positive blood culture bottles using probes that discriminated between staphylococci, streptococci, and enterococci. This study included 428 positive blood culture bottles and found an overall sensitivity of 98.7% and a specificity of 99% for FISH compared with conventional identification methods.

FISH has also been used to identify larger numbers of organisms, including gram-negative bacteria, in positive blood culture bottles. Jansen and colleagues[26] developed FISH probes against variable regions of the 16S rRNA to identify *Streptococcus* spp, *E faecalis*, *S aureus*, coagulase-negative staphylococci, *E coli*, *P aeruginosa*, and the entire Enterobacteriaceae family. These probes were used to analyze 182 positive blood culture bottles. The testing took only 25 to 45 minutes and, with the exception of the *S aureus* probe, demonstrated a sensitivity and specificity of 100%.

Among the most recent technologies being used to detect bacteria from positive blood culture bottles is matrix-assisted laser desorption ionization time-of-flight mass spectrometry (MALDI-TOF MS). In 1 study, of the 562 positive blood culture bottles containing a single pathogen, 370 (66%) were correctly identified using MALDI-TOF MS.[27] Of the 240 positive blood culture bottles processed, 181 (76%)

were correctly identified compared with conventional phenotypic identification; 87 of 100 (87%) gram-negative rods and 94 of 140 (67%) gram-positive cocci were correctly identified. The most common reason for erroneous identification was polymicrobial growth.

Another study using MALDI-TOF MS to identify bacteria involved analysis of 212 positive blood culture bottles.[28] Of these bottles, 170 of 212 (80.2%) bottles generated good spectral scores ($\geq$1.7); of these, 162 (95.3%) were correctly identified. Those 42 (19.8%) with poor spectral scores were not successfully identified, most likely because of low numbers of pathogens present in the bottles. Polymicrobial growth was seen in 10 (4.7%) of the positive blood culture bottles. The investigators were able to identify at least 1 organism from 9 of 10 bottles. Although misidentification did not occur in the polymicrobial bottles, not all pathogens were detected using MALDI-TOF MS. An important observation made by these investigators was that all 8 *Streptococcus mitis* were misidentified as *Streptococcus pneumoniae* even though they had good spectral scores of more than 1.9. This finding was also made by other investigators. In summary, the MALDI-TOF MS technology seems to provide accurate results for BSI with single pathogens from positive blood culture bottles in about 1 hour's time, making it potentially clinically useful.

Currently, none of the molecular approaches described earlier replace standard blood culture techniques. With the exception of a few antibiotic resistance genes (*mecA*, *vanA*, and *vanB*), most antimicrobial susceptibility testing requires purified bacterial isolates. However, many of these molecular methods can reduce the amount of time it takes to identify the organisms growing in culture compared with phenotypic identification. Whereas culture-based techniques require several days to complete, molecular methods can yield results in hours. The time saved can translate into improved patient outcome; for example, an infant could receive fewer doses of unnecessary or ineffective antibiotics or receive a more effective antibiotic sooner.

SUMMARY

Many recent technological developments in molecular biology can be applied to diagnosing BSI. The major advantage of a molecular test is speed, with just hours required to generate a result compared with days for conventional blood culture techniques. Although the specificity of molecular tests is high, the sensitivity when using whole blood directly has been suboptimal. Improvements in whole blood DNA extraction techniques are needed, especially when the number of microorganisms is low (which is usually the case for BSI). Extraction methods should be designed to handle larger volumes of blood, enrich for microorganism nucleic acid over human genomic DNA, and concentrate the purified nucleic acid in a small elution volume suitable for PCR or hybridization. Pending development of better whole blood molecular diagnostic methods, many investigators have included a short preenrichment incubation step or tested fluids from positive blood culture bottles to identify microorganisms and perform antibiotic resistance testing. The obvious trade-off for enhanced sensitivity of these strategies is increased time to obtain results. These methods may nonetheless confer some time savings over conventional culture, subculture, identification, and sensitivity testing protocols.

Industry-academic partnerships are critical to translate the discoveries made in individual research laboratories into kit-based in vitro diagnostics that can be manufactured in bulk and made widely available in clinical laboratories. When performing broad-range target amplification assays, it is imperative that reagents be free of nucleic acid, which requires extensive quality control measures. With these collaborations and focus on quality control, well-controlled, large-scale clinical trials can provide crucial data to resolve discordant results between traditional culture and molecular methods. In designing these trials it will be critical to first determine how discordant results will be interpreted.

A major practical consideration in translating molecular diagnostics to clinical use is routine availability of the assay in hospital laboratories. Manufacturers developing automated platforms must consider that, for optimal utility, this testing should be available around the clock and be easy to use by technicians with little molecular training. Once these hurdles are overcome, outcome-based studies can determine the clinical effectiveness and cost-effectiveness of rapid molecular diagnostics of BSI. The final step will be to educate clinicians on the test's strengths and weaknesses so that they can have confidence in the results. These arduous efforts are worthwhile; benefits would include reducing morbidity and mortality by more rapidly instituting appropriate antibiotic therapy, reducing unnecessary antibiotics, and decreasing length of NICU stay.

REFERENCES

1. Klein JO, Marcy SM. Bacterial sepsis and meningitis. Infectious diseases of the fetus and newborn. Philadelphia: WB Saunders; 1990.
2. Gerdes JS. Diagnosis and management of bacterial infections in the neonate. Pediatr Clin North Am 2004;51:939–59.
3. Brown DR, Kutler K, Rai B, et al. Perinatal neonatal clinical presentation: bacterial concentration and blood volume required for a positive blood culture. J Perinatol 1995;15:157–9.
4. Connell TG, Rele M, Cowley D, et al. How reliable is a negative blood culture result? Volume of blood submitted for culture in routine practice in a children's hospital. Pediatrics 2009;119(5):891–6.
5. Schuchat A, Whitney C, Zangwill K. Prevention of perinatal group B streptococcal disease: a public health perspective. MMWR Recomm Rep 1996;45:1–24.
6. Mothershed EA, Whitney AM. Nucleic acid-based methods for the detection of bacterial pathogens: present and future considerations for the clinical laboratory. Clin Chim Acta 2006;363:206–20.
7. Buhimschi CS, Bhandari V, Han YW. Using proteomics in perinatal and neonatal sepsis: hopes and challenges for the future. Curr Opin Infect Dis 2009;22: 235–43.
8. Gebert S, Siegel D, Wellinghausen N. Rapid detection of pathogens in blood culture bottles by real-time PCR in conjunction with the pre-analytic tool MolYsis. J Infect 2008;57:307–16.
9. Jordan JA, Durso MB. Real-time polymerase chain reaction for detecting bacterial DNA directly from blood of neonates being evaluated for sepsis. J Mol Diagn 2005;7(5):575–81.
10. Reier-Nilsen T, Farstad T, Nakstad B, et al. Comparison of broad range 16S rDNA PCR and conventional blood culture for diagnosis of sepsis in the newborn: a case control study. BMC Pediatr 2009;9:5–12.
11. Chan KY, Lam HS, Cheung HM, et al. Rapid identification and differentiation of Gram-negative and Gram-positive bacterial bloodstream infections by quantitative polymerase chain reaction in preterm infants. Crit Care Med 2009;37(8): 2441–7.
12. Jordan JA, Durso MB. Comparison of 16S rRNA gene PCR and BACTEC 9240 for detection of neonatal bacteremia. J Clin Microbiol 2000;8(7):2574–8.

13. Jordan JA, Durso MB, Butchko AR, et al. Evaluating the near-term infant for early onset sepsis: progress and challenges to consider with 16S rDNA polymerase chain reaction testing. J Mol Diagn 2006;8(3):357–63.

14. Eigner U, Weizenegger M, Fahr AM. Evaluation of a rapid direct assay for identification of bacteria and the mecA and van genes from positive-testing blood cultures. J Clin Microbiol 2005;43(10):5256–62.

15. Wellinghausen N, Wirths B, Essig A, et al. Evaluation of the Hyplex BloodScreen multiplex PCR–enzyme-linked immunosorbent assay system for direct identification of Gram-positive cocci and Gram-negative bacilli from positive blood cultures. J Clin Microbiol 2004;42(7):3147–52.

16. Jordan JA, Jones-Laughner J, Durso MB. Utility of pyrosequencing in identifying bacteria directly from positive blood culture bottles. J Clin Microbiol 2009;47(2): 368–72.

17. Fenollar F, Raoult D. Molecular genetic methods for the diagnosis of fastidious microorganisms. APMIS 2004;112:785–807.

18. Fenollar F, Raoult D. Molecular diagnosis of bloodstream infections caused by non-cultivable bacteria. Int J Antimicrob Agents 2007;30S:S7–15.

19. Qian Q, Tang YW, Kolbert CP, et al. Direct identification of bacteria from positive blood cultures by amplification and sequencing of the 16S rRNA gene: evaluation of BACTEC 9240 instrument true-positive and false-positive results. J Clin Microbiol 2001;39(10):3578–82.

20. Fredricks DN, Relman DA. Improved amplification of microbial DNA from blood cultures by removal of the PCR inhibitor sodium polyanetholesulfonate. J Clin Microbiol 1998;36(10):2810–6.

21. Karahan ZC, Mumcuoglu I, Guriz H, et al. PCR evaluation of false-positive signals from two automated blood-culture systems. J Med Microbiol 2006;55:53–7.

22. Zhao Y, Park S, Kreiswirth BN, et al. Rapid real-time nucleic acid sequence-based amplification–molecular beacon platform to detect fungal and bacterial bloodstream infections. J Clin Microbiol 2009;47(7):2067–78.

23. Cleven BEE, Palka-Santini M, Gielen J, et al. Identification and characterization of bacterial pathogens causing bloodstream infections by DNA microarray. J Clin Microbiol 2006;44(7):2389–97.

24. Waar K, Degener JE, van Luyn MJ, et al. Fluorescent in situ hybridization with specific DNA probes offers adequate detection of *Enterococcus faecalis* and *Enterococcus faecium* in clinical samples. J Med Microbiol 2005;54:937–44.

25. Gescher DM, Kovacevic D, Schmiedel D, et al. Fluorescence in situ hybridization (FISH) accelerates identification of Gram-positive cocci in positive blood cultures. Int J Antimicrob Agents 2008;325:551–9.

26. Jansen GJ, Mooibroek M, Idema J, et al. Rapid identification of bacteria in blood cultures by using fluorescently labeled oligonucleotide probes. J Clin Microbiol 2000;38(2):814–7.

27. La Scola B, Raoult D. Direct identification of bacteria in positive blood culture bottles by matrix-assisted laser desorption ionization time-of-flight mass spectrometry. PloS One 2009;4(11):e8041, 1–6.

28. Stevenson LG, Drake SK, Murray PR. Rapid identification of bacteria in positive blood culture broths by MALDI-TOF mass spectrometry. J Clin Microbiol 2010; 48(2):444–7.

Adjunct Laboratory Tests in the Diagnosis of Early-Onset Neonatal Sepsis

William E. Benitz, MD[a,b,*]

KEYWORDS

- Neonatal sepsis • Bacterial cultures • Blood counts
- Acute-phase reactants • Cytokines

Definitive diagnosis of sepsis rests upon isolation of pathogenic bacteria in cultures of specimens obtained from normally sterile spaces within the body. Because of the close relationship between sepsis (as reflected in a systemic inflammatory response) and bacteremia (bacteria in the bloodstream), recovery of bacteria from a blood culture is often considered to be sine qua non for diagnosis of sepsis. Whereas such a strict criterion is certainly appropriate for clinical research, a positive blood culture should not be required for diagnosis of sepsis in everyday practice. Patients with sepsis may not have any positive cultures, or cultures may be positive only from sites other than blood. Conversely, isolation of bacteria in a blood culture may reflect asymptomatic bacteremia or contamination. Supplemental diagnostic tests based on evaluation of the immune response often can help resolve ambiguities in these situations.

Diagnostic tests for neonatal sepsis have two distinct but complementary functions. Ascertainment of infants who have serious bacterial infection, with identification of the causative organism, allows selection of the optimal antimicrobial agent and duration of treatment. Because tests for which results are quickly available have low sensitivity, their utility for making decisions about initiation of treatment is limited. It is typically necessary to rely upon the greater sensitivity (and corresponding negative predictive value) of delayed testing (eg, serial hematological or acute-phase reactant measurements) or results (eg, cultures) to guide discontinuation of antibiotic therapy initiated empirically. Both aspects are addressed below.

This article reviews the role of conventional diagnostic tests—cultures, blood counts, acute-phase reactants, and inflammatory mediator levels—in diagnosis of

a Division of Neonatal and Developmental Medicine, Stanford University School of Medicine, 750 Welch Road, Suite 315, Stanford, Palo Alto, CA 94304, USA
b Packard Children's Hospital, 725 Welch Road, Palo Alto, CA 94304, USA
* Division of Neonatal and Developmental Medicine, Stanford University School of Medicine, 750 Welch Road, Suite 315, Stanford, Palo Alto, CA 94304.
E-mail address: benitzwe@stanford.edu

Clin Perinatol 37 (2010) 421–438
doi:10.1016/j.clp.2009.12.001
0095-5108/10/$ – see front matter © 2010 Elsevier Inc. All rights reserved.

early-onset neonatal sepsis. The developing roles of molecular methods for detection of bacterial DNA and other novel diagnostic methods such as proteomics are addressed elsewhere in this issue.

CULTURES
Blood

Samples of blood for culture may be obtained by arterial or venous puncture after preparation of the site with an antibacterial solution (alcoholic solutions of chlorhexidine, iodine, or povidone-iodine are preferable to aqueous povidone-iodine).[1–3] Data regarding sterilization of intravenous catheter sites indicate that cleansing for 30 seconds or two consecutive cleansings are superior to a single, brief (5–10 seconds) disinfection.[4] Specimens obtained from newly placed intravenous or umbilical catheters[5] are also suitable. Specimens from catheters that have been in place for hours or days may also be informative,[6] but isolation of an organism (particularly coagulase-negative *Staphylococci*) often reflects colonization of the catheter or infusion tubing rather than bacteremia.[7]

The volume of blood required to achieve optimal sensitivity of neonatal blood cultures has not been precisely defined. Historically, sample volumes much smaller than those considered appropriate for older patients have been used to minimize development of anemia from large or repeated phlebotomies. Use of small volumes was supported by data on circulating colony counts in infants with *Escherichia coli* sepsis, which suggested that an inoculum as small as 0.2 to 0.5 mL may be sufficient.[8] The only prospective comparison of isolation rates from small (0.2 mL) and larger (2 mL) inocula found a sensitivity of 96% and specificity of 99%.[9] Other reports indicate that larger volumes of blood are required to identify cases of low-level bacteremia, which may account for up to two-thirds of the cases of neonatal sepsis.[10] In vitro studies simulating inocula with low (1–3 colony-forming units [CFU]/mL) and ultralow (<1 CFU/mL) levels of bacteremia indicate that microorganism recovery should be increased using volumes of 1 to 2 mL for each culture.[11] Therefore, inoculation of at least 1 mL of blood into a single culture bottle is recommended. Because anaerobic organisms are rarely implicated in early-onset sepsis,[12] the entire specimen should be used for aerobic culture. There is little or no increase in ascertainment of bacteremia when multiple cultures are obtained from different sites.[13,14] However, recovery of identical organisms from replicate, independent specimens provides unequivocal evidence of a true bacteremia, and multiple negative cultures may provide stronger evidence of clearance of a previously documented bacteremia.[15]

Experience with manual methods, relying on development of turbidity in the culture broth, demonstrated that 96% of the cultures obtained before antibiotic administration were positive after 48 hours and 98% were positive at 72 hours.[16] Automated systems for detection of bacterial growth substantially decreased the time to detection of positive cultures.[17] One such system detected 94% of true positive bacterial cultures obtained before antibiotic therapy (excluding those yielding coagulase-negative *Staphylococci*, *Corynebacteria*, or yeast) within 24 hours and 97% within 36 hours. Few additional positive results developed between 36 and 72 hours.[18] Other investigators have reported similar results.[19–21] For asymptomatic term infants with suspected early-onset sepsis, negative cultures after 36 hours of incubation are sufficient to exclude sepsis and permit discontinuation of empiric antibiotic therapy.

In the sick neonate, negative cultures are of less value in excluding sepsis. There are few data on paired simultaneous blood cultures in neonates, so the sensitivity of blood culture in detection of bacteremia is difficult to assess. Although at least one series suggests a sensitivity of 100%,[13] it is important to recognize that this performance may not be representative. Some of the most informative data is provided by Pourcyrous and colleagues,[6] who compared yields of peripheral and umbilical blood specimens with sample volumes of 1 to 2 mL. Excluding possible contaminants (discordant organisms, *Staphylococcus epidermidis*), cultures obtained from umbilical catheters and by venipuncture were concordant (ie, each positive) in only 14 of 22 paired samples, implying a sensitivity of only 78%. Among infants in whom bacterial sepsis was confirmed at autopsy, 18% to 33% have negative premortem blood cultures.[22–24] These data suggest a false-negative rate of approximately 20%. In a sick infant, factors beyond a negative blood culture, including clinical signs and the results of hematological and acute-phase reactant measurements, should be considered before empiric antibiotic therapy is discontinued.

A limited evaluation, including a blood culture and observation without treatment has been suggested for asymptomatic infants thought to be at increased but moderate risk of bacterial sepsis.[25] The logic underlying this recommendation should be questioned. A probability of a positive blood culture sufficient to justify obtaining one should also merit timely initiation of empiric antibiotic therapy to prevent deterioration of the infant's condition due to untreated bacteremia. Conversely, development of clinical signs of infection in an untreated infant requires re-evaluation—including a new blood culture, which is much more likely to be diagnostic in a symptomatic infant—and initiation of treatment. The probability that a report of a positive culture will be the initial or sole stimulus for initiation of therapy appears to be very low.[26]

Spinal Fluid

The role of spinal fluid cultures in neonates with suspected sepsis remains controversial. Culture-proven bacterial meningitis occurs in approximately 0.25 of every 1000 live-born infants.[27,28] Blood cultures fail to yield the causative organism in 15% to 50% of infants with bacterial meningitis.[29,30] This is not an historical artifact, as blood cultures were negative in 38% (35 of 92) of infants diagnosed between 1997 and 2002 in a large multicenter series.[31] Conversely, up to 13% of infants with early-onset sepsis also have meningitis.[32–34] Therefore, culture of spinal fluid obtained before or soon after administration of antibiotics[35] may be essential to bacteriologic diagnosis.[27,36]

Because the prevalence of meningitis is low, some have advocated omission of lumbar puncture in apparently well, term infants undergoing evaluation solely because of maternal risk factors.[37] Fielkow and colleagues[38] observed no meningitis cases among 284 neonates evaluated because of maternal risk factors (attack rate upper 95% confidence limit 1.1%). Among 712 infants evaluated for maternal risk factors alone, Schwersenski and colleagues[39] found only 1 with meningitis (attack rate upper 95% confidence limit 0.4%). Because of the low yield and large number of infants who would need lumbar puncture to detect one additional infant with meningitis without bacteremia, it may be reasonable to omit lumbar puncture in such infants.

Similarly, the low rate of meningitis among preterm infants who present with signs of respiratory distress syndrome (RDS) have led some to recommend omission of lumbar in those infants.[37] The data supporting that recommendation are less compelling. In 203 neonates with RDS who had successful lumbar punctures, Eldadah and colleagues[40] observed no positive cerebrospinal fluid cultures. Hendricks-Munoz and Shapiro[41] reviewed the records of 1390 infants with RDS who did not have lumbar punctures and found no evidence of missed cases of meningitis. Those studies reported patient experiences before 1990. The clinical contexts for RDS and early-onset sepsis have changed substantially since then, owing to use of antepartum steroids and intrapartum antibiotic prophylaxis, respectively. RDS and bacterial pneumonia are clinically indistinguishable,[42] so additional, more current data are needed to support omission of lumbar puncture in preterm infants with signs of RDS.

In summary, although it is rare in asymptomatic term infants, meningitis is still seen as a complication of neonatal sepsis. Evaluation of sick newborn infants should include performance of a lumbar puncture for cerebrospinal fluid culture.

Tracheal Aspirates

Culture of tracheal aspirate specimens is a useful supplement to blood cultures in diagnosis of early-onset sepsis. Sherman and colleagues[43] identified 25 infants with positive Gram stains of tracheal aspirates among 320 infants less than 8 hours of age who were either not intubated or had been intubated for less than 30 minutes, had perinatal risk factors for infection, and had respiratory signs and an abnormal chest radiograph. All had positive cultures of the tracheal aspirate, but blood cultures were positive in only 14 (56%) of these infants. Tracheal aspirate cultures yielded useful diagnostic information, otherwise not available, in at least 3.4% of these infants. In a subsequent series, cultures were positive in 106 of 733 tracheal aspirate specimens obtained from infants with respiratory distress in the first 12 hours after birth.[44] Blood cultures were positive in only 53 (50%) of these infants, suggesting that tracheal aspirate culture provides unique diagnostic information in 7.2% of the infants evaluated. In a more recent report, 18 of 139 (6.5%) tracheal aspirate cultures obtained from intubated infants less than 12 hours of age yielded bacterial growth.[45] Nine of the positive cultures were considered to represent contaminants, on the basis of light growth of nonpathogenic organisms (bacillus, diphtheroids, *Streptococcus sanguis*, micrococci, nonpathogenic *Neisseria*, *Streptococcus viridans*) or of multiple species of coagulase-negative *Staphylococcus*. Only two of the nine infants with presumed tracheal infection had a positive blood culture, implying an incremental diagnostic yield of 5% (7 of 139 cultures). Therefore, culture of tracheal aspirate specimens obtained in the first 12 hours after birth adds significant diagnostic information. Because the trachea quickly becomes colonized after intubation,[46] however, such cultures are not useful after prolonged tracheal intubation.

Urine

Cultures of urine rarely provide useful diagnostic information for infants undergoing evaluation for early-onset neonatal sepsis. In 1979, Visser and Hall[47] suggested that the risk of suprapubic aspiration was not justified by the low yield (2 of 188) of urine cultures obtained in infants less than 72 hours of age. Subsequent data have confirmed those conclusions. Among 280 infants greater than or equal to 35 weeks gestation for whom urine cultures were obtained in the first 24 hours after birth, the urine culture was positive in only 1, who was also bacteremic.[48] No positive cultures were found in 349 preterm infants (<1500 g birth weight) evaluated in the first 24 hours.[49] Urine culture is neither necessary nor helpful in infants less than 72 hours of age.

Superficial Cultures

Cultures obtained from superficial sites such as the axilla, umbilical stump, external ear canal, nasopharynx, and indwelling orogastric or endotracheal tubes correlate poorly with pathogens isolated from nonpermissive, normally sterile sites.[50,51] They, therefore, have low positive predictive value and may lead to erroneous assumptions about the identity of the causative agent. Use of these cultures to guide management should be strongly discouraged.[52]

HEMATOLOGICAL TESTS

Early observations that neonates with bacterial sepsis often have abnormal white blood cell counts led to the hypothesis that hematologic studies might allow diagnosis of sepsis before results of cultures become available. Because the imperfect sensitivity of any single measurement, including the total white cell count, total neutrophil count, neutrophil count, immature-to-total (I:T) or immature-to-mature neutrophil ratios, soon became apparent, several strategies for combining multiple observations have been proposed.[53–55] The advantages of this approach have been demonstrated by Rodwell and colleagues[55] (**Table 1**). Combination of multiple hematological determinations into a single score, using a cutoff value of three or greater, achieves a modest

Table 1
Performance of hematological findings and a hematological scoring system in 298 neonates evaluated for sepsis during the first postnatal month[55]

Hematological Finding	Sensitivity (%)	Specificity (%)	Positive Predictive Value (%)	Negative Predictive Value (%)
↑ I:T ratio[a]	96	71	25	99
↓ or ↑ neutrophil count[a]	96	61	20	99
Immature:mature ratio ≥0.3	93	81	32	99
↑ immature neutrophil count[a]	63	69	17	95
↓ or ↑ white cell count[b]	44	92	36	94
Neutrophil degenerative changes ≥3+[c]	33	95	39	93
Platelet count ≤150,000/mm^3	22	99	60	93
Hematological score[d]				
≥1	100	41	14	100
≥2	100	63	21	100
≥3	96	78	31	99
≥4	89	89	45	99
≥5	41	96	52	94
≥6	22	100	86	93
Hematological score ≥3				
Preterm infants ≤24 hours of age[e]	100	82	34	100
Term infants ≤24 hours of age[f]	100	74	8	100
Infants >24 hours of age[g]	93	83	65	97

[a] As defined by the reference ranges of Manroe et al.[53]
[b] ≤5000 or ≥25,000, 30,000 or 21,000 per mm^3 at birth, 12–24 hours and day 2 or after, respectively.
[c] ≥3+ for vacuolization, toxic granulation, or Dohle bodies according to the 0 to 4+ scale of Zipurksy et al.[56]
[d] Assign one point for each individual abnormal hematological finding listed above (2 points for an abnormal total neutrophil count if no neutrophils are present on the blood smear) and sum to determine the score.
[e] Ten sepsis cases among 113 preterm infants.
[f] Three sepsis cases among 130 term infants.
[g] Fourteen sepsis cases among 55 infants.
Data from Manroe BL, Weinberg AG, Rosenfeld CR, et al. The neonatal blood count in health and disease. I. Reference values for neutrophilic cells. J Pediatr 1979;95(1):89–98.

improvement in specificity and positive predictive value without a reduction in sensitivity. Unless the score is very high (≥ 5), however, most infants with elevated scores will not prove to have bacterial infection. When infants being evaluated for early-onset sepsis are considered separately, all 13 with culture-proven sepsis had a hematological score greater than or equal to three, providing sensitivity and negative predictive values of 100%. Two-thirds of the preterm infants and more than 90% of the term infants with a hematological score greater than or equal to three on the first postnatal day did not have confirmed sepsis—giving the test a low positive predictive value. Inclusion of infants with probable infection increased the positive predictive value of scores greater than or equal to three in these infants to only 33% for preterm and 62% for term infants. Because the number of babies with sepsis in these subgroups is small, the confidence intervals on these test performance characteristics are wide. Greenberg and Yoder found that the sensitivity and negative predictive values of hematological scores obtained at 1 to 7 hours of age are much lower than for those obtained at 12 to 24 hours of age (**Table 2**),[57] confirming earlier observations that hematological results are often initially reassuring in infants with proven sepsis.[58,59]

More recently, Ottolini and colleagues[26] assessed the utility of early blood counts in evaluation of 1665 asymptomatic infants greater than or equal to 35 weeks gestational age deemed at risk for early-onset sepsis because of maternal or intrapartum risk factors (maternal group B streptococcal colonization, intrapartum fever $\geq 38.0°C$, rupture of membranes >18 hours before birth, or a previous infant with invasive group B streptococcal disease, and either no intrapartum antibiotic prophylaxis or only a single dose <4 hours before birth). Only 7 of the 454 at-risk infants who had abnormal blood counts (white blood cell >30,000 or <5000/mm3; absolute neutrophil count <1,500/mm3, or an I:T ratio >0.2) developed clinical signs of sepsis; none had a positive blood culture. In this group of patients, the sensitivity, specificity, and positive and negative predictive values of an abnormal white blood cell count were 41%, 73%, 1.5%, and 99%, respectively. Of the other 17,655 term infants born at their center during the study period, 1996 to 1999, 283 were diagnosed with clinical sepsis: 134 had clinical signs evident at the initial examination and 149 developed clinical signs of sepsis within the first 48 hours. Blood cultures yielded pathogenic organisms in 8 of these infants, all of whom had both clinical signs and abnormal white blood cell

Table 2
Performance of hematological scoring systems for diagnosis of early-onset group B streptococcal sepsis in the first 24 hours after birth[57]

Hematological Scoring System	Sensitivity (%)	Specificity (%)	Positive Predictive Value (%)	Negative Predictive Value (%)
Initial blood counts (1–7 hours of age)				
Manroe et al[53]	68	45	43	70
Rodwell et al[55]	63	55	46	71
Spector et al[54]	31	90	67	68
Blood counts at 12–24 hours of age				
Manroe et al[53]	100	50	56	100
Rodwell et al[55]	100	73	73	100
Spector et al[54]	53	83	67	73

Data from Greenberg DN, Yoder BA. Changes in the differential white blood cell count in screening for group B streptococcal sepsis. Pediatr Infect Dis J 1990;9(12):886–9.

indices. These data suggest that an early complete blood count adds little diagnostic information to clinical assessment in the evaluation of either asymptomatic or symptomatic neonates with possible bacterial infection.

Normal hematological findings in infants with clinical findings consistent with sepsis should not provide sufficient reassurance to support a decision to defer initiation of antibiotic therapy. Symptomatic infants should be treated with antibiotics until infection has been excluded by other methods. Screening blood counts in asymptomatic term or late preterm infants with maternal risk factors for sepsis are insensitive and have a very high false-positive rate, so they should not be relied upon to guide decisions about initiation of antibiotic therapy in such infants. Close monitoring for development of clinical signs of infection should replace reliance on blood counts in infants for whom antibiotic therapy is deferred. Asymptomatic infants at significant risk, such as those with multiple risk factors for sepsis,[60] are better managed with a complete diagnostic evaluation and empiric treatment while those studies are pending.

ACUTE-PHASE REACTANTS

Inflammatory stimuli of any sort, including infection, trauma, or ischemia, cause marginalization, extravasation, and activation of granulocytes and monocytes, with release of multiple proinflammatory cytokines, including interleukin (IL)-1β, IL-6, and tumor necrosis factor-α (TNF-α).[61] These mediators stimulate production of a variety of proteins referred to as acute-phase reactants. The time courses of these responses in adults have been well characterized (**Fig. 1**)[61] and follow a similar pattern in neonates. Several of these, including C-reactive protein (CRP), fibrinogen (for which the erythrocyte sedimentation rate may be a surrogate measurement), haptoglobin, orosomucoid, amyloid protein A, and procalcitonin (PCT) have been evaluated as diagnostic tools in neonatal sepsis.

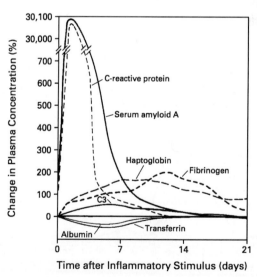

Fig. 1. Time course of acute-phase reactant responses to an inflammatory stimulus. (*From* Gabay C, Kushner I. Acute-phase proteins and other systemic responses to inflammation. N Engl J Med 1999;340(6):448–4; with permission.)

Erythrocyte Sedimentation Rate

The availability of a simple and inexpensive method for determination of the erythrocyte sedimentation rate using only few drops of capillary blood[62] led to consideration of this test for early diagnosis of neonatal sepsis. Adler and Denton[63] described a gradual increase in sedimentation rate over the first 2 weeks after birth, with the 95th percentile increasing from 2 mm per hour at 24 hours to 6 mm per hour at 48 hours of age. Evans and colleagues[64] noted that all four infants less than 3 days of age with confirmed sepsis in their series had microsedimentation rates greater than the 95% percentile for healthy infants (6 mm/hr). A subsequent report from Ibsen and colleagues confirmed that although an elevated initial sedimentation rate supports a diagnosis of serious bacterial infection, a low value does not exclude the diagnosis.[65] Because this test is easily performed even where access to laboratory technology is limited, it may still have some utility in such settings. In other situations, it has been replaced by more specific biochemical measurements, which also have been more extensively evaluated.

CRP

IL-6 released by activated granulocytes stimulates the liver to produce CRP, which takes its name from the observation that it forms an insoluble complex with the C-polysaccharide of *Streptococcus pneumoniae*. Serum levels may increase 100- to 1000-fold in response to bacterial infection or other inflammatory conditions. In infants with treated infections, serum levels begin to increase 6 to 8 hours after the onset of illness and peak after 2 to 3 days (**Fig. 2**).[66] Because of this typical delayed response, the sensitivity of CRP elevation at the time of evaluation for suspected

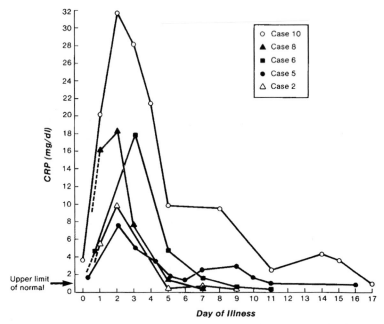

Fig. 2. Time course of CRP levels in neonates with group B streptococcal infection. (*From* Philip AGS. Response of C-reactive protein in neonatal Group B streptococcal infection. Pediatr Infect Dis 1985;4(2):145–8; with permission.)

sepsis is low, particularly with early-onset sepsis. In the author's experience in over 1000 infants, only 35% of infants with culture-proven early-onset sepsis and 39% of those with proven or probable early-onset sepsis had an elevated CRP ($\geq$10 mg/L).[67] Several smaller series had previously reported sensitivity values ranging from 29% to 90%,[68] and similar results have been described more recently.[69,70] Because many neonates with early-onset sepsis will not be identified by measurement of a serum CRP level, it should have no role in the initial evaluation of these infants.

Serial determinations of CRP levels over the first 2 to 3 days of illness may be quite useful in determining the duration of empiric antibiotic therapy, however.[67,71] Noting that at least one of three CRP levels obtained at the time of evaluation and 12 and 24 hours later was elevated in 92% of infants with gram-negative bacteremia and in 64% of those with gram-positive bacteremia (79% of those with organisms other than S epidermidis), Pourcyrous and colleagues[71] suggested that serial normal CRP values, in the absence of other clinical findings suggestive of infection, might indicate that it is safe to discontinue antibiotics. Benitz and colleagues[67] examined this question, using a different schedule for sample collection, with specimens obtained at the time of the initial evaluation, 8 to 24 hours after that, and again 24 hours after the second collection. The initial measurement added no information to the other two. Two delayed levels separated by 24 hours had a negative predictive value of 99.7% for both proven and for proven or probable sepsis and likelihood ratios of 0.15 and 0.03 for proven and proven or probable sepsis, respectively. Extending the interval of sampling into the second 24 hours enhances the negative predictive value of serial normal levels. Because persistently normal CRP levels correlate strongly with the absence of infection, they may be used to determine that antibiotics may be safely discontinued. This strategy may reduce the duration of empiric treatment of infants with nonspecific clinical findings and at-risk asymptomatic neonates.

Determination of the duration of therapy by monitoring for normalization of elevated CRP levels has also been suggested.[72,73] Although these preliminary observations suggest that a return of the serum CRP level to normal may be an indication that the duration of treatment has been adequate, the numbers of infants with proven infection with pathogenic bacteria in these series (eight and four, respectively, all of whom were treated for at least 5 days) are not sufficient to permit assessment of that hypothesis. Until data from a much larger sample of infants with demonstrated infection is available, this application of CRP levels cannot be recommended.

Many conditions other than bacterial infection may be associated with elevated CRP levels. Elevated levels may also be seen with viral infection, traumatic or ischemic tissue injuries, hemolysis, meconium aspiration, or chorioamnionitis without invasive fetal or neonatal disease. One or more elevated CRP levels, in the absence of other data indicating that the infant is infected, should not constitute a sole indication for continuation of empiric antibiotic therapy.

Procalcitonin

Considerable attention has recently been drawn to PCT as a potential alternative to CRP for diagnosis of neonatal sepsis. PCT is produced both in the liver and by macrophages, with serum levels rising 4 to 6 hours after exposure to bacterial products.[74] Because this PCT response is more rapid than elevation of CRP, this marker is an attractive alternative for detection of early-onset sepsis. Initial reports of its clinical application appeared to support this expectation, suggesting sensitivity of an elevated serum level might be as high as 100%.[75,76] This early promise has not been fully realized after more extensive evaluation. Three challenges, in particular, have limited the application of PCT levels in evaluation of newborn infants for possible sepsis: the need for detailed age-specific normative ranges, disappointing sensitivity early in the course of infection, and lack of specificity.

Early experience in newborn infants suggested a spontaneous increase in PCT levels over the first day after birth.[77] This observation was soon confirmed and extended by others. Data collected by Sachse and colleagues[78] indicated that PCT levels in healthy infants peaked at 24 to 36 hours after birth and decreased thereafter. Chiesa and colleagues[79] established normative reference ranges for PCT during the first 48 hours after birth, which include an increase for the upper 95th percentile from 0.7 ng/mL at birth to 20 ng/mL at 24 hours, followed by a decline to less than 2 ng/mL at 48 hours of age (**Fig. 3**A). Turner and colleagues[80] extended these observations to preterm infants, in whom serum PCT levels peak at approximately 28 hours of age, but at levels lower than those observed in term infants. Clinical utility of PCT in diagnosis of early-onset sepsis will depend upon establishment of normative ranges specific to both gestational and postnatal ages. The limitations of a single cutoff value during this interval may be exemplified by the results of Resch and colleagues,[81] who found a sensitivity of 77% and specificity of 91% using a cutoff value of 6 ng/mL for infants between 0 and 12 hours of age.

Applying age-specific reference values in a sample of 120 infants admitted to their neonatal intensive care unit, Chiesa and colleagues[82] found a sensitivity of 92.6% and a specificity of 97.5% for PCT concentrations for detection of early-onset sepsis. Sepsis was confirmed by positive blood cultures in 14 infants and presumed on the basis of clinical signs and ancillary laboratory studies in 14 more (all of whom were born to women who received intrapartum antibiotics). Notably, however, the sensitivity of elevated PCT levels during the first 6 hours after birth was only 50% (3 of 6 tested infants with sepsis; **Fig. 3**B). In a subsequent report, results were similar at 24 hours of age (sensitivity 95% and specificity 96%), but less favorable at birth (sensitivity 79% and specificity 95%).

Several reports have subsequently examined the performance of PCT levels at birth, using either cord blood specimens or samples obtained soon after birth. In a sample of 120 infants, 21 of whom were infected, Guibourdenche and colleagues[83] found that

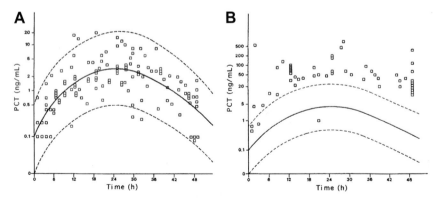

Fig. 3. (A) Reference range for procalcitonin levels in healthy neonates over the first 48 hours after birth. Broken lines represent upper and lower boundaries of the 95% confidence interval. Solid line represents the geometric mean. (B) Procalcitonin values among infants with culture-proven or presumed sepsis in the first 48 hours after birth. (*From* Chiesa C, Panero A, Rossi N, et al. Reliability of procalcitonin concentrations for the diagnosis of sepsis in critically ill neonates. Clin Infect Dis 1998;26(3):664–2; with permission.)

a PCT level greater than 2.5 ng/mL at birth had a sensitivity of 87% and specificity of 90%. Almost identical results were obtained by Joram and colleagues using a cord blood level cutoff of 0.5 ng/mL.[84] Kordek and colleagues[85] reported that the sensitivity and specificity of PCT levels in umbilical cord blood at an optimal cutoff value of less than or equal to 2.6 ng/mL were only 69% and 81%, respectively. In a subsequent series, that group found a sensitivity of 80% and a specificity of 72% using a cord blood cutoff value of 1.22 ng/mL. In each of these series, PCT was more sensitive than CRP. More recently, Lopez Sastre and colleagues, using a threshold PCT level of 0.55 ng/mL, reported a sensitivity of only 75% and specificity of only 72% at birth.[86] Therefore, the most appropriate threshold value of confirmation or exclusion of early-onset sepsis remains indeterminate, and neither the sensitivity nor specificity of an elevated PCT level at birth is sufficient to guide antibiotic therapy for an infant at risk for serious infection.

Moderately increased sensitivity of PCT, as compared with CRP, may be offset by lower specificity in the population of interest: infants with signs of possible sepsis who are not infected. Elevated levels of PCT are found in infants with respiratory distress syndrome,[87] hemodynamic instability,[87] asphyxia,[88] intracranial hemorrhage,[88] pneumothorax,[88] or resuscitation[88] and in those with infection. The positive predictive value of this measure is therefore limited by the many noninfectious causes of an elevated PCT level in a sick neonate, so it should not be used to justify continuation of antibiotic therapy in an infant who does not otherwise have convincing signs of sepsis.

ILS AND OTHER CYTOKINES

Because acute-phase reactants are produced in response to proinflammatory cytokines, direct measurement of serum cytokine levels promised to provide an earlier indication of infection than could be achieved by measurement of the secondary responses. Initial assessments of several cytokines, including IL-1β,[89] IL-6,[90–92] IL-8),[92–94] soluble IL-2 receptor (sIL2R),[95] and TNF-α[92] demonstrated early responses to bacterial infection in neonates. Initial reports of high sensitivity and specificity have not been consistently borne out by subsequent experience. Dollner and colleagues[96] evaluated several inflammatory mediators in cord blood specimens and found that IL-1β, IL-6, and IL-8 measurements were associated with the largest areas under the receiver-operator characteristic curves (**Fig. 4**). The sensitivities of these tests at the optimal cutoff values were only 74%, 84%, and 81%, respectively. Santana Reyes and colleagues[97] collected blood specimens at the time of admission of newborn infants with suspected infection. They found that sensitivity and specificity were 80% and 92% for CRP, 60% and 87% for IL-1β, 61% and 80% for IL-6, 62% and 96% for IL-8, 54% and 92% for TNF-α, and 63% and 94% for soluble receptor of IL-2. As an individual analyte, none of these mediators reliably identifies infected neonates or excludes infection in those at risk.

COMBINATION TESTS

Noting that serum levels of cytokines often return to normal as those of acute-phase reactants rise, several groups have proposed use of combinations of measurements to enhance the likelihood of an abnormal result in the face of uncertainty about the stage of illness at which an infant is evaluated for suspected infection. In concept, elevation of a cytokine level would permit detection of infants early in the course of infection, before CRP elevation is apparent, while the delayed elevation of CRP would identify infants later in the course, after a transient cytokine response has resolved. Franz and colleagues[98] found that the combination of IL-8 and CRP on admission

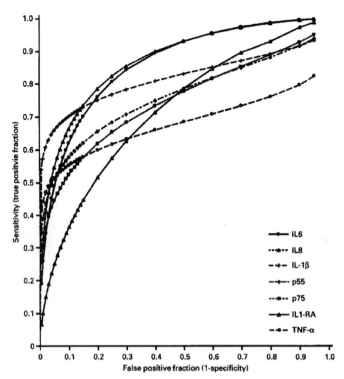

Fig. 4. Receiver-operator characteristic curves for cord blood serum cytokine determinations for diagnosis of early-onset neonatal sepsis in preterm infants. (*From* Dollner H, Vatten L, Linnebo I, et al. Inflammatory mediators in umbilical plasma from neonates who develop early-onset sepsis. Biol Neonate 2001;80(1):41–7; with permission.)

detected early-onset bacterial infection with a sensitivity of 92% and specificity of 74%. Because this combination was much more specific that the combination of I:T ratio and CRP level, they estimated a 40% reduction in the number of infants in whom treatment might be initiated using the former rather than latter criterion. Santana Reyes and colleagues[97] found the best combination for sepsis diagnosis to be CRP, IL-8, and sIL2R, with a sensitivity of 85% and a specificity of 97%. Others have confirmed enhanced performance of combined as compared with single markers, but no panel of analytes has been prospectively shown to have both excellent sensitivity and good specificity.

SUMMARY

Timely diagnosis of neonatal bacterial infection remains one of the most common and problematic tasks encountered in neonatal medicine. Evaluation of infants at risk for early-onset infection must be based on the pregnancy and intrapartum history and clinical manifestations of illness in the infant, which may be absent or nonspecific. While careful observation for development of clinical signs remains essential to management of these infants, the potential for reduction of morbidity and mortality with early initiation of antibiotic therapy for bacterial infection has stimulated an ongoing search for laboratory methods for diagnosis of infection before clinical signs become apparent. Cultures of normally sterile body fluids, and of blood in particular, remain crucial to definitive diagnosis of sepsis, but there are both false-positive and false-negative results, and results become available only after a day or two. Despite long-established use of hematological counts for identification of infected infants, these tests are neither sensitive nor specific, particularly at the beginning of an episode of early-onset sepsis. Over the past two decades, several acute-phase reactants, including CRP and PCT, have been evaluated. More recently, serum levels of inflammatory mediators have been considered. Of these, IL-6 and IL-8 appear most promising. However, because levels of these cytokines decrease quickly after the initial response, optimal utility may be obtained in combination with CRP or PCT, which increase more slowly but remain elevated for longer periods of time.

Ancillary diagnostic tests for early-onset infection have potential applications in three circumstances. First, in the case of an infant who is seriously ill, with shock, respiratory failure, lethargy, acidemia, or the like, the decision to initiate antibiotic therapy is not dependent on laboratory test results. The role of ancillary tests in these infants lies in retrospective ascertainment of those who were not infected and for whom antibiotics can be safely discontinued after some interval of empiric treatment. Negative culture results, particularly when supplemented by absence of signs of an acute-phase response, are most useful in this situation. Only CRP has been systematically evaluated for this purpose.[67,71,99] Second, a test that could identify infants who are septic among those with only historical risk factors (prolonged rupture of membranes, intrapartum fever, group B streptococcal colonization, etc) or with minor clinical signs (transient hypoglycemia, tachypnea, an oxygen requirement, etc) would be useful to ensure treatment of infected infants while allowing nontreatment of others. No currently available test or combination of tests has sufficient sensitivity and specificity to achieve these objectives. In these situations, the choices are either initiation of empiric therapy, followed by reliance on cultures and acute-phase reactants to identify infants for whom treatment was unnecessary, or close clinical observation, with initiation of therapy for infants who develop clinical signs of infection. Third, acute-phase reactants or cytokine levels may be of value for monitoring response to therapy or prognosis in infants in whom infection is confirmed. Failure of CRP levels to return to normal or recurrent elevation after an initial improvement may be an indication of a significant complication, such as subdural empyema complicating bacterial meningitis, for example. Although preliminary reports suggest that normalization of acute-phase reactants may indicate adequacy of a course of treatment, enabling discontinuation of therapy, experience in infants with culture-proven sepsis is not yet sufficient to support recommendation of this practice.

REFERENCES

1. Calfee DP, Farr BM. Comparison of four antiseptic preparations for skin in the prevention of contamination of percutaneously drawn blood cultures: a randomized trial. J Clin Microbiol 2002;40(5):1660–5.
2. Mimoz O, Karim A, Mercat A, et al. Chlorhexidine compared with povidone-iodine as skin preparation before blood culture. A randomized, controlled trial. Ann Intern Med 1999;131(11):834–7.
3. Trautner BW, Clarridge JE, Darouiche RO. Skin antisepsis kits containing alcohol and chlorhexidine gluconate or tincture of iodine are associated with low rates of blood culture contamination. Infect Control Hosp Epidemiol 2002;23(7):397–401.
4. Malathi I, Millar MR, Leeming JP, et al. Skin disinfection in preterm infants. Arch Dis Child 1993;69(3 Spec No):312–6.

5. Cowett RM, Peter G, Hakanson DO, et al. Reliability of bacterial culture of blood obtained from an umbilical artery catheter. J Pediatr 1976;88(6):1035–6.

6. Pourcyrous M, Korones SB, Bada HS, et al. Indwelling umbilical arterial catheter: a preferred sampling site for blood culture. Pediatrics 1988;81(6):821–5.

7. Ruderman JW, Morgan MA, Klein AH. Quantitative blood cultures in the diagnosis of sepsis in infants with umbilical and Broviac catheters. J Pediatr 1988;112(5): 748–51.

8. Dietzman DE, Fischer GW, Schoenknecht FD. Neonatal *Escherichia coli* septicemia—bacterial counts in blood. J Pediatr 1974;85(1):128–30.

9. Solorzano-Santos F, Miranda-Novales MG, Leanos-Miranda B, et al. A blood micro-culture system for the diagnosis of bacteremia in pediatric patients. Scand J Infect Dis 1998;30(5):481–3.

10. Kellogg JA, Ferrentino FL, Goodstein MH, et al. Frequency of low level bacteremia in infants from birth to two months of age. Pediatr Infect Dis J 1997;16(4): 381–5.

11. Schelonka RL, Chai MK, Yoder BA, et al. Volume of blood required to detect common neonatal pathogens. J Pediatr 1996;129(2):275–8.

12. Noel GJ, Laufer DA, Edelson PJ. Anaerobic bacteremia in a neonatal intensive care unit: an eighteen-year experience. Pediatr Infect Dis J 1988;7(12):858–62.

13. Sarkar S, Bhagat I, DeCristofaro JD, et al. A study of the role of multiple site blood cultures in the evaluation of neonatal sepsis. J Perinatol 2006;26(1):18–22.

14. Wiswell TE, Hachey WE. Multiple site blood cultures in the initial evaluation for neonatal sepsis during the first week of life. Pediatr Infect Dis J 1991;10(5):365–9.

15. Sarkar S, Bhagat I, Wiswell TE, et al. Multiple site blood cultures are mandatory to document the clearance of bacteremia in neonates with sepsis. Pediatr Res 2003;53(4) [abstract 2848].

16. Pichichero ME, Todd JK. Detection of neonatal bacteremia. J Pediatr 1979;94(6): 958–60.

17. Pauli I Jr, Shekhawat P, Kehl S, et al. Early detection of bacteremia in the neonatal intensive care unit using the new BACTEC system. J Perinatol 1999;19(2):127–31.

18. Garcia-Prats JA, Cooper TR, Schneider VF, et al. Rapid detection of microorganisms in blood cultures of newborn infants utilizing an automated blood culture system. Pediatrics 2000;105(3 Pt 1):523–7.

19. Kumar Y, Qunibi M, Neal TJ, et al. Time to positivity of neonatal blood cultures. Arch Dis Child Fetal Neonatal Ed 2001;85(3):F182–6.

20. Janjindamai W, Phetpisal S. Time to positivity of blood culture in newborn infants. Southeast Asian J Trop Med Public Health 2006;37(1):171–6.

21. Jardine L, Davies MW, Faoagali J. Incubation time required for neonatal blood cultures to become positive. J Paediatr Child Health 2006;42(12):797–802.

22. Eisenfeld L, Ermocilla R, Wirtschafter D, et al. Systemic bacterial infections in neonatal deaths. Am J Dis Child 1983;137(7):645–9.

23. Squire E, Favara B, Todd J. Diagnosis of neonatal bacterial infection: hematologic and pathologic findings in fatal and nonfatal cases. Pediatrics 1979;64(1):60–4.

24. Pierce JR, Merenstein GB, Stocker JT. Immediate postmortem cultures in an intensive care nursery. Pediatr Infect Dis 1984;3(6):510–3.

25. Schrag S, Gorwitz R, Fultz-Butts K, et al. Prevention of perinatal group B streptococcal disease. Revised guidelines from CDC. MMWR Recomm Rep 2002; 51(RR-11):1–22.

26. Ottolini MC, Lundgren K, Mirkinson LJ, et al. Utility of complete blood count and blood culture screening to diagnose neonatal sepsis in the asymptomatic at risk newborn. Pediatr Infect Dis J 2003;22(5):430–4.

27. Wiswell TE, Baumgart S, Gannon CM, et al. No lumbar puncture in the evaluation for early neonatal sepsis: will meningitis be missed? Pediatrics 1995; 95(6):803–6.
28. Holt DE, Halket S, de Louvois J, et al. Neonatal meningitis in England and Wales: 10 years on. Arch Dis Child Fetal Neonatal Ed 2001;84(2):F85–9.
29. Visser VE, Hall RT. Lumbar puncture in the evaluation of suspected neonatal sepsis. J Pediatr 1980;96(6):1063–7.
30. Shattuck KE, Chonmaitree T. The changing spectrum of neonatal meningitis over a fifteen-year period. Clin Pediatr (Phila) 1992;31(3):130–6.
31. Garges HP, Moody MA, Cotten CM, et al. Neonatal meningitis: what is the correlation among cerebrospinal fluid cultures, blood cultures, and cerebrospinal fluid parameters? Pediatrics 2006;117(4):1094–100.
32. Hamada S, Vearncombe M, McGeer A, et al. Neonatal group B streptococcal disease: incidence, presentation, and mortality. J Matern Fetal Neonatal Med 2008;21(1):53–7.
33. Grimwood K, Darlow BA, Gosling IA, et al. Early-onset neonatal group B streptococcal infections in New Zealand 1998–1999. J Paediatr Child Health 2002;38(3): 272–7.
34. Neto MT. Group B streptococcal disease in Portuguese infants younger than 90 days. Arch Dis Child Fetal Neonatal Ed 2008;93(2):F90–3.
35. Kanegaye JT, Soliemanzadeh P, Bradley JS. Lumbar puncture in pediatric bacterial meningitis: defining the time interval for recovery of cerebrospinal fluid pathogens after parenteral antibiotic pretreatment. Pediatrics 2001;108(5):1169–74.
36. Heath PT, Nik Yusoff NK, Baker CJ. Neonatal meningitis. Arch Dis Child Fetal Neonatal Ed 2003;88(3):F173–8.
37. McIntyre P, Isaacs D. Lumbar puncture in suspected neonatal sepsis. J Paediatr Child Health 1995;31(1):1–2.
38. Fielkow S, Reuter S, Gotoff SP. Cerebrospinal fluid examination in symptom-free infants with risk factors for infection. J Pediatr 1991;119(6):971–3.
39. Schwersenski J, McIntyre L, Bauer CR. Lumbar puncture frequency and cerebrospinal fluid analysis in the neonate. Am J Dis Child 1991;145(1):54–8.
40. Eldadah M, Frenkel LD, Hiatt IM, et al. Evaluation of routine lumbar punctures in newborn infants with respiratory distress syndrome. Pediatr Infect Dis J 1987; 6(3):243–6.
41. Hendricks-Munoz KD, Shapiro DL. The role of the lumbar puncture in the admission sepsis evaluation of the premature infant. J Perinatol 1990;10(1):60–4.
42. Vollman JH, Smith WL, Ballard ET, et al. Early-onset group B streptococcal disease: clinical, roentgenographic, and pathologic features. J Pediatr 1976; 89(2):199–203.
43. Sherman MP, Goetzman BW, Ahlfors CE, et al. Tracheal aspiration and its clinical correlates in the diagnosis of congenital pneumonia. Pediatrics 1980;65(2): 258–63.
44. Sherman MP, Chance KH, Goetzman BW. Gram's stains of tracheal secretions predict neonatal bacteremia. Am J Dis Child 1984;138(9):848–50.
45. Booth GR, Al-Hosni M, Ali A, et al. The utility of tracheal aspirate cultures in the immediate neonatal period. J Perinatol 2009;29(7):493–6.
46. Harris H, Wirtschafter D, Cassady G. Endotracheal intubation and its relationship to bacterial colonization and systemic infection of newborn infants. Pediatrics 1976;58(6):816–23.
47. Visser VE, Hall RT. Urine culture in the evaluation of suspected neonatal sepsis. J Pediatr 1979;94(4):635–8.

48. DiGeronimo RJ. Lack of efficacy of the urine culture as part of the initial workup of suspected neonatal sepsis. Pediatr Infect Dis J 1992;11(9):764–6.
49. Tamim MM, Alesseh H, Aziz H. Analysis of the efficacy of urine culture as part of sepsis evaluation in the premature infant. Pediatr Infect Dis J 2003;22(9): 805–8.
50. Evans ME, Schaffner W, Federspiel CF, et al. Sensitivity, specificity, and predictive value of body surface cultures in a neonatal intensive care unit. JAMA 1988; 259(2):248–52.
51. Finelli L, Livengood JR, Saiman L. Surveillance of pharyngeal colonization: detection and control of serious bacterial illness in low birth weight infants. Pediatr Infect Dis J 1994;13(10):854–9.
52. Fulginiti VA, Ray CG. Body surface cultures in the newborn infant. An exercise in futility, wastefulness, and inappropriate practice. Am J Dis Child 1988;142(1): 19–20.
53. Manroe BL, Weinberg AG, Rosenfeld CR, et al. The neonatal blood count in health and disease. I. Reference values for neutrophilic cells. J Pediatr 1979; 95(1):89–98.
54. Spector SA, Ticknor W, Grossman M. Study of the usefulness of clinical and hematologic findings in the diagnosis of neonatal bacterial infections. Clin Pediatr (Phila) 1981;20(6):385–92.
55. Rodwell RL, Leslie AL, Tudehope DI. Early diagnosis of neonatal sepsis using a hematologic scoring system. J Pediatr 1988;112(5):761–7.
56. Zipursky A, Palko J, Milner R, et al. The hematology of bacterial infections in premature infants. Pediatrics 1976;57(6):839–53.
57. Greenberg DN, Yoder BA. Changes in the differential white blood cell count in screening for group B streptococcal sepsis. Pediatr Infect Dis J 1990;9:886–9.
58. Christensen RD, Rothstein G, Hill HR, et al. Fatal early-onset group B streptococcal sepsis with normal leukocyte counts. Pediatr Infect Dis 1985;4(3): 242–5.
59. Rozycki HJ, Stahl GE, Baumgart S. Impaired sensitivity of a single early leukocyte count in screening for neonatal sepsis. Pediatr Infect Dis J 1987;6(5):440–2.
60. Benitz WE, Gould JB, Druzin ML. Risk factors for early-onset group B streptococcal sepsis: estimation of odds ratios by critical literature review. Pediatrics 1999;103(6):e77.
61. Gabay C, Kushner I. Acute-phase proteins and other systemic responses to inflammation. N Engl J Med 1999;340(6):448–54.
62. Barrett BA, Hill PI. A micromethod for the erythrocyte sedimentation rate suitable for use on venus or capillary blood. J Clin Pathol 1980;33(11):1118–20.
63. Adler SM, Denton RL. The erythrocyte sedimentation rate in the newborn period. J Pediatr 1975;86(6):942–8.
64. Evans HE, Glass L, Mercado C. The micro-erythrocyte sedimentation rate in newborn infants. J Pediatr 1970;76(3):448–51.
65. Ibsen KK, Nielsen M, Prag J, et al. The value of the micromethod erythrocyte sedimentation rate in the diagnosis of infections in newborns. Scand J Infect Dis Suppl 1980;(Suppl 23):143–5.
66. Philip AG. Response of C-reactive protein in neonatal Group B streptococcal infection. Pediatr Infect Dis 1985;4(2):145–8.
67. Benitz WE, Han MY, Madan A, et al. Serial serum C-reactive protein levels in the diagnosis of neonatal infection. Pediatrics 1998;102(4):E41.
68. Fowlie PW, Schmidt B. Diagnostic tests for bacterial infection from birth to 90 days—a systematic review. Arch Dis Child Fetal Neonatal Ed 1998;78(2):F92–8.

69. Dollner H, Vatten L, Austgulen R. Early diagnostic markers for neonatal sepsis: comparing C-reactive protein, interleukin-6, soluble tumour necrosis factor receptors and soluble adhesion molecules. J Clin Epidemiol 2001;54(12):1251–7.
70. Garland SM, Bowman ED. Reappraisal of C-reactive protein as a screening tool for neonatal sepsis. Pathology 2003;35(3):240–3.
71. Pourcyrous M, Bada HS, Korones SB, et al. Significance of serial C-reactive protein responses in neonatal infection and other disorders. Pediatrics 1993;92(3):431–5.
72. Ehl S, Gering B, Bartmann P, et al. C-reactive protein is a useful marker for guiding duration of antibiotic therapy in suspected neonatal bacterial infection. Pediatrics 1997;99(2):216–21.
73. Philip AG, Mills PC. Use of C-reactive protein in minimizing antibiotic exposure: experience with infants initially admitted to a well-baby nursery. Pediatrics 2000;106(1):E4.
74. Dandona P, Nix D, Wilson MF, et al. Procalcitonin increase after endotoxin injection in normal subjects. J Clin Endocrinol Metab 1994;79(6):1605–8.
75. Assicot M, Gendrel D, Carsin H, et al. High serum procalcitonin concentrations in patients with sepsis and infection. Lancet 1993;341(8844):515–8.
76. Gendrel D, Assicot M, Raymond J, et al. Procalcitonin as a marker for the early diagnosis of neonatal infection. J Pediatr 1996;128(4):570–3.
77. Monneret G, Labaune JM, Isaac C, et al. Procalcitonin and C-reactive protein levels in neonatal infections. Acta Paediatr 1997;86(2):209–12.
78. Sachse C, Dressler F, Henkel E. Increased serum procalcitonin in newborn infants without infection. Clin Chem 1998;44(6 Pt 1):1343–4.
79. Chiesa C, Panero A, Rossi N, et al. Reliability of procalcitonin concentrations for the diagnosis of sepsis in critically ill neonates. Clin Infect Dis 1998;26(3):664–72.
80. Turner D, Hammerman C, Rudensky B, et al. Procalcitonin in preterm infants during the first few days of life: introducing an age related nomogram. Arch Dis Child Fetal Neonatal Ed 2006;91(4):F283–6.
81. Resch B, Gusenleitner W, Muller WD. Procalcitonin and interleukin-6 in the diagnosis of early-onset sepsis of the neonate. Acta Paediatr 2003;92(2):243–5.
82. Chiesa C, Pellegrini G, Panero A, et al. C-reactive protein, interleukin-6, and procalcitonin in the immediate postnatal period: influence of illness severity, risk status, antenatal and perinatal complications, and infection. Clin Chem 2003; 49(1):60–8.
83. Guibourdenche J, Bedu A, Petzold L, et al. Biochemical markers of neonatal sepsis: value of procalcitonin in the emergency setting. Ann Clin Biochem 2002;39(Pt 2):130–5.
84. Joram N, Boscher C, Denizot S, et al. Umbilical cord blood procalcitonin and C reactive protein concentrations as markers for early diagnosis of very early-onset neonatal infection. Arch Dis Child Fetal Neonatal Ed 2006;91:F65–6.
85. Kordek A, Halasa M, Podraza W. Early detection of an early-onset infection in the neonate based on measurements of procalcitonin and C-reactive protein concentrations in cord blood. Clin Chem Lab Med 2008;46(8):1143–8.
86. Lopez Sastre JB, Solis DP, Serradilla VR, Colomer BF, Cotallo GD. Evaluation of procalcitonin for diagnosis of neonatal sepsis of vertical transmission. BMC Pediatr 2007;7:9.
87. Lapillonne A, Basson E, Monneret G, et al. Lack of specificity of procalcitonin for sepsis diagnosis in premature infants. Lancet 1998;351(9110):1211–2.
88. Bonac B, Derganc M, Wraber B, et al. Interleukin-8 and procalcitonin in early diagnosis of early severe bacterial infection in critically ill neonates. Pflugers Arch 2000;440(Suppl 5):R72–4.

89. Berner R, Csorba J, Brandis M. Different cytokine expression in cord blood mono-nuclear cells after stimulation with neonatal sepsis or colonizing strains of *Streptococcus agalactiae*. Pediatr Res 2001;49(5):691–7.
90. Buck C, Bundschu J, Gallati H, et al. Interleukin-6: a sensitive parameter for the early diagnosis of neonatal bacterial infection. Pediatrics 1994;93(1):54–8.
91. Messer J, Eyer D, Donato L, et al. Evaluation of interleukin-6 and soluble receptors of tumor necrosis factor for early diagnosis of neonatal infection. J Pediatr 1996;129(4):574–80.
92. Berner R, Niemeyer CM, Leititis JU, et al. Plasma levels and gene expression of granulocyte colony-stimulating factor, tumor necrosis factor-alpha, interleukin (IL)-1beta, IL-6, IL-8, and soluble intercellular adhesion molecule-1 in neonatal early-onset sepsis. Pediatr Res 1998;44(4):469–77.
93. Franz AR, Kron M, Pohlandt F, et al. Comparison of procalcitonin with interleukin 8, C-reactive protein and differential white blood cell count for the early diagnosis of bacterial infections in newborn infants. Pediatr Infect Dis J 1999;18(8):666–71.
94. Franz AR, Steinbach G, Kron M, et al. Reduction of unnecessary antibiotic therapy in newborn infants using interleukin-8 and C-reactive protein as markers of bacterial infections. Pediatrics 1999;104(3 Pt 1):447–53.
95. Spear ML, Stefano JL, Fawcett P, et al. Soluble interleukin-2 receptor as a predictor of neonatal sepsis. J Pediatr 1995;126(6):982–5.
96. Dollner H, Vatten L, Linnebo I, et al. Inflammatory mediators in umbilical plasma from neonates who develop early-onset sepsis. Biol Neonate 2001;80(1):41–7.
97. Santana Reyes C, Garcia-Munoz F, Reyes D, et al. Role of cytokines (interleukin-1beta, 6, 8, tumour necrosis factor-alpha, and soluble receptor of interleukin-2) and C-reactive protein in the diagnosis of neonatal sepsis. Acta Paediatr 2003;92(2):221–7.
98. Franz AR, Steinbach G, Kron M, et al. Interleukin-8: a valuable tool to restrict antibiotic therapy in newborn infants. Acta Paediatr 2001;90(9):1025–32.
99. Bomela HN, Ballot DE, Cory BJ, et al. Use of C-reactive protein to guide duration of empiric antibiotic therapy in suspected early neonatal sepsis. Pediatr Infect Dis J 2000;19(6):531–5.

Pathophysiology and Treatment of Septic Shock in Neonates

James L. Wynn, MD[a],*, Hector R. Wong, MD[b]

KEYWORDS

• Neonate • Sepsis • Shock • Treatment • Pathophysiology

Sepsis or serious infection within the first 4 weeks of life kills more than 1 million newborns globally every year.[1] The attack rate for neonatal sepsis is variable (from <1% to >35% of live births) based on gestational age and time of onset (early [<72 hours after birth] or late [>72 hours after birth]).[2–5] Neonates with sepsis may present in or progress to septic shock, exemplified initially by cardiovascular dysfunction requiring fluid resuscitation or inotropic support.[6] If the progression of infection cannot be stopped, end-organ damage and death become much more likely. Although the true incidence is not known, a recent retrospective cohort study of 3800 neonates admitted to the neonatal intensive care unit (NICU) in a 6-year period reported septic shock in 1.3% with an associated mortality peaking at 71% for extremely low birth weight (ELBW) neonates less than 1000 g.[7] There are few published data regarding the pathophysiology of septic shock in neonates. Previous clinical investigations into neonatal sepsis and shock have largely focused on diagnostic markers. Descriptions of septic shock are predominantly case reports on very small numbers, mixed populations with severe respiratory distress syndrome (RDS) and sepsis, or pediatric studies that included neonates who were not evaluated as a separate group.[8–24]

DEFINITIONS OF THE SEPSIS CONTINUUM

In 2005, definitions for pediatric infection, systemic inflammatory response syndrome (SIRS), sepsis, severe sepsis, septic shock, and organ dysfunction were suggested that included term neonates (0–7 days), newborns (1 week to 1 month) and infants (1 month to 1 year) (**Tables 1** and **2**).[25] Working definitions for the sepsis continuum specific for preterm neonates are needed to provide a uniform basis for clinicians and researchers to study and diagnose severe sepsis in this particularly vulnerable

[a] Division of Neonatal-Perinatal Medicine, Department of Pediatrics, Duke University, 2424 Hock Plaza, Suite 504, DUMC Box 2739, Durham, NC 27710, USA
[b] Division of Critical Care Medicine, Cincinnati Children's Hospital Medical Center, 3333 Burnet Avenue, Cincinnati, OH 45229, USA
* Corresponding author.
E-mail address: james.wynn@duke.edu

Clin Perinatol 37 (2010) 439–479
doi:10.1016/j.clp.2010.04.002
0095-5108/10/$ – see front matter © 2010 Elsevier Inc. All rights reserved.

Table 1
Definition of systemic inflammatory response syndrome (SIRS), infection, sepsis, severe sepsis, and septic shock

Consensus Definitions	Suggested Modifications for Premature Infants
SIRS	**SIRS**
The presence of at least 2 of the following 4 criteria, 1 of which must be abnormal temperature or leukocyte count: • Core[a] temperature of >38.5°C or <36°C • Tachycardia, defined as a mean heart rate >2SD more than normal for age in the absence of external stimulus, chronic drugs, or painful stimuli; or otherwise unexplained persistent increase in a 0.5- to 4-h time period OR for children <1 y old: bradycardia, defined as a mean heart rate <10th percentile for age in the absence of external vagal stimulus, β-blocker drugs, or congenital heart disease; or otherwise unexplained persistent depression in a 0.5-h time period • Mean respiratory rate >2SD more than normal for age or mechanical ventilation for an acute process not related to underlying neuromuscular disease or the receipt of general anesthesia • Leukocyte count increased or decreased for age (not secondary to chemotherapy-induced leukopenia) or >10% immature neutrophils	The presence of at least 2 of the following 4 criteria, 1 of which must be abnormal temperature or leukocyte count: • Core temperature of >38.0°C[b] or <36°C • Tachycardia, defined as a mean heart rate >2SD more than normal for age in the absence of external stimulus, chronic drugs, or painful stimuli; or otherwise unexplained persistent increase in a 0.5- to 4-h time period OR bradycardia, defined as a mean heart rate <10th percentile for age in the absence of β-blocker drugs or congenital heart disease[c], or otherwise unexplained persistent bradycardia[d] • Mean respiratory rate >2SD more than normal for age or mechanical ventilation for an acute process not related to underlying neuromuscular disease or the receipt of general anesthesia • Leukocyte count increased or decreased for age or >20% immature to total neutrophil ratio[e] or C-reactive protein >10 mg/dL
Infection	No change suggested
A suspected or proven (by positive culture, tissue stain, or polymerase chain reaction test) infection caused by any pathogen OR a clinical syndrome associated with a high probability of infection. Evidence of infection includes positive findings on clinical examination, imaging, or laboratory tests (eg, white blood cells in a normally sterile body fluid, perforated viscus, chest radiograph consistent with pneumonia, petechial or purpuric rash, or purpura fulminans)	

Sepsis	No change suggested
SIRS in the presence of or as a result of suspected or proven infection	
Severe sepsis	No change suggested
Sepsis plus 1 of the following: cardiovascular organ dysfunction OR ARDS OR 2 or more other organ dysfunctions	
Septic shock	No change suggested
Sepsis and cardiovascular organ dysfunction	

a Core temperature must be measured by rectal, bladder, oral, or central catheter probe.
b Neonatal fever is considered greater than 38°C.
c External vagal stimulus use is uncommon in preterm infants.
d Infrequent self-resolving bradycardic episodes can be common in premature neonates in the absence of sepsis.
e More commonly accepted ratio is greater than 20% immature to total ratio and chemotherapy-induced leukopenia is uncommon in premature infants.

From Goldstein B, Giroir B, Randolph A. International pediatric sepsis consensus conference: definitions for sepsis and organ dysfunction in pediatrics. Pediatr Crit Care Med 2005;6(1):2–8; with permission.

Table 2
Definitions of organ dysfunction

Consensus Definitions of Organ Dysfunction[25]	Suggested Modifications for Premature Infants
Cardiovascular dysfunction Despite administration of isotonic intravenous fluid bolus >40 mL/kg in 1 h • Decrease in BP (hypotension) <5th percentile for age or systolic BP >2SD less than normal for age OR • Need for vasoactive drug to maintain BP in normal range (dopamine >5 μg/kg/min or dobutamine, epinephrine, or norepinephrine at any dose) OR • Two of the following: Unexplained metabolic acidosis: base deficit >5.0 mEq/L Increased arterial lactate >2 times upper limit of normal Oliguria: urine output <0.5 mL/kg/h Prolonged capillary refill >5 s Core to peripheral temperature gap >3°C	Cardiovascular dysfunction Despite administration of isotonic intravenous fluid bolus >40 mL/kg in 1 h (>10 ml/kg in infants <32 weeks)[d] • Decrease in BP (hypotension) <5th percentile for age or systolic BP >2SD less than normal for age or MAP <30 mm Hg with poor capillary refill time (>4 s)[e] OR • Need for vasoactive drug to maintain BP in normal range (dopamine >5 μg/kg/min or dobutamine, or epinephrine at any dose)[f] OR • Two of the following: Unexplained metabolic acidosis: base deficit >5.0 mEq/L Increased arterial lactate >2 times upper limit of normal Oliguria: urine output <0.5 mL/kg/h Prolonged capillary refill >4 s[g] Simultaneous measurement of core and peripheral temperature not common in premature neonates
Pulmonary[a] • PaO_2/FiO_2 <300 in absence of cyanotic heart disease or preexisting lung disease OR • $PaCO_2$ >65 torr or 20 mm Hg more than baseline $PaCO_2$ OR • Proven need[b] for >50% FiO_2 to maintain saturation >92% OR • Need for nonelective invasive or noninvasive mechanical ventilation[c]	Pulmonary • Excessive oxygen should be limited to avoid complications including retinopathy of prematurity • $PaCO_2$ >65 torr or 20 mm Hg more than baseline $PaCO_2$ OR • Proven need for >50% FiO_2 to maintain saturation >92% (88% for <32 weeks) OR • Need for nonelective invasive or noninvasive mechanical ventilation

Neurologic
- Glasgow Coma Score >11

OR

- Acute change in mental status with a decrease in Glasgow Coma Score >3 points from abnormal baseline

Hematologic
- Platelet count <80,000/mm^3 or a decline of 50% in platelet count from highest value recorded in the past 3 days (for chronic hematology/oncology patients)

OR

- International normalized ratio >2

Renal
- Serum creatinine >2 times upper limit of normal for age or 2-fold increase in baseline creatinine

Hepatic
- Total bilirubin >4 mg/dL (not applicable for newborn)

OR

- ALT 2 times upper limit of normal for age

Neurologic
- Acute change in mental status[h]

Hematologic
- Platelet count <80,000/mm^3 or a decline of 50% in platelet count from highest value recorded in the past 3 days[i]

OR

- International normalized ratio >2

Renal
- Serum creatinine >2 times upper limit of normal for age or 2-fold increase in baseline creatinine

Hepatic
- ALT 2 times upper limit of normal for age[j] or 50% increase over patient's baseline[k]

Abbreviations: ALT, alanine transaminase; BP, blood pressure.

[a] ARDS must include a Pao_2/Fio_2 ratio ≤200 mm Hg, bilateral infiltrates, acute onset, and no evidence of left heart failure. Acute lung injury is defined identically except the Pao_2/Fio_2 ratio must be ≥300 mm Hg.

[b] Proven need assumes oxygen requirement was tested by decreasing flow with subsequent increase in flow if required.

[c] In postoperative patients, this requirement can be met if the patient has developed an acute inflammatory or infectious process in the lungs that prevents them from being extubated.

[d] Rapid large volume expansion can be associated with intraventricular hemorrhage.

[e] 30 mm Hg suggested as minimum MAP.

[f] Norepinephrine not commonly used in premature neonates.

[g] Greater than 4 s may reflect a low systemic blood flow.[264]

[h] Glasgow Coma Score not applicable to term or preterm neonates.

[i] Neonates not frequently chronic hematology-oncology patients.

[j] Indirect hyperbilirubinemia is common in newborns.

[k] Transaminases are commonly increased in preterm neonates on long-term intravenous hyperalimentation.

From Goldstein B, Giroir B, Randolph A. International pediatric sepsis consensus conference: definitions for sepsis and organ dysfunction in pediatrics. Pediatr Crit Care Med 2005;6(1):2–8; with permission.

population. The authors have proposed modifications to the consensus definitions to incorporate preterm infants that are also presented in **Tables 1** and **2**.

Why have definitions of sepsis and septic shock not been established for preterm neonates? These patients present diagnostic challenges that are clouded by immaturity of organ systems and transitional physiology. For example, normal blood pressure values for gestational and postnatal age have not been established, particularly in the very low birth weight neonate (VLBW, <1500 g), largely because blood pressure alone cannot identify abnormal cardiac output, organ perfusion, and oxygen delivery.[26] In the absence of normative values, it is nearly impossible to establish parameters that are associated with poor outcome. Perhaps the most obvious limitation is the differences in monitoring capabilities between the preterm neonate and older, physically larger patients. For example, pulmonary artery catheterization may be used in children or adults to monitor the course of septic shock, but this is not feasible in small neonates. For these reasons, the hemodynamic response to septic shock and optimum clinical interventions in preterm neonates are not well understood.

RISK FACTORS FOR DEVELOPMENT OF NEONATAL SEPTIC SHOCK

Risk factors for a neonate developing sepsis have been well described. Although risk factors for septic shock overlap those for sepsis, specific antenatal and postnatal risks for the development of neonatal septic shock have not been described in detail.

Maternal factors contributing to the risk of neonatal sepsis are shown in **Box 1** and include prematurity, low birth weight, rectovaginal colonization with group B streptococcus (GBS), prolonged rupture of membranes, maternal intrapartum fever, and chorioamnionitis.[2,3,27–33]

Factors in the postnatal period associated with an increased risk of sepsis or septic shock include male gender, birth weight less than 1000 g, hypogammaglobulinemia, intravenous alimentation, central venous catheters, use of steroids or drugs that decrease gastric acid acidity, and prolonged duration of mechanical ventilation. The development of severe necrotizing enterocolitis (NEC) is also associated with severe sepsis, shock, multi-organ system failure, and death.[34,35] Genetic evaluations in children and adults have identified several polymorphisms in cytokines and their receptors as well as other host defense proteins that may either increase or decrease risk for sepsis or poor outcome from sepsis.[36–41] However, gene polymorphism studies in neonates have not yielded consistent results because of relatively small sample sizes and a general lack of formal prospective validation studies.[42–56]

MICROBIOLOGY OF SEPSIS AND SEPTIC SHOCK IN NEONATES

Several pathogens have been associated with sepsis in the neonatal period. The predominant agents are bacterial, but viruses including herpes simplex and enteroviruses have been associated with fulminant neonatal sepsis with high mortality.[57–59] In 1 study, gram-negative infection accounted for 38% of cases of septic shock and 62.5% of sepsis mortality.[7] These results are similar to those from a previous study that showed gram-negative infection was associated with 69% of cases of fulminant septic shock (death within 48 hours).[60] Gram-positive causes of sepsis are dominated by GBS and coagulase-negative staphylococcus (CoNS).[3,61] Although lethality and shock from GBS have been well described, mortality associated with CoNS is extremely low[3,4] and septic shock is rare.[60] Fungi (primarily *Candida albicans*) may also lead to fulminant neonatal sepsis and predominantly affect ELBW infants.[3,62,63] Studies of neonatal sepsis are confounded by the limitations of sensitivity of the current diagnostic gold standard blood culture. Sample volume constraints in

---

Box 1
Risk factors for the development of neonatal sepsis and septic shock

Maternal factors

- Maternal age (>30 years)
- Lack of prenatal care
- High gravidity
- Premature or prolonged (>6 hours) rupture of membrane (PROM)
- Meconium-stained amniotic fluid
- Foul-smelling amniotic fluid
- Premature labor
- Chorioamnionitis
- GBS rectovaginal colonization
- Urinary tract infection
- Intrapartum fever
- Multiple courses of prenatal steroids or tocolytic agents
- Prolonged duration of internal monitoring

Delivery room

- Prematurity <37 weeks
- Low birth weight ≤2500 g
- 5-minute Apgar score <5
- Resuscitation in delivery room
- Male gender

Neonatal

- Vascular catheterization
- Mechanical ventilation (continuous positive airway pressure or endotracheal tube)
- Lack of enteral feeding
- Gastrointestinal tract pathology
- Medications (H2 blockers, proton pump inhibitors; postnatal steroids, cephalosporins)
- Neutropenia
- Decreased baseline serum IgG concentrations
- Hyperalimentation
- Prolonged hospital stay
- Delay in time to regain birth weight

---

newborns may undermine the identification of organisms causing shock, particularly in preterm infants.[64] For this reason, many studies combine the entities culture-proven sepsis and clinical sepsis (cultures negative but strong clinical suspicion leading to long-term antibiotic treatment). Improved techniques such as molecular diagnostics, see the article by Benitz elsewhere in this issue for further exploration of this topic, may help to delineate which patients with clinical sepsis truly have sepsis versus other causes of clinical deterioration.

PATHOPHYSIOLOGY OF SEPSIS AND SHOCK: MOLECULAR AND CELLULAR EVENTS
Molecular Signaling: Pattern Recognition Receptors, Pathogen-associated Molecular Patterns, and Damage- or Danger-associated Molecular Patterns

Pathogen recognition by local immune sentinel cells is the first step toward the development of an immune response once local barrier function has been compromised (**Fig. 1**). Recognition is initiated via the activation of pattern recognition receptors (PRRs)[65] including Toll-like receptors (TLRs). There are 10 known TLRs in humans, and each receptor has a specific molecular activation trigger.[66,67] TLRs, present on and within multiple cell types, recognize extracellular and intracellular pathogens by their signature microbial products known as pathogen-associated molecular patterns (PAMPs). Lipopolysaccharide (LPS, endotoxin) on gram-negative bacteria is the prototypic PAMP and a key mediator of systemic inflammation, septic shock, and multi-organ failure and death.[68] LPS signals primarily through TLR4 in conjunction with the cell surface adaptor proteins CD14 and MD-2.[65] Gram-positive bacterial PAMPS such as lipoteichoic acid signal primarily through TLR2, whereas viral PAMPS such as double-stranded RNA signal through TLR3. Microorganisms often stimulate more than 1 TLR simultaneously allowing for initiation of a pathogen-specific host response.[67,69] Ligand-receptor binding results in downstream production of cytokines and chemokines as well as activation of other antimicrobial effector mechanisms.[66]

Intracellular non-TLR PRRs include NOD-like receptors (NLRs) and RIG-like receptors (RLRs). Nucleotide-binding oligomerization domain (an NLR) detects peptidoglycan of gram-positive bacteria in the cytosol, and retinoic acid–inducible protein I (RIG-I) detects viral double-stranded RNA and induces type I interferon production.[67] Once engaged by pathogens, these PRRs initiate an immune response including the production of proinflammatory cytokines via mitogen-activated protein kinase (MAPK) and the transcription factor nuclear factor κB (NF-κB). To date, RLR and NLR function have not been examined in neonates with sepsis.

Because TLRs play an essential role in recognition and response to pathogens, alterations in their expression, structure, signaling pathways, and function can have consequences to host defense. Polymorphisms or mutations in TLRs are associated with increased risk for infection in adults[70–73] and in children[74–76] but are less well characterized in neonates. Upregulation of TLR2 and TLR4 mRNA in leukocytes of neonates occurs during gram-positive and gram-negative infection, respectively, across gestational ages.[77] Dysregulation or overexpression of TLR4 is involved in the development of necrotizing enterocolitis in experimental animal models,[78] demonstrating the importance of TLRs in the initial immune response to pathogens and their role in neonatal sepsis and septic shock. Mutations have been identified in NLRs that are involved in the pathogenesis of neonatal-onset multisystem inflammatory disease (cryopyrin).[79] Investigation for mutations in specific domains of NLRs has been performed to identify causes of abnormal inflammatory signaling leading to NEC, but no associations have been identified.[80] RLR mutations have been identified but are of unknown clinical significance.[81] The role that intracellular PRR play is of particular interest with respect to defense against *Listeria monocytogenes*, a pathogen particularly virulent in neonates, which can be recognized by NLRs.[82]

Mutations or decreased expression of costimulatory molecules necessary for TLR activation are also associated with an increased risk for infection. For example, the lipopolysaccharide (LPS, endotoxin) coreceptor CD14 and LPS-binding protein (LBP, which binds intravascular LPS and facilitates its attachment to CD14) are both increased during neonatal sepsis.[83–85] Genetic variations in these proteins have been associated with increased risk for sepsis in adults.[47,49,50] Gene

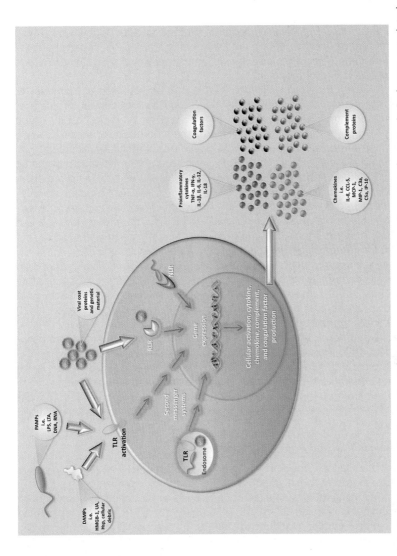

Fig. 1. Activation of sentinel immune cells. Sentinel cells (e.g. monocyte, macrophage) sense pathogens via Pathogen-associated molecular patterns (PAMPs) or damage-/danger-associated molecular patterns (DAMPs) binding to PRRs. PRRs include Toll-like receptors (TLRs), Rig-1-like receptors (RLRs), and NOD-like receptors (NLRs). PAMPs include lipopolysaccharide (LPS), lipotechoic acid (LTA), DNA, and RNA. DAMPs can also be sensed through TLRs and include uric acid (UA), heat shock proteins (Hsp), and HMGB-1. Signaling occurs through a series of second messengers and results in transcription and translation of cytokines and chemokines that amplify the immune response.

polymorphisms in myeloid differentiation-2 (MD-2), a small protein involved in LPS signaling through TLR4, increase the risk for organ dysfunction and sepsis in adults[86] but the significance in neonates is unknown. Polymorphisms in select cytokines (IL-6 and IL-10) or their receptors (IL-4ra[53]), and constituents of their signaling pathways, may be associated with increased risk of infection,[42,43,46,51] although there is not complete agreement on these findings.[44,52,54] Polymorphisms in post-TLR activation intracellular signaling molecules including myeloid differentiation factor 88 (MyD88),[87] IL-1 receptor–associated kinase 4 (IRAK-4),[88] and NF-κB essential modulator (NEMO)[89] are associated with invasive bacterial infection in older populations. These genetic factors predisposing to sepsis are likely just the tip of the iceberg because evaluation of intracellular second messenger inflammatory signaling systems is a relatively new and active area of research.

In addition to being activated by PAMPs, TLRs can be activated by damage- or danger-associated molecular patterns (DAMPs), such as intracellular proteins or mediators released by dying or damaged cells (see **Fig. 1**). High-mobility group box-1 (HMGB-1), an important DAMP, is involved in the progression of sepsis to septic shock.[68,90] HMGB-1 is produced by macrophages or endothelial cells stimulated with LPS or TNF-α and signals through TLR2, TLR4, and receptor for advanced glycation end products (RAGE).[91] Important actions of HMGB-1 include cytokine production, activation of coagulation, and neutrophil recruitment.[90,92] HMGB-1 mediates disruption of epithelial junctions within the gut via the induction of reactive nitrogen intermediates (RNI) leading to increased bacterial translocation.[93] The role of HMGB-1 and RAGE signaling in septic shock in human neonates has not been well studied, but has been linked to the pathophysiology of NEC in a preclinical model.[94]

Other DAMPs including heat shock proteins (Hsps) and uric acid may also contribute to the pathophysiology of septic shock. Hsps activate proinflammatory signaling through TLRs, regulate neutrophil function, are immune adjuvants, and are increased in adults and children with sepsis.[95] Increased Hsp60 and Hsp70 measured within 24 hours of pediatric intensive care unit admission was associated with pediatric septic shock and there was a strong trend toward a significant association with death.[96,97] Hsp production in septic neonates has not been evaluated. Uric acid can increase cytokine production, polymorphonuclear leukocyte (PMN) recruitment, and dendritic cell stimulation,[98] and may also serve as an antioxidant.[99] Uric acid is reduced in the serum of septic neonates compared with control neonates.[100] The importance of DAMPs in neonatal sepsis and shock has yet to be determined.

Cytokines, Chemokines, and Adhesion Molecules

Following PRR stimulation, production of cytokines and chemokines results in amplification of the innate response directed at the invading organisms (see **Fig. 1**). Increases of proinflammatory cytokines during sepsis and septic shock have been identified including interleukin (IL)-1β, IL-6, IL-8, IL-12, IL-18, interferon gamma (IFN-γ), and tumor necrosis factor-alpha (TNF-α).[101] Compared with septic adults, septic neonates produce less IL-1β, TNF-α, IFN-γ, and IL-12.[102–107] The decreased cytokine production is due in part to decreased production of important intracellular mediators of TLR signaling including myeloid differentiation factor 88 (MyD88), interferon regulatory factor 5 (IRF5), and p38, which exhibit gestational age-specific diminution.[108] In a recent comprehensive study (>140 analytes) of serum from neonates evaluated for late-onset sepsis, IL-18 emerged as a predictive biomarker to differentiate infected from noninfected neonates,[109] similar to data from adults with sepsis.[110] IL-18 reduces PMN apoptosis,[111] potentiates IFN-γ production,[112] and induces production of TNF-α, IL-1β, and IL-8.[113] IL-18 primes PMNs for degranulation with production of reactive oxygen intermediates (ROI) on subsequent stimulation.[114] Dysregulation of many of these functions linked to IL-18 are seen in sepsis and septic shock.

Proinflammatory cytokine production leads to activation of endothelial cells including increased expression of cell adhesion molecules (CAMs) that facilitate leukocyte recruitment and diapedesis (**Fig. 2**). Upregulation of CAMs (soluble ICAM, VCAM, L-, P-, and E-selectins, and CD11b/CD18) during sepsis facilitates rolling and extravascular migration of leukocytes.[115–118] Decreased neonatal PMN and monocyte L-selectin and MAC-1 expression impair accumulation at sites of inflammation.[119,120] Chemokine gradients produced by endothelial cells and local macrophages are necessary in addition to CAM interactions for effective and specific leukocyte attraction and accumulation. Without adequate leukocyte recruitment, there is increased risk for propagation from a local to a systemic infection. Although poor cellular chemotaxis in the neonate has been observed, it is not likely a result of reduced serum concentrations of chemokines.[121] Suboptimal chemotaxis may be related to other mechanisms such as poor complement receptor upregulation following stimulation,[122] deficiencies in another downstream signaling process,[123] or inhibition by bacterial products.[124]

A wide variety of chemokines are increased during sepsis including IP-10, CCL5 (RANTES), MCP-1, MIP-1, and IL-8.[125] Other chemoattractive molecules are also increased in sepsis including complement proteins C3a and C5a, host defense proteins or peptides such as cathelicidins and defensins, and components of invading bacteria themselves.[101,109] The role of chemoattractive substances in the pathogenesis of severe sepsis is highlighted by recent studies showing IL-8 can be used as a stratifying factor for survival in children[126] and C5a is implicated in sepsis-associated organ dysfunction in adults.[68] Studies of chemokines in neonates with sepsis have shown that IP-10 is a sensitive early marker of infection,[125] and decreased levels of CCL5 help predict development of disseminated intravascular coagulation (DIC).[127]

Antiinflammatory Response

If inflammatory homeostasis is not restored, the consequences can include SIRS, which is associated with multi-organ failure and death (**Fig. 3**). The careful interplay between anti- and proinflammatory stimuli serves to govern the immune response to allow local pathogen containment but prevent systemic activation leading to excessive inflammatory damage through SIRS.[128] Near simultaneous increases in antiinflammatory cytokine production occur during infection, with TGF-β, IL-4, IL-10, IL-11, and IL-13 countering the actions of proinflammatory cytokines (see **Fig. 2**).[101,129,130] These mediators blunt the activation of phagocytic cells, block fever, modify coagulation factor expression, and decrease production of ROI/RNI, NO, and other vasoactive mediators.[131–135] In addition to the antiinflammatory cytokines, specific soluble cytokines and receptor antagonists produced during sepsis modulate proinflammatory mediator action, including TNFR2 (which regulates the concentration of TNF-α), sIL-6R, sIL2, and IL-1ra. Increases in these inhibitors have been documented in neonatal sepsis with resolution following effective treatment.[130,136,137] The role of these regulatory cytokine inhibitors in the immune response to neonatal sepsis and septic shock has been incompletely characterized. Soluble RAGE (sRAGE) competes with cell-bound RAGE for the binding of HMGB-1 and other RAGE ligands,[138] reduces the intensity of the inflammatory response, and is increased in adults during sepsis.[139] In addition, administration of exogenous sRAGE improved survival and reduced inflammation in infected adult rodents.[140]

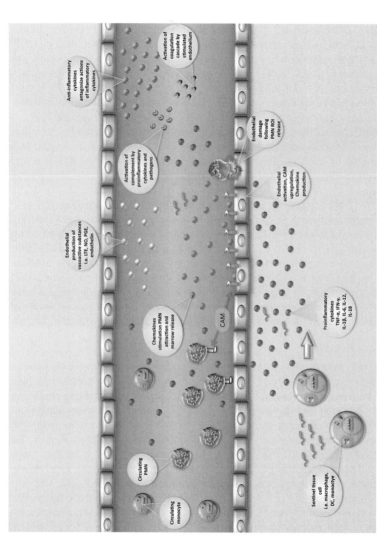

Fig. 2. Cellular recruitment and endothelial activation following pathogen detection. Pathogen-stimulated tissue/blood monocytes, dendritic cells (DC), and macrophages release proinflammatory cytokines that activate the surrounding endothelium. Endothelial activation results in upregulation of CAM, production of chemokines and vasoactive substances, activation of complement, and development of a procoagulant state. Recruitment of PMNs occurs along the chemokine gradient surrounding the area of inflammation. Antiinflammatory cytokines counter the actions of proinflammatory cytokines to prevent excessive cellular activation and recruitment that can result in tissue damage and systemic inflammation. Endothelium can be damaged when PMNs release ROI. LTE, leukotriene; NO, nitric oxide; PMN, neutrophil.

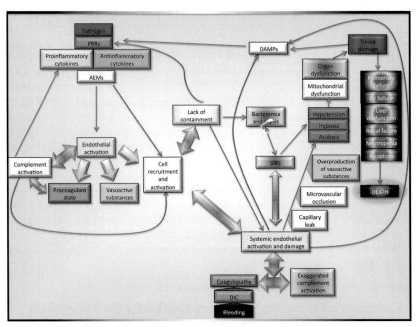

Fig. 3. Pathophysiology of neonatal sepsis and septic shock. AEM, antimicrobial effector mechanisms; CV, cardiovascular; DAMP, danger-/damage-associated molecular patterns; DIC, disseminated intravascular coagulation; PRR, pattern recognition receptors; SIRS, systemic inflammatory response syndrome.

Role of Complement in Host Defense and Sepsis Pathophysiology

Complement is an extraordinarily important component of early innate immunity that facilitates killing of bacteria through opsonization and direct microbicidal activity. Complement components also possess chemotactic or anaphylactic activity that increases leukocyte aggregation and local vascular permeability at the site of invasion. In addition, complement components reciprocally activate several other important processes such as coagulation, proinflammatory cytokine production, and leukocyte activation (see **Fig. 3**).[68] Dysregulation of complement activation may participate in the untoward effects seen in neonates with severe sepsis or septic shock. Neonates, particularly the very premature, exhibit decreased basal levels of complement proteins and function for the alternative and classic pathways.[141,142] In addition, complement-mediated opsonization is poor in premature neonates and limited in term neonates.[143,144]

Complement-mediated activation of leukocytes during sepsis occurs via up-regulated cell surface receptors (CR1 [CD35], CR3 [Mac-1, CD11b/CD18]).[145,146] For example, stimulation of CR1 and C5aR, the receptors for C3b and C5a, respectively, facilitate opsonization (CR1-C3b), redistribution of blood flow, increased inflammation, platelet aggregation, and release of ROI (C5a-C5aR).[147,148] In addition, activation of the multifunctional CR3 facilitates leukocyte adhesion, phagocytosis, migration and activation, as well as recognition of a broad range of microbial products.[149] Upregulation of CR3 on neutrophils following stimulation is blunted in neonates compared with adults and is believed to play a significant role in diminished chemotaxis and transmigration.[122] Similar to the effects of TLR stimulation, C5a-mediated local leukocyte activation also results in increased cytokine production with subsequent upregulation of adhesion molecules on vascular endothelium allowing for increased cell recruitment to the site of infection.[150] Deficiencies in C5aR found in term neonates compared with adults may limit the ability to respond to C5a and therefore increase the likelihood of infection.[151] The expression of C5aR on neutrophils of preterm infants has not been quantified.

Complement regulatory proteins modify the effects of complement and prevent potential damage caused by over activation. In particular, CD59 blocks formation of C9 polymerization and target lysis, CD55 destabilizes CR1 and C3 and C5 convertases, and CD35 (CR1) accelerates the deactivation of C3b.[152] The role of these regulators in the neonatal response to sepsis and septic shock is presently unknown. Dysregulation of complement activation can lead to a vicious activation cycle that results in excessive cellular stimulation, cytokine production, endothelial cell activation, and local tissue damage. Dysregulation likely contributes to the development of SIRS and shock (see **Fig. 3**).[153]

Data in adults link increased C5a levels with multiple facets of sepsis-associated pathology such as the development of DIC via increased tissue factor expression, cardiomyopathy, increased proinflammatory cytokine levels and the development of SIRS, adrenal insufficiency, and neutrophil dysfunction.[68] Whether or not C5a or other complement proteins play a role in the development of these phenomena in septic neonates remains to be determined.

Other Host Defense Proteins, Acute Phase Reactants, and Opsonins

In addition to the initial inflammatory response and complement activation following pathogen recognition, the presence of microbes result in increases in other innate proteins that possess valuable immune function.[154] These components serve to reduce bacterial load and include collectins (eg, surfactant proteins A and D), lactoferrin, cathelicidins, bacteriocidal permeability increasing protein (BPI), and phospholipase A_2.[155] Acute phase reactant proteins such as CRP (opsonin), haptoglobin and lactoferrin (reduce available iron/antimicrobial peptide-lactoferricin), serum amyloid A (cellular recruitment), procalcitonin (unknown function), and others increase during sepsis and provide useful ancillary immune functions.[101] Neutrophils from term neonates are deficient in BPI, potentially contributing to the increased risk for infection.[156] Polymorphisms in BPI increase the risk for gram-negative sepsis in children,[157] although the effect of these polymorphisms in neonates is unknown. Sepsis results in an increase in other serum components with opsoninic function including fibronectin and natural antibodies (predominantly IgM) produced by circulating B1 lymphocytes.[158–160] Despite these increases, neonatal plasma has significantly impaired opsonizing activity compared with adults that increases the likelihood of progression to systemic infection.[161]

Role of Dysregulated Coagulation in Severe Sepsis

Development of a procoagulant state in the microvasculature surrounding a focal site of infection is a natural host defense mechanism, trapping invading pathogens and preventing further dissemination (see **Fig. 2**). However, like the inflammatory response, if the procoagulant response to infection escalates unchecked, it can lead to DIC resulting in severe tissue and organ damage (see **Fig. 3**).[162] Neonates with early increased ratios of serum inflammatory to antiinflammatory cytokines during sepsis have an increased risk of developing DIC.[127] This finding is consistent with the increased serum levels of IL-6[59] and high frequency of DIC seen with disseminated HSV infection.[163]

Initiation of coagulation cascades during infection may begin with activated neutrophils, monocytes, or endothelium, which express increased tissue factor apoprotein.[164,165]Activation of tissue factor leads to increased clotting proteins including thrombin-antithrombin complex (TAT), plasminogen activator inhibitor

(PAI), and plasmin-α2-antiplasmin complex.[166] There is also a shift toward inactivation of protein S and depletion of anticoagulant proteins including antithrombin III (ATIII) and protein C.[167,168] A small study reported that low protein C levels in preterm neonates with sepsis predicted death.[169] In DIC, platelets are consumed in micro-thrombi creating a state of thrombocytopenia; a common finding in infected neonates.[170] The longest duration and lowest initial and nadir platelet levels have been noted during neonatal gram-negative and fungal infections,[171] and this thrombo-cytopenia may or may not be associated with DIC. Decreased platelet function in preterm neonates with sepsis further increases the risk for bleeding.[172] In ELBW infants, platelets are hyporeactive for the first few days after birth, complicating the ability of the immune system to contain a microbiological threat and increasing the risk for hemorrhage.[173]

Role of the Neutrophil in Septic Shock

The most important means of early innate cellular defense against bacterial invasion in neonates is the neutrophil or PMN. Neonatal PMNs exhibit quantitative and qualitative deficits compared with adult cells.[174,175] A complete discussion of these deficits is presented elsewhere in this issue. Three aspects of PMN function with particular rele-vance to neonatal severe sepsis and septic shock deserve brief mention: neutropenia, decreased deformability, and delayed apoptosis.

Rapid depletion of neonatal marrow PMN reserves during infection[176] can lead to neutropenia with consequent impaired antimicrobial defenses and significantly increased risk for death.[177] Neutropenia is particularly common in gram-negative sepsis in neonates.[178] Release of immature neutrophil forms (bands), which have even greater dysfunction than mature neonatal neutrophils,[179] can further predispose to adverse outcomes. PMN respiratory burst activity is also suppressed during sepsis and may contribute to poor microbicidal activity.[180–182]

PMNs of neonates have reduced deformability compared with PMNs of adults, which, combined with the low blood pressure/flow state associated with septic shock, increases the risk of microvascular occlusion.[174,183] Irreversible aggregation of newborn PMNs in the vascular space leads to decreased diapedesis, rapid depletion of bone marrow reserves, vascular crowding,[183] and increased likelihood of compro-mised tissue perfusion[184] leading to organ dysfunction.

Neutrophils, although essential for combating pathogens, can also cause significant tissue damage and thus play a role in progression from sepsis to multi-organ system dysfunction. Reactive oxygen and nitrogen intermediates and proteolytic enzymes produced by PMNs can be released extracellularly, via activation of membrane-asso-ciated NADPH oxidase. Extracellular release of these reactive intermediates and enzymes can lead to destruction of nonphagocytized bacteria but can also cause local tissue destruction.[185] Increased levels of neutrophil elastase as well as the neutrophil activators urokinase plasminogen activator, and urokinase plasminogen activator receptor have been described in infected neonates.[109] Compared with adult PMNs, neonatal PMNs exhibit delayed apoptosis[186,187] as well as sustained capacity for acti-vation (CD11b upregulation) and cytotoxic function (ROI production) that contributes to tissue damage.[188] Neutrophil-mediated damage may include endothelial and lung injury (including surfactant inactivation[189]) (see **Fig. 2**) in addition to other organ dysfunction (see **Fig. 3**).

Other Innate Cellular Contributions to Sepsis

Many other cells besides neutrophils are involved in the development of an immune response to infection, but the role that these cells play in the development of neonatal septic shock is incompletely characterized. Monocytes, macrophages, and dendritic cells amplify cellular recruitment through production of inflammatory mediators, phagocytosis and killing of pathogens, and antigen presentation to cells of the adaptive immune system. Important substances produced by stimulated monocytes that may contribute to septic shock include complement components, cytokines (pro- and antiinflammatory), coagulation factors, and extracellular matrix proteins (see **Fig. 1**).[190] The role of NK cells in neonatal bacterial sepsis is incompletely defined. Despite activation,[191] NK cytotoxicity is deficient in sepsis and recurrent infections.[192,193] Circulating NK cells are decreased with neonatal shock.[194] Further studies are necessary to more clearly define the role of NK cells in neonatal sepsis and shock.

Mast cells play a role in the response to pathogen invasion via production of histamines (which promote vasodilation and upregulation of P-selectin) and cytokines (TNF-α, IL-1α/β), and by promoting neutrophil recruitment, direct bacterial phagocytosis, and antigen presentation.[195] The production of histamine by mast cells likely contributes to the vasodilation associated with septic shock. Like eosinophils and PMNs, mast cells of adults are also capable of bacterial killing via generation of extracellular traps, like the neutrophil extracellular traps described previously.[196] This means of immune protection has not been investigated in neonates. Mast cells may also alter adaptive immune function by patterning the T_H2 immunosuppressive phenotype seen in the neonate and therefore contribute to the increased risk of infection. Immature dendritic cells exposed to histamine and LPS during maturation exhibit altered T-cell polarizing activity with predominance of T_H2 phenotype via increased production of IL-10 and decreased production of IL-12.[197] Furthermore, compared with mast cells of adults[198] stimulated mast cells from neonates secrete significantly more histamine, which may contribute to vasodilation and the development of shock.[199]

Role of the Endothelium and Vasoactive Mediators in Septic Shock

Vascular endothelium has not historically been considered part of the innate cellular defenses, but recent studies have shown the importance of these sentinel cells in the early recognition and containment of microbial invasion. The endothelium can be a 2-edged sword, however, as excessive activation can lead to vascular dilation and leak, which are a driving forces behind the severe consequences of septic shock (see **Fig. 3**).[124,200]

Expression of TLRs allows endothelium to become activated in the presence of microbial components, leading to production of cytokines, chemokines, and adhesion molecules that attract circulating leukocytes and facilitate adherence.[124] Vasoactive substances released from activated leukocytes, platelets, and endothelial cells are shown in **Fig. 2** and include platelet-activating factor (PAF), thromboxane (TBX), leukotrienes (LTE), nitric oxide (NO), histamine, bradykinin, and prostaglandins (PGE).[201,202] Activated PMNs produce phospholipase A2 (PLA$_2$), which is increased in the serum of neonates with sepsis[203] and leads to generation of vasoactive substances including PGE and LTE. Thromboxane produced by activated platelets and endothelin produced by activated endothelium[204] are potent vasoconstrictors that participate in the development of pulmonary hypertension (PPHN).[205–208] Systemic overproduction of cytokines and vasoactive substances is associated with circulatory alterations and organ failure seen in severe sepsis and septic shock (see **Fig. 3**).[25,209–212] For example, the balance of NO and endothelin-1 (ET-1) may be disrupted with endothelial damage, favoring the constrictive effects of ET-1 leading to ischemia and injury. This may explain in part why NO inhibitors increased mortality in adults with septic shock.[213]

Activated or damaged endothelium establishes a prothrombotic environment that can result in local microvascular occlusion[165] or progress to DIC.[214] Endothelial cell apoptosis, detachment from the lamina, and alterations in vascular tone combine to promote capillary leak of proteins and fluid leading to hypovolemia and shock.[215] The role of endothelial activation during sepsis and septic shock in neonates, particularly in the premature infant, has not been thoroughly investigated. Adhesion molecules E- and P-selectin, expressed and secreted by activated endothelium, are increased in the serum of septic neonates[109] and likely reflect significant endothelial activation. Toxins from GBS have been shown to damage pulmonary endothelium[216] and likely participate in pulmonary complications associated with GBS pneumonia such as acute respiratory distress syndrome (ARDS) and PPHN.[217] Using transgenic mice, it was recently shown that pulmonary endothelial cells sense blood-borne bacteria and their products,[124] whereas alveolar macrophages patrol the airspaces for pathogens.[218] These data help to explain in part the occurrence of ARDS and PPHN associated with severe sepsis in the absence of a primary pulmonary infectious focus.

PATHOPHYSIOLOGY OF SEPTIC SHOCK: CARDIOVASCULAR AND OTHER ORGAN EFFECTS
Cardiovascular Effects

The hemodynamic response to sepsis has been less well characterized in premature and term neonates compared with children and adults, and the hemodynamic abnormalities are significantly more variable.[219] Factors contributing to developmental differences in hemodynamic responses include altered structure and function of cardiomyocytes, limited ability to increase stroke volume and contractility, and contributions of the transition from fetal to neonatal circulation.[220] A patent ductus arteriosus (PDA) and the presence of PPHN are significant modifying factors for the management of hypotension and hypoxia. In preterm infants with a PDA, aggressive volume administration to treat low blood pressure may lead to fluid overload, pulmonary edema, or heart failure. In the term infant with severe PPHN, on the other hand, aggressive volume and vasoactive medication administration to maintain a normal blood pressure may be beneficial by reducing right to left shunting and improving oxygenation. Although cardiomyopathy and heart failure may occasionally complicate sepsis in neonates, underlying coronary artery disease or other chronic cardiac conditions often present in septic adults do not complicate septic shock in the neonate.

In adults, septic shock is most commonly characterized by reduced systemic vascular resistance and increased cardiac index.[221] In children, a nonhyperdynamic state with reduced cardiac output and increased systemic vascular resistance is most common.[219,222–224] The hemodynamic presentation in neonates is much more variable[219] and complicated by an unclear association between a normal blood pressure and adequate systemic blood flow.[225,226] Abnormal peripheral vasoregulation with or with out myocardial dysfunction are the primary mechanisms for the hypotension accompanying septic shock in the neonate.[227] Neonates with sepsis may present with tachycardia, poor perfusion and normal blood pressure (high systemic vascular resistance) or with hypotension and either adequate perfusion (warm shock, vasodilation) or inadequate perfusion (cold shock, vasoconstriction). These distinctions may be important for directing appropriate therapy to restore tissue perfusion, as discussed later.

Multi-organ Dysfunction Syndrome

Septic shock that leads to multi-organ failure or MODS carries a dismal prognosis. Poor cardiac output and microcirculatory failure, sometimes combined with formation of microthrombi and DIC, can lead to compromised perfusion to the kidney,[228,229] liver,[230] gut,[231] and central nervous system[232] (see **Fig. 3**).[59,210,233,234] Recent studies suggest that the mechanism of organ failure in sepsis may relate to decreased oxygen use associated with mitochondrial dysfunction rather than or in addition to poor oxygen delivery to tissues.[235,236] Many other organ systems can be compromised in the setting of septic shock. Pulmonary complications include ARDS,[237] secondary surfactant deficiency,[238] pulmonary edema, pneumonia,[23] and PPHN.[220,237] Endocrine abnormalities may include adrenal insufficiency associated with refractory hypotension[239] and altered thyroid function.[240] Lymphocyte loss secondary to thymic involution and splenocyte apoptosis may also be present and may lead to a state of immune compromise following the acute phase of sepsis.[241–246] The importance of this finding has been shown in infected adults,[247–249] but the effect in neonates in whom adaptive immune function is immature is unknown. In a transgenic mouse model, neonatal animals lacking an adaptive immune system showed no difference in survival with polymicrobial sepsis compared with wild-type controls. This is in stark contrast to findings in adult mice.[250] Hematologic findings during severe sepsis may include thrombocytopenia,[170] neutropenia,[177] and coagulation abnormalities including DIC.[162] Sepsis can lead to metabolic and nutritional consequences. Increased energy expenditure and oxygen consumption[251] and decreased mitochondrial oxidative function precipitated by hypoxia and the presence of damaging free radicals may lead to impaired growth and energy failure.[252,253] The importance of providing optimum nutritional support in septic adults and children is increasingly recognized and should also be considered in septic neonates.

TREATMENT OF SEPSIS AND SEPTIC SHOCK
Initial Resuscitation

Treatment guidelines for the management of severe sepsis and septic shock have been established for adults,[254] children, and term neonates,[255] but no such consensus guidelines exist for preterm neonates. The authors have attempted to incorporate the special circumstances related to premature physiology into the framework of treatment guidelines for term infants (**Fig. 4**). Development, testing, and acceptance of consensus guidelines for classification and management of preterm neonates with sepsis and septic shock are urgently needed to more systematically assess, diagnose, and treat these conditions.

As with all emergencies in neonatology, management of septic shock begins with airway, breathing, and circulation. Septic neonates often present with apnea or severe respiratory distress and may require intubation.[3,4] Following establishment of a secure airway and maintenance of lung volume for adequate gas exchange, administration of antibiotics and continuing assessment for cardiovascular dysfunction is critical. Shortly after birth, an umbilical vein catheter can be used for resuscitation but beyond this time, other peripheral or central venous access is essential for volume resuscitation, antibiotic administration, and pressor therapy. Timely therapy, including rapid restoration of adequate tissue perfusion, has been shown to improve outcomes in adults and children with sepsis, and should be the goal in neonates.

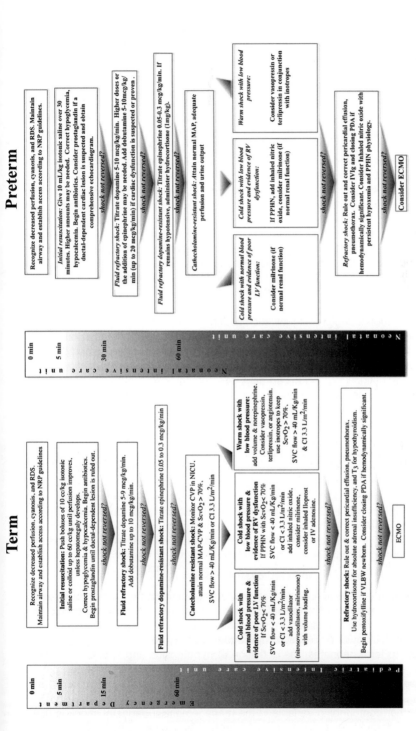

Fig. 4. American College of Critical Care Medicine consensus guidelines for treatment of shock in term infants and suggested modifications for preterm infants. CI, cardiac index; CVP, central venous pressure; MAP, mean arterial pressure; NRP, Neonatal Resuscitation Program; PDA, patent ductus arteriosus; PPHN, persistent pulmonary hypertension of the newborn; RDS, respiratory distress syndrome; S_{CVO_2}, central venous oxygen saturation; SVC, superior vena cava; VLBW, very low birth weight. (*From* Brierley J, Carcillo JA, Choong K, et al. Clinical practice parameters for hemodynamic support of pediatric and neonatal septic shock: 2007 update from the American College of Critical Care Medicine. Crit Care Med 2009 Feb;37:666–88; with permission.)

Therapeutic Endpoints

In the absence of widely available or well-tested methods for quantifying hemodynamic compromise in septic shock in neonates, clinicians generally rely on vital signs and physical examination for decisions about therapy. Although mean arterial pressure (MAP) may not reflect systemic blood flow, monitoring blood pressure and other measures such as capillary refill time and urine output provide indirect information on the adequacy of organ blood flow. Suggestions for cardiovascular therapeutic end points in term neonates include a capillary refill time of less than 2 seconds, normal pulses without differential between peripheral and central pulses, warm extremities, urine output greater than 1 ml/kg/h, low serum lactate, and mixed venous saturation of more than 70%.[256] Therapeutic end points in premature neonates have not been established but the goals for term infants seem reasonable. ELBW infants present the greatest challenge for determination of therapeutic end points in septic shock. Assessment of MAP, urine output, and capillary refill may not be particularly useful determinates of systemic blood flow in ELBW infants, particularly in the first 72 hours of life.[257] In addition, the contribution of fetal hemoglobin may complicate accurate determination of central venous oxygen saturation (Scvo$_2$) in neonates. Scvo$_2$ obtained using hemoglobin A calibration is 4% to 7% higher compared with Scvo$_2$ that accounts for fetal hemoglobin[258] implying that perhaps the goal Scvo$_2$ should be different in neonates than in older patients for optimum tissue oxygen delivery.

In the future, monitoring techniques such as functional echocardiography (FE) and near-infrared spectroscopy (NIRS) may provide physiologic data to optimize management of septic shock. FE provides a bedside means to assess cardiac output, peripheral vascular resistance, and organ blood flow in response to volume, colloid, and vasoactive medications.[259,260] FE can also be used to assess superior vena cava (SVC) flow, which has been suggested as a surrogate marker for cerebral blood flow[261] and should be maintained at 40 ml/kg/min or higher.[262] Prolonged decreases in SVC flow are associated with impaired neurodevelopmental outcome in very preterm neonates.[263] In the absence of FE to monitor SVC flow, a capillary refill time of more than 4 seconds combined with a serum lactate concentration of more than 4 mmol/L had a specificity of 97% for identifying VLBW infants with a low SVC flow state on the first day of life.[264] NIRS can be used to monitor end-organ perfusion noninvasively[265] and is used often in neonates with congenital heart disease.[266] A combination of FE and NIRS, in conjunction with traditional measures (MAP, Spo$_2$, capillary refill, urine output) as well as intermittent laboratory evaluations of tissue perfusion such as pH, mixed venous saturation, lactate, and base deficit would be ideal for monitoring severity of septic shock and response to therapy.

Management of Hypotension and Cardiovascular Support

An algorithm for time-sensitive, goal-directed stepwise management of hemodynamic support for the term newborn with septic shock has been established and should be followed.[255] Preterm neonates require specific caveats to this algorithm because of their unique physiology and risk for complications (see **Fig. 4**).

In contrast to term neonates, the definition of hypotension and shock in preterm neonates is less clear, particularly in the immediate newborn period.[26] Blood pressure may be a poor indicator of systemic blood flow in preterm neonates,[225] yet objective measures of adequacy of tissue perfusion and oxygenation delivery are lacking. Another confounding variable in the management of neonatal shock is that inotrope use (dopamine, dobutamine) in hypotensive preterm neonates has not been shown to significantly improve short- or long-term outcomes.[227,267,268] These considerations notwithstanding, and in absence of evidence of harm, some neonatologists advocate treating hypotension in preterm neonates to achieve a MAP of greater than or equal to 30 mm Hg. This goal MAP is based in part on a small study showing improved cerebral blood flow autoregulation above this threshold.[269] However, a gestational age-based cutoff for normal blood pressure (goal MAP > GA) is used at many tertiary centers, especially in the first 3 days after birth. Clearly, more studies are required to determine whether targeting a specific blood pressure improves outcomes in preterm infants.

Once a decision is made to treat hypotension with or without shock in a neonate, the recommended initial step is a fluid bolus (crystalloid). Although there is less data in neonates to support this intervention, it remains the accepted clinical practice to treat and monitor closely for signs of intravascular volume depletion.[227] In term infants or older preterm infants, aggressive volume expansion (20–40 mL/kg) should be considered. In contrast to outcomes with early aggressive fluid resuscitation in older populations,[270] there is insufficient evidence to support early volume expansion in very preterm neonates,[271] and there is a significant risk of intracranial hemorrhage associated with rapid volume expansion in the first few days after birth.[272] In hypotensive preterm neonates, it is recommended that a single bolus of saline (10–20 ml/kg over 30–60 minutes) be given and if further intervention is necessary to begin vasoactive medications.[268] In cases of obvious acute volume loss in preterm infants, more volume may be needed.

Dopamine is generally the first-line vasoactive drug, with a starting dose of 5 to 10 μg/kg/min[227] and dose escalation as needed. For neonates with shock, which is unresolved with volume resuscitation and dopamine, several possibilities exist for additional therapy, including glucocorticoids (see later discussion), other catecholamines, and inotropes/vasodilators. Epinephrine or norepinephrine infusions for refractory shock in neonates have been studied to a limited extent. Neonates with vasodilatory shock may have a positive response to the α-adrenergic vasoconstrictive effect of these agents. A recent report in term neonates showed the addition of noradrenaline to existing therapy (after fluid loading and dopamine or dobutamine infusion) resulted in increased blood pressure and decreased tissue lactate.[18] In another study, low-dose epinephrine was found to be as effective as low-/moderate-dose dopamine for increasing blood pressure, cerebral blood volume, and cerebral oxygen delivery in VLBW infants.[273] Patients with depressed myocardial function may benefit from infusion of dobutamine for inotropy and vasodilation. In a study of 42 preterm neonates with low systemic blood flow (as determined by low SVC flow[262]) in the first 24 hours after birth, dobutamine treatment improved and maintained systemic blood flow better than dopamine.[274,275] As a caution, dobutamine, particularly in high doses, can increase myocardial oxygen demand caused by β1 adrenergic stimulation. Dobutamine also has chronotropic actions and severe tachycardia may lead to decreased cardiac output that may be corrected by decreasing the dose. Milrinone, a phosphodiesterase inhibitor and inodilator, has not been studied in neonatal septic shock but has been used in pediatric patients with septic shock.[276,277] In a study of patients aged 9 months to 15 years with volume-resuscitated catecholamine-resistant nonhyperdynamic septic shock, milrinone increased cardiac index, stroke volume, and oxygen delivery, and decreased systemic vascular resistance without increasing heart rate or blood pressure.[276] Another alternative agent for treating septic shock is the vasoconstrictor arginine-vasopressin (AVP) or its longer half-life analogue terlipressin.[278] In a report of 6 ELBW infants, AVP improved MAP and urine output in patients with septic shock but not in those with nonseptic shock.[279]

Hydrocortisone Treatment in Neonatal Septic Shock

Induced by proinflammatory cytokines, endogenous cortisol attenuates the intensity of the systemic inflammatory response associated with severe sepsis and septic shock.[280] Studies in adults have shown that high-dose glucocorticoid therapy does not affect sepsis mortality although low-dose therapy may be beneficial.[254] In 1 randomized clinical trial, low-dose cortisol treatment in conjunction with standard of care measures was associated with a reduction in mortality in adults with septic shock and adrenal insufficiency.[281] In another study in adults, cortisol treatment sped the reversal of septic shock but had no effect on mortality.[282]

Cortisol production in the neonate is significantly increased early in septic shock.[283] However, very preterm neonates can have relative adrenal insufficiency that may contribute to hemodynamic instability and hypotension. In many clinical practices, hydrocortisone is the third-line agent in treatment of neonatal shock after volume resuscitation and dopamine.[227,268,284] In addition to its cytokine-suppressing effects, hydrocortisone has been shown to increase the sensitivity of the cardiovascular system to endogenous or exogenous catecholamines, resulting in improvements in myocardial contractility, stroke volume, effective circulating blood volume, systemic vascular resistance, and urine output. Hydrocortisone has not been evaluated in prospective randomized clinical trials for the treatment of septic shock in the neonate, but it has been shown to increase blood pressure, decrease heart rate, and decrease vasoactive medication requirements in preterm and term neonates.[284,285] If hydrocortisone treatment is considered, obtaining a pretreatment serum cortisol level is prudent to differentiate contributing causes of hypotension. The reader is referred to a recent review on the diagnosis and treatment of adrenal insufficiency in the premature neonate.[286]

Pulmonary Support

Increased inspired oxygen may be necessary in the setting of neonatal septic shock to maximize tissue oxygen delivery. Decreased pulmonary function (RDS) and/or respiratory failure (apnea) in conjunction with increased tissue demand (increased respiratory and metabolic activity associated with acidosis) contribute to tissue hypoxia. Mechanical ventilation can improve gas exchange through maintenance of lung volume and decreased work of breathing. Administration of exogenous surfactant to neonates with severe pneumonia has been shown to improve oxygenation and gas exchange and reduce the need for extracorporeal membrane oxygenation (ECMO).[238] In extremely sick neonates, consideration should be given to maintaining a normal or near-normal pH and oxygen saturations in the 90s rather than allowing permissive hypercapnia and lower saturations, which is standard practice in healthy preterm neonates. Normalizing pH and arterial oxygen content may improve cardiac contractility and improve tissue oxygen content, thus decreasing the risk of multi-organ dysfunction and the risk of pulmonary hypertension. Infants with sepsis and PPHN may require inhaled nitric oxide (iNO) in addition to optimized ventilation strategies such as high frequency oscillatory ventilation.[287] If oxygenation or tissue perfusion remain severely compromised despite optimal medical management, ECMO should be considered in neonates greater than 2 kg without contraindications such as the presence of or high risk for acute hemorrhage.[288,289]

OTHER SUPPORTIVE CARE OF NEONATES WITH SEPTIC SHOCK

Avoidance of hypothermia and hypoglycemia is important in neonates with septic shock. With the exception of patients with acute perinatal hypoxic ischemic encephalopathy,[290] normothermia should be maintained on a radiant warmer. Use of a 10% glucose solution delivering 4 to 6 mg/kg/min of glucose combined with frequent monitoring to ensure normoglycemia is recommended. Correction of a significant coagulopathy and anemia (hemoglobin $\leq$ 10 g/dL) through the transfusion of fresh frozen plasma or packed red blood cells may also serve to improve blood pressure[291] and oxygen delivery. The importance of providing adequate protein and calories to the infant with sepsis and septic shock cannot be overstated. Increased energy demands promote catabolism if adequate nutrition is not provided. Premature neonates have decreased muscles mass and energy reserves as well as higher baseline nutritional requirements compared with term neonates.[292] Increase in serum triglyceride levels during sepsis[293] and increased serum oxygen-derived free radicals associated with infusions of lipid have prompted some clinicians to withhold or decrease intralipid infusions. A recent study showed concurrent administration of intralipids in neonates with infection is not associated with hypertriglyceridemia in the absence of liver dysfunction or fetal growth restriction.[294] It is suggested that intralipid infusions during sepsis or septic shock in neonates be accompanied by careful monitoring of serum triglycerides to avoid hypertriglyceridemia. Maintenance of a carbohydrate to lipid ratio of ~3:1 increases fat use and decreases production of oxygen-derived free radicals to levels seen with fat exclusion.[295] Protein intakes of 2 to 3 g/kg/d are generally not associated with azotemia, hyperammonemia, or metabolic acidosis[296] in the setting of sepsis, but monitoring of blood urea nitrogen is recommended. Monitoring liver and renal function is important for assessing the effectiveness of therapies to improve tissue perfusion and for making decisions about dosing medications that require modification for elimination.

ALTERNATIVE IMMUNOLOGIC AND PHARMACOTHERAPIES FOR NEONATAL SEPSIS/SHOCK

There have been many attempts directed at improving outcomes of sepsis and septic shock in neonates via immunomodulation. A complete review of adjunct immunologic therapies in neonatal sepsis, see the article by Tarnow-Mordi and colleagues elsewhere in this issue for further exploration of this topic.

OUTCOMES WITH SEPSIS AND SEPTIC SHOCK

The outcome of septic shock in the neonate is dismal. One study reported death or severe sequelae in 52% of infants, with only 28% of infants less than 1000 g alive and free of disability at 18 months of age.[7] Variables predictive of mortality include cardiac dysfunction manifested as refractory shock, acute renal failure, neutropenia, increased prothrombin time, excessive bleeding, metabolic acidosis, and hypothermia.[231,297]

Neurodevelopmental outcomes following neonatal sepsis, without stratification for shock, have been studied in some detail and demonstrate significant risk for impairment, particularly in the most premature neonates.[298] VLBW infants with sepsis, compared with those without, have been reported to have significantly increased mortality (21% vs 9%), longer hospital stay (98 vs 58 days), and a higher risk of chronic lung disease.[31] ELBW infants are at especially high risk for sepsis-associated adverse neurodevelopmental outcomes, including deafness, cerebral palsy, lower mental and psychomotor development scores, and vision impairment.[299,300] In a study of preterm infants, white matter abnormality on magnetic resonance imaging at term corrected age-predicted neurodevelopmental impairment in those with sepsis compared with those without.[301] Surgical NEC, which is often accompanied by SIRS or shock, has been associated with significant growth delay and adverse neurodevelopmental outcomes at 18 to 22 months.[302] A study of ELBW infants with systemic candidiasis found that 73% died or developed a neurodevelopmental impairment[63] including retinopathy.[303] These data show that the toll of neonatal sepsis and septic shock reaches far beyond the acute complications of organ dysfunction and mortality.

FUTURE CONSIDERATIONS

Neonatal sepsis requires translational and clinical research. Definitions for the sepsis continuum and treatment algorithms specific for preterm infants should be developed to improve the quality of clinical trials and facilitate meta-analyses of prophylactic and therapeutic interventions. Systems biology and genomic and proteomic studies have yielded important data on septic shock in older populations[304–312] and the use of these modern techniques in the study of neonatal inflammation and response to pathogen challenge has begun.[109,138,313] With further research, real-time sampling using only microliters of blood will allow rapid identification of highest-risk patients, pathogen-specific responses, and sepsis-staging biomarkers.[314] Immaturities of immune function and physiology in the neonate necessitate developmental stage-specific evaluations of sepsis pathophysiology and treatment. Exploration of adjuvant treatments including LPS-binding proteins (rBPI,[315] sCD14, or anti-CD14[316]), antiinflammatory therapies (pentoxifylline,[317] nicotinic stimulation,[318] statins[319]), synthetic host defense peptides (rhSP-D,[320] lactoferrin[321,322]), combination therapies[323] (ie, IVIg and colony-stimulating factor), and innate immune priming using TLR agonists[250] may yield improved outcomes. Advances in these areas are urgently needed and are likely to substantially improve long-term outcomes.

SUMMARY

Neonatal septic shock is a devastating condition associated with high morbidity and mortality, Definitions for the sepsis continuum and treatment algorithms specific for premature neonates are needed to improve studies of septic shock and assess benefit from clinical interventions. Unique features of the immature immune system and pathophysiologic responses to sepsis, particularly those of extremely preterm infants, necessitate that clinical trials consider them as a separate group. Keen clinical suspicion and knowledge of risk factors will help to identify those neonates at greatest risk for development of septic shock. Genomic and proteomic approaches, particularly those that use very small sample volumes, will increase our understanding of the pathophysiology and direct the development of novel agents for prevention and treatment of severe sepsis and shock in the neonate. Although at present antimicrobial therapy and supportive care remain the foundation of treatment, in the future immunomodulatory agents are likely to improve outcomes for this vulnerable population.

ACKNOWLEDGMENTS

The authors thank Associate Professor C. Michael Cotten, MD, MHS for his review of this manuscript.

REFERENCES

1. Lawn JE, Cousens S, Zupan J. 4 million neonatal deaths: when? Where? Why? Lancet 2005;365(9462):891–900.
2. Stoll BJ, Hansen N, Fanaroff AA, et al. Changes in pathogens causing early-onset sepsis in very-low-birth-weight infants. N Engl J Med 2002;347(4):240–7.

3. Stoll BJ, Hansen N, Fanaroff AA, et al. Late-onset sepsis in very low birth weight neonates: the experience of the NICHD Neonatal Research Network. Pediatrics 2002;110(2 Pt 1):285–91.
4. Stoll BJ, Hansen NI, Higgins RD, et al. Very low birth weight preterm infants with early onset neonatal sepsis: the predominance of Gram-negative infections continues in the National Institute of Child Health and Human Development Neonatal Research Network, 2002–2003. Pediatr Infect Dis J 2005; 24(7):635–9.
5. Haque KN, Khan MA, Kerry S, et al. Pattern of culture-proven neonatal sepsis in a district general hospital in the United Kingdom. Infect Control Hosp Epidemiol 2004;25(9):759–64.
6. Haque KN. Defining common infections in children and neonates. J Hosp Infect 2007;65(Suppl 2):110–4.
7. Kermorvant-Duchemin E, Laborie S, Rabilloud M, et al. Outcome and prognostic factors in neonates with septic shock. Pediatr Crit Care Med 2008;9(2):186–91.
8. Furman WL, Menke JA, Barson WJ, et al. Continuous naloxone infusion in two neonates with septic shock. J Pediatr 1984;105(4):649–51.
9. Togari H, Mikawa M, Iwanaga T, et al. Endotoxin clearance by exchange blood transfusion in septic shock neonates. Acta Paediatr Scand 1983;72(1):87–91.
10. Fenton LJ, Strunk RC. Complement activation and group B streptococcal infection in the newborn: similarities to endotoxin shock. Pediatrics 1977;60(6):901–7.
11. Tollner U, Pohlandt F. Septicemia in the newborn due to Gram-negative bacilli. Risk factors, clinical symptoms, and hematologic changes. Eur J Pediatr 1976;123(4):243–54.
12. Frommhold D, Birle A, Linderkamp O, et al. Drotrecogin alpha (activated) in neonatal septic shock. Scand J Infect Dis 2005;37(4):306–8.
13. Miyairi I, Berlingieri D, Protic J, et al. Neonatal invasive group A streptococcal disease: case report and review of the literature. Pediatr Infect Dis J 2004; 23(2):161–5.
14. Ahmed K, Sein PP, Shahnawaz M, et al. *Pasteurella gallinarum* neonatal meningitis. Clin Microbiol Infect 2002;8(1):55–7.
15. Roll C, Schmid EN, Menken U, et al. Fatal *Salmonella enteritidis* sepsis acquired prenatally in a premature infant. Obstet Gynecol 1996;88(4 Pt 2):692–3.
16. Wolfler A, Silvani P, Musicco M, et al. Incidence of and mortality due to sepsis, severe sepsis and septic shock in Italian Pediatric Intensive Care Units: a prospective national survey. Intensive Care Med 2008;34(9):1690–7.
17. Rodriguez-Nunez A, Lopez-Herce J, Gil-Anton J, et al. Rescue treatment with terlipressin in children with refractory septic shock: a clinical study. Crit Care 2006;10(1):R20.
18. Tourneux P, Rakza T, Abazine A, et al. Noradrenaline for management of septic shock refractory to fluid loading and dopamine or dobutamine in full-term newborn infants. Acta Paediatr 2008;97(2):177–80.
19. Filippi L, Poggi C, Serafini L, et al. Terlipressin as rescue treatment of refractory shock in a neonate. Acta Paediatr 2008;97(4):500–2.
20. Meyer S, Loffler G, Polcher T, et al. Vasopressin in catecholamine-resistant septic and cardiogenic shock in very-low-birthweight infants. Acta Paediatr 2006;95(10):1309–12.
21. McAdams RM, Garza-Cox S, Yoder BA. Early-onset neonatal pneumococcal sepsis syndrome. Pediatr Crit Care Med 2005;6(5):595–7.
22. Matok I, Leibovitch L, Vardi A, et al. Terlipressin as rescue therapy for intractable hypotension during neonatal septic shock. Pediatr Crit Care Med 2004;5(2):116–8.

23. Aikio O, Vuopala K, Pokela ML, et al. Diminished inducible nitric oxide synthase expression in fulminant early-onset neonatal pneumonia. Pediatrics 2000; 105(5):1013–9.
24. Duke TD, Butt W, South M. Predictors of mortality and multiple organ failure in children with sepsis. Intensive Care Med 1997;23(6):684–92.
25. Goldstein B, Giroir B, Randolph A. International pediatric sepsis consensus conference: definitions for sepsis and organ dysfunction in pediatrics. Pediatr Crit Care Med 2005;6(1):2–8.
26. Cayabyab R, McLean CW, Seri I. Definition of hypotension and assessment of hemodynamics in the preterm neonate. J Perinatol 2009;29(Suppl 2):S58–62.
27. Shah GS, Budhathoki S, Das BK, et al. Risk factors in early neonatal sepsis. Kathmandu Univ Med J (KUMJ) 2006;4(2):187–91.
28. Salem SY, Sheiner E, Zmora E, et al. Risk factors for early neonatal sepsis. Arch Gynecol Obstet 2006;274(4):198–202.
29. Yancey MK, Duff P, Kubilis P, et al. Risk factors for neonatal sepsis. Obstet Gynecol 1996;87(2):188–94.
30. Benitz WE, Gould JB, Druzin ML. Risk factors for early-onset group B streptococcal sepsis: estimation of odds ratios by critical literature review. Pediatrics 1999;103(6):e77.
31. Fanaroff AA, Korones SB, Wright LL, et al. Incidence, presenting features, risk factors and significance of late onset septicemia in very low birth weight infants. The National Institute of Child Health and Human Development Neonatal Research Network. Pediatr Infect Dis J 1998;17(7):593–8.
32. Schuchat A, Zywicki SS, Dinsmoor MJ, et al. Risk factors and opportunities for prevention of early-onset neonatal sepsis: a multicenter case-control study. Pediatrics 2000;105(1 Pt 1):21–6.
33. Escobar GJ, Li DK, Armstrong MA, et al. Neonatal sepsis workups in infants >/=2000 grams at birth: a population-based study. Pediatrics 2000;106(2 Pt 1):256–63.
34. Sharma R, Tepas JJ 3rd, Hudak ML, et al. Neonatal gut barrier and multiple organ failure: role of endotoxin and proinflammatory cytokines in sepsis and necrotizing enterocolitis. J Pediatr Surg 2007;42(3):454–61.
35. Sonntag J, Wagner MH, Waldschmidt J, et al. Multisystem organ failure and capillary leak syndrome in severe necrotizing enterocolitis of very low birth weight infants. J Pediatr Surg 1998;33(3):481–4.
36. Dahmer MK, Randolph A, Vitali S, et al. Genetic polymorphisms in sepsis. Pediatr Crit Care Med 2005;6(Suppl 3):S61–73.
37. Cogulu O, Onay H, Uzunkaya D, et al. Role of angiotensin-converting enzyme gene polymorphisms in children with sepsis and septic shock. Pediatr Int 2008;50(4):477–80.
38. Lyons EJ, Amos W, Berkley JA, et al. Homozygosity and risk of childhood death due to invasive bacterial disease. BMC Med Genet 2009;10:55.
39. Liangos O, Jaber BL. Multiple organ dysfunction syndrome in children with sepsis: role of genetic factors. Semin Nephrol 2008;28(5):499–509.
40. Kumpf O, Schumann RR. Genetic influence on bloodstream infections and sepsis. Int J Antimicrob Agents 2008;32(Suppl 1):S44–50.
41. Sutherland AM, Walley KR. Bench-to-bedside review: association of genetic variation with sepsis. Crit Care 2009;13(2):210.
42. Ahrens P, Kattner E, Kohler B, et al. Mutations of genes involved in the innate immune system as predictors of sepsis in very low birth weight infants. Pediatr Res 2004;55(4):652–6.

43. Baier RJ, Loggins J, Yanamandra K. IL-10, IL-6 and CD14 polymorphisms and sepsis outcome in ventilated very low birth weight infants. BMC Med 2006;4:10.

44. Chauhan M, McGuire W. Interleukin-6 (-174C) polymorphism and the risk of sepsis in very low birth weight infants: meta-analysis. Arch Dis Child Fetal Neonatal Ed 2008;93(6):F427–9.

45. Dzwonek AB, Neth OW, Thiebaut R, et al. The role of mannose-binding lectin in susceptibility to infection in preterm neonates. Pediatr Res 2008;63(6):680–5.

46. Gopel W, Hartel C, Ahrens P, et al. Interleukin-6-174-genotype, sepsis and cerebral injury in very low birth weight infants. Genes Immun 2006;7(1):65–8.

47. Hartel C, Rupp J, Hoegemann A, et al. 159C>T CD14 genotype–functional effects on innate immune responses in term neonates. Hum Immunol 2008; 69(6):338–43.

48. Hartel C, Schultz C, Herting E, et al. Genetic association studies in VLBW infants exemplifying susceptibility to sepsis–recent findings and implications for future research. Acta Paediatr 2007;96(2):158–65.

49. Hubacek JA, Stuber F, Frohlich D, et al. Gene variants of the bactericidal/permeability increasing protein and lipopolysaccharide binding protein in sepsis patients: gender-specific genetic predisposition to sepsis. Crit Care Med 2001;29(3):557–61.

50. Mollen KP, Gribar SC, Anand RJ, et al. Increased expression and internalization of the endotoxin coreceptor CD14 in enterocytes occur as an early event in the development of experimental necrotizing enterocolitis. J Pediatr Surg 2008; 43(6):1175–81.

51. Reiman M, Kujari H, Ekholm E, et al. Interleukin-6 polymorphism is associated with chorioamnionitis and neonatal infections in preterm infants. J Pediatr 2008;153(1):19–24.

52. Schueller AC, Heep A, Kattner E, et al. Prevalence of two tumor necrosis factor gene polymorphisms in premature infants with early onset sepsis. Biol Neonate 2006;90(4):229–32.

53. Treszl A, Heninger E, Kalman A, et al. Lower prevalence of IL-4 receptor alpha-chain gene G variant in very-low-birth-weight infants with necrotizing enterocolitis. J Pediatr Surg 2003;38(9):1374–8.

54. Treszl A, Kocsis I, Szathmari M, et al. Genetic variants of TNF-[FC12]a, IL-1beta, IL-4 receptor [FC12]a-chain, IL-6 and IL-10 genes are not risk factors for sepsis in low-birth-weight infants. Biol Neonate 2003;83(4):241–5.

55. Treszl A, Kocsis I, Szathmari M, et al. Genetic variants of the tumour necrosis factor-alpha promoter gene do not influence the development of necrotizing enterocolitis. Acta Paediatr 2001;90(10):1182–5.

56. Treszl A, Tulassay T, Vasarhelyi B. Genetic basis for necrotizing enterocolitis–risk factors and their relations to genetic polymorphisms. Front Biosci 2006;11: 570–80.

57. Verboon-Maciolek MA, Krediet TG, Gerards LJ, et al. Clinical and epidemiologic characteristics of viral infections in a neonatal intensive care unit during a 12-year period. Pediatr Infect Dis J 2005;24(10):901–4.

58. Verboon-Maciolek MA, Krediet TG, Gerards LJ, et al. Severe neonatal parechovirus infection and similarity with enterovirus infection. Pediatr Infect Dis J 2008; 27(3):241–5.

59. Kawada J, Kimura H, Ito Y, et al. Evaluation of systemic inflammatory responses in neonates with herpes simplex virus infection. J Infect Dis 2004; 190(3):494–8.

60. Karlowicz MG, Buescher ES, Surka AE. Fulminant late-onset sepsis in a neonatal intensive care unit, 1988–1997, and the impact of avoiding empiric vancomycin therapy. Pediatrics 2000;106(6):1387–90.

61. Hyde TB, Hilger TM, Reingold A, et al. Trends in incidence and antimicrobial resistance of early-onset sepsis: population-based surveillance in San Francisco and Atlanta. Pediatrics 2002;110(4):690–5.

62. Benjamin DK, DeLong E, Cotten CM, et al. Mortality following blood culture in premature infants: increased with Gram-negative bacteremia and candidemia, but not Gram-positive bacteremia. J Perinatol 2004;24(3):175–80.

63. Benjamin DK Jr, Stoll BJ, Fanaroff AA, et al. Neonatal candidiasis among extremely low birth weight infants: risk factors, mortality rates, and neurodevelopmental outcomes at 18 to 22 months. Pediatrics 2006;117(1):84–92.

64. Schelonka RL, Chai MK, Yoder BA, et al. Volume of blood required to detect common neonatal pathogens. J Pediatr 1996;129(2):275–8.

65. Kawai T, Akira S. The roles of TLRs, RLRs and NLRs in pathogen recognition. Int Immunol 2009;21(4):317–37.

66. Kumagai Y, Takeuchi O, Akira S. Pathogen recognition by innate receptors. J Infect Chemother 2008;14(2):86–92.

67. Trinchieri G, Sher A. Cooperation of Toll-like receptor signals in innate immune defence. Nat Rev Immunol 2007;7(3):179–90.

68. Rittirsch D, Flierl MA, Ward PA. Harmful molecular mechanisms in sepsis. Nat Rev Immunol 2008;8(10):776–87.

69. Krumbiegel D, Zepp F, Meyer CU. Combined Toll-like receptor agonists synergistically increase production of inflammatory cytokines in human neonatal dendritic cells. Hum Immunol 2007;68(10):813–22.

70. Bochud PY, Chien JW, Marr KA, et al. Toll-like receptor 4 polymorphisms and aspergillosis in stem-cell transplantation. N Engl J Med 2008;359(17):1766–77.

71. Wurfel MM, Gordon AC, Holden TD, et al. Toll-like receptor 1 polymorphisms affect innate immune responses and outcomes in sepsis. Am J Respir Crit Care Med 2008;178(7):710–20.

72. Agnese DM, Calvano JE, Hahm SJ, et al. Human toll-like receptor 4 mutations but not CD14 polymorphisms are associated with an increased risk of Gram-negative infections. J Infect Dis 2002;186(10):1522–5.

73. Lorenz E, Mira JP, Cornish KL, et al. A novel polymorphism in the toll-like receptor 2 gene and its potential association with staphylococcal infection. Infect Immun 2000;68(11):6398–401.

74. Zhang SY, Jouanguy E, Ugolini S, et al. TLR3 deficiency in patients with herpes simplex encephalitis. Science 2007;317(5844):1522–7.

75. Mockenhaupt FP, Cramer JP, Hamann L, et al. Toll-like receptor (TLR) polymorphisms in African children: common TLR-4 variants predispose to severe malaria. J Commun Dis 2006;38(3):230–45.

76. Faber J, Meyer CU, Gemmer C, et al. Human toll-like receptor 4 mutations are associated with susceptibility to invasive meningococcal disease in infancy. Pediatr Infect Dis J 2006;25(1):80–1.

77. Zhang JP, Chen C, Yang Y. [Changes and clinical significance of Toll-like receptor 2 and 4 expression in neonatal infections]. Zhonghua Er Ke Za Zhi 2007;45(2):130–3 [in Chinese].

78. Leaphart CL, Cavallo J, Gribar SC, et al. A critical role for TLR4 in the pathogenesis of necrotizing enterocolitis by modulating intestinal injury and repair. J Immunol 2007;179(7):4808–20.

79. Goldbach-Mansky R, Dailey NJ, Canna SW, et al. Neonatal-onset multisystem inflammatory disease responsive to interleukin-1beta inhibition. N Engl J Med 2006;355(6):581–92.
80. Szebeni B, Szekeres R, Rusai K, et al. Genetic polymorphisms of CD14, toll-like receptor 4, and caspase-recruitment domain 15 are not associated with necrotizing enterocolitis in very low birth weight infants. J Pediatr Gastroenterol Nutr 2006;42(1):27–31.
81. Shigemoto T, Kageyama M, Hirai R, et al. Identification of loss of function mutations in human genes encoding RIG-I and mda5: implications for resistance to type I diabetes. J Biol Chem 2009;284(20):13348–54.
82. Warren SE, Mao DP, Rodriguez AE, et al. Multiple Nod-like receptors activate caspase 1 during Listeria monocytogenes infection. J Immunol 2008;180(11): 7558–64.
83. Behrendt D, Dembinski J, Heep A, et al. Lipopolysaccharide binding protein in preterm infants. Arch Dis Child Fetal Neonatal Ed 2004;89(6):F551–4.
84. Berner R, Furll B, Stelter F, et al. Elevated levels of lipopolysaccharide-binding protein and soluble CD14 in plasma in neonatal early-onset sepsis. Clin Diagn Lab Immunol 2002;9(2):440–5.
85. Blanco A, Solis G, Arranz E, et al. Serum levels of CD14 in neonatal sepsis by Gram-positive and Gram-negative bacteria. Acta Paediatr 1996;85(6):728–32.
86. Gu W, Shan YA, Zhou J, et al. Functional significance of gene polymorphisms in the promoter of myeloid differentiation-2. Ann Surg 2007;246(1):151–8.
87. von Bernuth H, Picard C, Jin Z, et al. Pyogenic bacterial infections in humans with MyD88 deficiency. Science 2008;321(5889):691–6.
88. Picard C, Puel A, Bonnet M, et al. Pyogenic bacterial infections in humans with IRAK-4 deficiency. Science 2003;299(5615):2076–9.
89. Ku CL, Picard C, Erdos M, et al. IRAK4 and NEMO mutations in otherwise healthy children with recurrent invasive pneumococcal disease. J Med Genet 2007;44(1):16–23.
90. Lotze MT, Tracey KJ. High-mobility group box 1 protein (HMGB1): nuclear weapon in the immune arsenal. Nat Rev Immunol 2005;5(4):331–42.
91. Mullins GE, Sunden-Cullberg J, Johansson AS, et al. Activation of human umbilical vein endothelial cells leads to relocation and release of high-mobility group box chromosomal protein 1. Scand J Immunol 2004;60(6):566–73.
92. van Zoelen MA, Yang H, Florquin S, et al. Role of toll-like receptors 2 and 4, and the receptor for advanced glycation end products in high-mobility group box 1-induced inflammation in vivo. Shock 2009;31(3):280–4.
93. Sappington PL, Yang R, Yang H, et al. HMGB1 B box increases the permeability of Caco-2 enterocytic monolayers and impairs intestinal barrier function in mice. Gastroenterology 2002;123(3):790–802.
94. Zamora R, Grishin A, Wong C, et al. High-mobility group box 1 protein is an inflammatory mediator in necrotizing enterocolitis: protective effect of the macrophage deactivator semapimod. Am J Physiol Gastrointest Liver Physiol 2005;289(4):G643–52.
95. Pack CD, Kumaraguru U, Suvas S, et al. Heat-shock protein 70 acts as an effective adjuvant in neonatal mice and confers protection against challenge with herpes simplex virus. Vaccine 2005;23(27):3526–34.
96. Wheeler DS, Lahni P, Odoms K, et al. Extracellular heat shock protein 60 (Hsp60) levels in children with septic shock. Inflamm Res 2007;56(5):216–9.
97. Wheeler DS, Fisher LE Jr, Catravas JD, et al. Extracellular hsp70 levels in children with septic shock. Pediatr Crit Care Med 2005;6(3):308–11.

98. Kono H, Rock KL. How dying cells alert the immune system to danger. Nat Rev Immunol 2008;8(4):279–89.

99. Batra S, Kumar R, Seema, et al. Alterations in antioxidant status during neonatal sepsis. Ann Trop Paediatr 2000;20(1):27–33.

100. Kapoor K, Basu S, Das BK, et al. Lipid peroxidation and antioxidants in neonatal septicemia. J Trop Pediatr 2006;52(5):372–5.

101. Ng PC. Diagnostic markers of infection in neonates. Arch Dis Child Fetal Neonatal Ed 2004;89(3):F229–35.

102. Ng PC, Li K, Wong RP, et al. Proinflammatory and anti-inflammatory cytokine responses in preterm infants with systemic infections. Arch Dis Child Fetal Neonatal Ed 2003;88(3):F209–13.

103. Levy O, Zarember KA, Roy RM, et al. Selective impairment of TLR-mediated innate immunity in human newborns: neonatal blood plasma reduces mono-cyte TNF-alpha induction by bacterial lipopeptides, lipopolysaccharide, and imiquimod, but preserves the response to R-848. J Immunol 2004;173(7):4627–34.

104. Bozza FA, Salluh JI, Japiassu AM, et al. Cytokine profiles as markers of disease severity in sepsis: a multiplex analysis. Crit Care 2007;11(2):R49.

105. Hodge G, Hodge S, Haslam R, et al. Rapid simultaneous measurement of multiple cytokines using 100 microl sample volumes–association with neonatal sepsis. Clin Exp Immunol 2004;137(2):402–7.

106. Heper Y, Akalin EH, Mistik R, et al. Evaluation of serum C-reactive protein, pro-calcitonin, tumor necrosis factor alpha, and interleukin-10 levels as diagnostic and prognostic parameters in patients with community-acquired sepsis, severe sepsis, and septic shock. Eur J Clin Microbiol Infect Dis 2006;25(8):481–91.

107. Atici A, Satar M, Cetiner S, et al. Serum tumor necrosis factor-alpha in neonatal sepsis. Am J Perinatol 1997;14(7):401–4.

108. Sadeghi K, Berger A, Langgartner M, et al. Immaturity of infection control in preterm and term newborns is associated with impaired toll-like receptor signaling. J Infect Dis 2007;195(2):296–302.

109. Kingsmore SF, Kennedy N, Halliday HL, et al. Identification of diagnostic biomarkers for infection in premature neonates. Mol Cell Proteomics 2008; 7(10):1863–75.

110. Grobmyer SR, Lin E, Lowry SF, et al. Elevation of IL-18 in human sepsis. J Clin Immunol 2000;20(3):212–5.

111. Hirata J, Kotani J, Aoyama M, et al. A role for IL-18 in human neutrophil apoptosis. Shock 2008;30(6):628–33.

112. Cusumano V, Midiri A, Cusumano VV, et al. Interleukin-18 is an essential element in host resistance to experimental group B streptococcal disease in neonates. Infect Immun 2004;72(1):295–300.

113. Puren AJ, Fantuzzi G, Gu Y, et al. Interleukin-18 (IFNgamma-inducing factor) induces IL-8 and IL-1beta via TNFalpha production from non-CD14+ human blood mononuclear cells. J Clin Invest 1998;101(3):711–21.

114. Elbim C, Guichard C, Dang PM, et al. Interleukin-18 primes the oxidative burst of neutrophils in response to formyl-peptides: role of cytochrome b558 transloca-tion and N-formyl peptide receptor endocytosis. Clin Diagn Lab Immunol 2005; 12(3):436–46.

115. Dollner H, Vatten L, Austgulen R. Early diagnostic markers for neonatal sepsis: comparing C-reactive protein, interleukin-6, soluble tumour necrosis factor recep-tors and soluble adhesion molecules. J Clin Epidemiol 2001;54(12):1251–7.

116. Turunen R, Andersson S, Nupponen I, et al. Increased CD11b-density on circulating phagocytes as an early sign of late-onset sepsis in extremely low-birthweight infants. Pediatr Res 2005;57(2):270–5.

117. Figueras-Aloy J, Gomez-Lopez L, Rodriguez-Miguelez JM, et al. Serum soluble ICAM-1, VCAM-1, L-selectin, and P-selectin levels as markers of infection and their relation to clinical severity in neonatal sepsis. Am J Perinatol 2007;24(6):331–8.

118. Kourtis AP, Lee FK, Stoll BJ. Soluble L-selectin, a marker of immune activation, in neonatal infection. Clin Immunol 2003;109(2):224–8.

119. McEvoy LT, Zakem-Cloud H, Tosi MF. Total cell content of CR3 (CD11b/CD18) and LFA-1 (CD11a/CD18) in neonatal neutrophils: relationship to gestational age. Blood 1996;87(9):3929–33.

120. Buhrer C, Graulich J, Stibenz D, et al. L-selectin is down-regulated in umbilical cord blood granulocytes and monocytes of newborn infants with acute bacterial infection. Pediatr Res 1994;36(6):799–804.

121. Sullivan SE, Staba SL, Gersting JA, et al. Circulating concentrations of chemokines in cord blood, neonates, and adults. Pediatr Res 2002;51(5):653–7.

122. Anderson DC, Rothlein R, Marlin SD, et al. Impaired transendothelial migration by neonatal neutrophils: abnormalities of Mac-1 (CD11b/CD18)-dependent adherence reactions. Blood 1990;76(12):2613–21.

123. Meade VM, Barese CN, Kim C, et al. Rac2 concentrations in umbilical cord neutrophils. Biol Neonate 2006;90(3):156–9.

124. Hickey MJ, Kubes P. Intravascular immunity: the host-pathogen encounter in blood vessels. Nat Rev Immunol 2009;9(5):364–75.

125. Ng PC, Li K, Chui KM, et al. IP-10 is an early diagnostic marker for identification of late-onset bacterial infection in preterm infants. Pediatr Res 2007;61(1):93–8.

126. Wong HR, Cvijanovich N, Wheeler DS, et al. Interleukin-8 as a stratification tool for interventional trials involving pediatric septic shock. Am J Respir Crit Care Med 2008;178(3):276–82.

127. Ng PC, Li K, Leung TF, et al. Early prediction of sepsis-induced disseminated intravascular coagulation with interleukin-10, interleukin-6, and RANTES in preterm infants. Clin Chem 2006;52(6):1181–9.

128. Sriskandan S, Altmann DM. The immunology of sepsis. J Pathol 2008;214(2): 211–23.

129. Hartel C, Osthues I, Rupp J, et al. Characterisation of the host inflammatory response to *Staphylococcus epidermidis* in neonatal whole blood. Arch Dis Child Fetal Neonatal Ed 2008;93(2):F140–5.

130. Sikora JP, Chlebna-Sokol D, Krzyzanska-Oberbek A. Proinflammatory cytokines (IL-6, IL-8), cytokine inhibitors (IL-6sR, sTNFRII) and anti-inflammatory cytokines (IL-10, IL-13) in the pathogenesis of sepsis in newborns and infants. Arch Immunol Ther Exp (Warsz) 2001;49(5):399–404.

131. Opal SM, Esmon CT. Bench-to-bedside review: functional relationships between coagulation and the innate immune response and their respective roles in the pathogenesis of sepsis. Crit Care 2003;7(1):23–38.

132. Wang P, Wu P, Siegel MI, et al. Interleukin (IL)-10 inhibits nuclear factor kappa B (NF kappa B) activation in human monocytes. IL-10 and IL-4 suppress cytokine synthesis by different mechanisms. J Biol Chem 1995;270(16):9558–63.

133. Brubaker JO, Montaner LJ. Role of interleukin-13 in innate and adaptive immunity. Cell Mol Biol (Noisy-le-grand) 2001;47(4):637–51.

134. Trepicchio WL, Bozza M, Pedneault G, et al. Recombinant human IL-11 attenuates the inflammatory response through down-regulation of proinflammatory cytokine release and nitric oxide production. J Immunol 1996;157(8):3627–34.

135. Koj A. Termination of acute-phase response: role of some cytokines and anti-inflammatory drugs. Gen Pharmacol 1998;31(1):9–18.
136. Spear ML, Stefano JL, Fawcett P, et al. Soluble interleukin-2 receptor as a predictor of neonatal sepsis. J Pediatr 1995;126(6):982–5.
137. Dollner H, Vatten L, Linnebo I, et al. Inflammatory mediators in umbilical plasma from neonates who develop early-onset sepsis. Biol Neonate 2001; 80(1):41–7.
138. Buhimschi CS, Bhandari V, Han YW, et al. Using proteomics in perinatal and neonatal sepsis: hopes and challenges for the future. Curr Opin Infect Dis 2009;22(3):235–43.
139. Bopp C, Hofer S, Weitz J, et al. sRAGE is elevated in septic patients and associated with patients outcome. J Surg Res 2008;147(1):79–83.
140. Liliensiek B, Weigand MA, Bierhaus A, et al. Receptor for advanced glycation end products (RAGE) regulates sepsis but not the adaptive immune response. J Clin Invest 2004;113(11):1641–50.
141. Wolach B, Dolfin T, Regev R, et al. The development of the complement system after 28 weeks' gestation. Acta Paediatr 1997;86(5):523–7.
142. Notarangelo LD, Chirico G, Chiara A, et al. Activity of classical and alternative pathways of complement in preterm and small for gestational age infants. Pediatr Res 1984;18(3):281–5.
143. Drossou V, Kanakoudi F, Diamanti E, et al. Concentrations of main serum opsonins in early infancy. Arch Dis Child Fetal Neonatal Ed 1995;72(3):F172–5.
144. Miller ME, Stiehm ER. Phagocytic, opsonic and immunoglobulin studies in newborns. Calif Med 1973;119(2):43–63.
145. Nupponen I, Andersson S, Jarvenpaa AL, et al. Neutrophil CD11b expression and circulating interleukin-8 as diagnostic markers for early-onset neonatal sepsis. Pediatrics 2001;108(1):E12.
146. Berger M, O'Shea J, Cross AS, et al. Human neutrophils increase expression of C3bi as well as C3b receptors upon activation. J Clin Invest 1984;74(5):1566–71.
147. Snyderman R, Goetzl EJ. Molecular and cellular mechanisms of leukocyte chemotaxis. Science 1981;213(4510):830–7.
148. Vogt W. Anaphylatoxins: possible roles in disease. Complement 1986;3(3): 177–88.
149. Ehlers MR. CR3: a general purpose adhesion-recognition receptor essential for innate immunity. Microbes Infect 2000;2(3):289–94.
150. Markiewski MM, Lambris JD. The role of complement in inflammatory diseases from behind the scenes into the spotlight. Am J Pathol 2007;171(3):715–27.
151. Nybo M, Sorensen O, Leslie R, et al. Reduced expression of C5a receptors on neutrophils from cord blood. Arch Dis Child Fetal Neonatal Ed 1998;78(2): F129–32.
152. Lothian C, Dahlgren C, Lagercrantz H, et al. Different expression and mobilisation of the complement regulatory proteins CD35, CD55 and CD59 in neonatal and adult neutrophils. Biol Neonate 1997;72(1):15–21.
153. Castellheim A, Lindenskov PH, Pharo A, et al. Meconium aspiration syndrome induces complement-associated systemic inflammatory response in newborn piglets. Scand J Immunol 2005;61(3):217–25.
154. Wong HR, Doughty LA, Wedel N, et al. Plasma bactericidal/permeability-increasing protein concentrations in critically ill children with the sepsis syndrome. Pediatr Infect Dis J 1995;14(12):1087–91.
155. Levy O. Innate immunity of the newborn: basic mechanisms and clinical correlates. Nat Rev Immunol 2007;7(5):379–90.

156. Levy O, Martin S, Eichenwald E, et al. Impaired innate immunity in the newborn: newborn neutrophils are deficient in bactericidal/permeability-increasing protein. Pediatrics 1999;104(6):1327–33.
157. Michalek J, Svetlikova P, Fedora M, et al. Bactericidal permeability increasing protein gene variants in children with sepsis. Intensive Care Med 2007;33(12): 2158–64.
158. Dyke MP, Forsyth KD. Decreased plasma fibronectin concentrations in preterm infants with septicaemia. Arch Dis Child 1993;68(5 Spec No):557–60.
159. Romeo MG, Tina LG, Sciacca A, et al. [Decreased plasma fibronectin (pFN) level in preterm infants with infections]. Pediatr Med Chir 1995;17(6):563–6 [in Italian].
160. Kalayci AG, Adam B, Yilmazer F, et al. The value of immunoglobulin and complement levels in the early diagnosis of neonatal sepsis. Acta Paediatr 1997;86(9):999–1002.
161. Madden NP, Levinsky RJ, Bayston R, et al. Surgery, sepsis, and nonspecific immune function in neonates. J Pediatr Surg 1989;24(6):562–6.
162. Hathaway WE, Mull MM, Pechet GS. Disseminated intravascular coagulation in the newborn. Pediatrics 1969;43(2):233–40.
163. Kimberlin DW, Lin CY, Jacobs RF, et al. Natural history of neonatal herpes simplex virus infections in the acyclovir era. Pediatrics 2001;108(2):223–9.
164. Rivers RP, Cattermole HE, Wright I. The expression of surface tissue factor apoprotein by blood monocytes in the course of infections in early infancy. Pediatr Res 1992;31(6):567–73.
165. Markiewski MM, Nilsson B, Ekdahl KN, et al. Complement and coagulation: strangers or partners in crime? Trends Immunol 2007;28(4):184–92.
166. Aronis S, Platokouki H, Photopoulos S, et al. Indications of coagulation and/or fibrinolytic system activation in healthy and sick very-low-birth-weight neonates. Biol Neonate 1998;74(5):337–44.
167. Lauterbach R, Pawlik D, Radziszewska R, et al. Plasma antithrombin III and protein C levels in early recognition of late-onset sepsis in newborns. Eur J Pediatr 2006;165(9):585–9.
168. Roman J, Velasco F, Fernandez F, et al. Coagulation, fibrinolytic and kallikrein systems in neonates with uncomplicated sepsis and septic shock. Haemostasis 1993;23(3):142–8.
169. Venkataseshan S, Dutta S, Ahluwalia J, et al. Low plasma protein C values predict mortality in low birth weight neonates with septicemia. Pediatr Infect Dis J 2007;26(8):684–8.
170. Sola MC, Del Vecchio A, Rimsza LM. Evaluation and treatment of thrombocytopenia in the neonatal intensive care unit. Clin Perinatol 2000;27(3):655–79.
171. Guida JD, Kunig AM, Leef KH, et al. Platelet count and sepsis in very low birth weight neonates: is there an organism-specific response? Pediatrics 2003; 111(6 Pt 1):1411–5.
172. Finkelstein Y, Shenkman B, Sirota L, et al. Whole blood platelet deposition on extracellular matrix under flow conditions in preterm neonatal sepsis. Eur J Pediatr 2002;161(5):270–4.
173. Bednarek FJ, Bean S, Barnard MR, et al. The platelet hyporeactivity of extremely low birth weight neonates is age-dependent. Thromb Res 2009;124(1):42–5.
174. Urlichs F, Speer C. Neutrophil function in preterm and term infants. Neoreviews 2004;5:e417–30.
175. Marodi L. Innate cellular immune responses in newborns. Clin Immunol 2006; 118(2–3):137–44.

176. Christensen RD, Rothstein G. Exhaustion of mature marrow neutrophils in neonates with sepsis. J Pediatr 1980;96(2):316–8.

177. Engle WA, McGuire WA, Schreiner RL, et al. Neutrophil storage pool depletion in neonates with sepsis and neutropenia. J Pediatr 1988;113(4):747–9.

178. Sarkar S, Bhagat I, Hieber S, et al. Can neutrophil responses in very low birth weight infants predict the organisms responsible for late-onset bacterial or fungal sepsis? J Perinatol 2006;26(8):501–5.

179. Christensen RD, Bradley PP, Rothstein G. The leukocyte left shift in clinical and experimental neonatal sepsis. J Pediatr 1981;98(1):101–5.

180. Drossou V, Kanakoudi F, Tzimouli V, et al. Impact of prematurity, stress and sepsis on the neutrophil respiratory burst activity of neonates. Biol Neonate 1997;72(4):201–9.

181. Shigeoka AO, Santos JI, Hill HR. Functional analysis of neutrophil granulocytes from healthy, infected, and stressed neonates. J Pediatr 1979;95(3): 454–60.

182. Wright WC Jr, Ank BJ, Herbert J, et al. Decreased bactericidal activity of leukocytes of stressed newborn infants. Pediatrics 1975;56(4):579–84.

183. Linderkamp O, Ruef P, Brenner B, et al. Passive deformability of mature, immature, and active neutrophils in healthy and septicemic neonates. Pediatr Res 1998;44(6):946–50.

184. Mease AD, Burgess DP, Thomas PJ. Irreversible neutrophil aggregation. A mechanism of decreased newborn neutrophil chemotactic response. Am J Pathol 1981;104(1):98–102.

185. Ohman L, Tullus K, Katouli M, et al. Correlation between susceptibility of infants to infections and interaction with neutrophils of Escherichia coli strains causing neonatal and infantile septicemia. J Infect Dis 1995;171(1):128–33.

186. Allgaier B, Shi M, Luo D, et al. Spontaneous and Fas-mediated apoptosis are diminished in umbilical cord blood neutrophils compared with adult neutrophils. J Leukoc Biol 1998;64(3):331–6.

187. Hanna N, Vasquez P, Pham P, et al. Mechanisms underlying reduced apoptosis in neonatal neutrophils. Pediatr Res 2005;57(1):56–62.

188. Koenig JM, Stegner JJ, Schmeck AC, et al. Neonatal neutrophils with prolonged survival exhibit enhanced inflammatory and cytotoxic responsiveness. Pediatr Res 2005;57(3):424–9.

189. Nupponen I, Pesonen E, Andersson S, et al. Neutrophil activation in preterm infants who have respiratory distress syndrome. Pediatrics 2002;110(1 Pt 1):36–41.

190. Nathan CF. Secretory products of macrophages. J Clin Invest 1987;79(2): 319–26.

191. Hodge G, Hodge S, Han P, et al. Multiple leucocyte activation markers to detect neonatal infection. Clin Exp Immunol 2004;135(1):125–9.

192. Georgeson GD, Szony BJ, Streitman K, et al. Natural killer cell cytotoxicity is deficient in newborns with sepsis and recurrent infections. Eur J Pediatr 2001; 160(8):478–82.

193. el-Sameea ER, Metwally SS, Mashhour E, et al. Evaluation of natural killer cells as diagnostic markers of early onset neonatal sepsis: comparison with C-reactive protein and interleukin-8. Egypt J Immunol 2004;11(1):91–102.

194. Mazur B, Godula-Stuglik U, Domarecki A, et al. [The influence of severe infections on the natural killer cells in neonates with vary gestational age]. Ginekol Pol 2000;71(6):542–9 [in Polish].

195. Marshall JS, Jawdat DM. Mast cells in innate immunity. J Allergy Clin Immunol 2004;114(1):21–7.

196. von Kockritz-Blickwede M, Goldmann O, Thulin P, et al. Phagocytosis-independent antimicrobial activity of mast cells by means of extracellular trap formation. Blood 2008;111(6):3070–80.
197. Mazzoni A, Young HA, Spitzer JH, et al. Histamine regulates cytokine production in maturing dendritic cells, resulting in altered T cell polarization. J Clin Invest 2001;108(12):1865–73.
198. Damsgaard TE, Nielsen BW, Henriques U, et al. Histamine releasing cells of the newborn. Mast cells from the umbilical cord matrix and basophils from cord blood. Pediatr Allergy Immunol 1996;7(2):83–90.
199. Schneider LA, Schlenner SM, Feyerabend TB, et al. Molecular mechanism of mast cell mediated innate defense against endothelin and snake venom sarafotoxin. J Exp Med 2007;204(11):2629–39.
200. Peters K, Unger RE, Brunner J, et al. Molecular basis of endothelial dysfunction in sepsis. Cardiovasc Res 2003;60(1):49–57.
201. Marshall JC. Such stuff as dreams are made on: mediator-directed therapy in sepsis. Nat Rev Drug Discov 2003;2(5):391–405.
202. Marom D, Yuhas Y, Sirota L, et al. Nitric oxide levels in preterm and term infants and in premature infants with bacteremia. Biol Neonate 2004;86(3):160–4.
203. Schrama AJ, de Beaufort AJ, Poorthuis BJ, et al. Secretory phospholipase A(2) in newborn infants with sepsis. J Perinatol 2008;28(4):291–6.
204. Siauw C, Kobsar A, Dornieden C, et al. Group B streptococcus isolates from septic patients and healthy carriers differentially activate platelet signaling cascades. Thromb Haemost 2006;95(5):836–49.
205. Figueras-Aloy J, Gomez-Lopez L, Rodriguez-Miguelez JM, et al. Plasma endothelin-1 and clinical manifestations of neonatal sepsis. J Perinat Med 2004;32(6): 522–6.
206. Kuhl PG, Cotton RB, Schweer H, et al. Endogenous formation of prostanoids in neonates with persistent pulmonary hypertension. Arch Dis Child 1989;64(7 Spec No):949–52.
207. Rosenberg AA, Kennaugh J, Koppenhafer SL, et al. Elevated immunoreactive endothelin-1 levels in newborn infants with persistent pulmonary hypertension. J Pediatr 1993;123(1):109–14.
208. Rossi P, Persson B, Boels PJ, et al. Endotoxemic pulmonary hypertension is largely mediated by endothelin-induced venous constriction. Intensive Care Med 2008;34(5):873–80.
209. Bulger EM, Maier RV. Lipid mediators in the pathophysiology of critical illness. Crit Care Med 2000;28(Suppl 4):N27–36.
210. Gotsch F, Romero R, Kusanovic JP, et al. The fetal inflammatory response syndrome. Clin Obstet Gynecol 2007;50(3):652–83.
211. Shi Y, Li HQ, Shen CK, et al. Plasma nitric oxide levels in newborn infants with sepsis. J Pediatr 1993;123(3):435–8.
212. Kultursay N, Kantar M, Akisu M, et al. Platelet-activating factor concentrations in healthy and septic neonates. Eur J Pediatr 1999;158(9):740–1.
213. Lopez A, Lorente JA, Steingrub J, et al. Multiple-center, randomized, placebo-controlled, double-blind study of the nitric oxide synthase inhibitor 546C88: effect on survival in patients with septic shock. Crit Care Med 2004;32(1):21–30.
214. Nimah M, Brilli RJ. Coagulation dysfunction in sepsis and multiple organ system failure. Crit Care Clin 2003;19(3):441–58.
215. Cribbs SK, Martin GS, Rojas M. Monitoring of endothelial dysfunction in critically ill patients: the role of endothelial progenitor cells. Curr Opin Crit Care 2008; 14(3):354–60.

216. Gibson RL, Nizet V, Rubens CE. Group B streptococcal beta-hemolysin promotes injury of lung microvascular endothelial cells. Pediatr Res 1999;45(5 Pt 1):626–34.
217. Dakshinamurti S. Pathophysiologic mechanisms of persistent pulmonary hypertension of the newborn. Pediatr Pulmonol 2005;39(6):492–503.
218. Arai H, Matsuda T, Goto R, et al. Increased numbers of macrophages in tracheal aspirates in premature infants with funisitis. Pediatr Int 2008;50(2):184–8.
219. McKiernan CA, Lieberman SA. Circulatory shock in children: an overview. Pediatr Rev 2005;26(12):451–60.
220. Luce WA, Hoffman TM, Bauer JA. Bench-to-bedside review: developmental influences on the mechanisms, treatment and outcomes of cardiovascular dysfunction in neonatal versus adult sepsis. Crit Care 2007;11(5):228.
221. Maeder M, Fehr T, Rickli H, et al. Sepsis-associated myocardial dysfunction: diagnostic and prognostic impact of cardiac troponins and natriuretic peptides. Chest 2006;129(5):1349–66.
222. Tabbutt S. Heart failure in pediatric septic shock: utilizing inotropic support. Crit Care Med 2001;29(Suppl 10):S231–6.
223. Ceneviva G, Paschall JA, Maffei F, et al. Hemodynamic support in fluid-refractory pediatric septic shock. Pediatrics 1998;102(2):e19.
224. Carcillo JA, Fields AI. Clinical practice parameters for hemodynamic support of pediatric and neonatal patients in septic shock. Crit Care Med 2002;30(6):1365–78.
225. Evans N. Which inotrope for which baby? Arch Dis Child Fetal Neonatal Ed 2006;91(3):F213–20.
226. Kluckow M, Evans N. Relationship between blood pressure and cardiac output in preterm infants requiring mechanical ventilation. J Pediatr 1996;129(4):506–12.
227. Seri I, Noori S. Diagnosis and treatment of neonatal hypotension outside the transitional period. Early Hum Dev 2005;81(5):405–11.
228. Cochat P, Bourgeois J, Gilly J, et al. [Anatomical study of the kidneys of newborn infants dying after a septic state]. Pediatrie 1986;41(1):7–15 [in French].
229. Csaicsich D, Russo-Schlaff N, Messerschmidt A, et al. Renal failure, comorbidity and mortality in preterm infants. Wien Klin Wochenschr 2008;120(5–6):153–7.
230. Spapen H. Liver perfusion in sepsis, septic shock, and multiorgan failure. Anat Rec (Hoboken) 2008;291(6):714–20.
231. Bhutta ZA, Yusuf K. Neonatal sepsis in Karachi: factors determining outcome and mortality. J Trop Pediatr 1997;43(2):65–70.
232. Faix RG, Donn SM. Association of septic shock caused by early-onset group B streptococcal sepsis and periventricular leukomalacia in the preterm infant. Pediatrics 1985;76(3):415–9.
233. Harris MC, D'Angio CT, Gallagher PR, et al. Cytokine elaboration in critically ill infants with bacterial sepsis, necrotizing enterocolitis, or sepsis syndrome: correlation with clinical parameters of inflammation and mortality. J Pediatr 2005;147(4):462–8.
234. Di Naro E, Cromi A, Ghezzi F, et al. Fetal thymic involution: a sonographic marker of the fetal inflammatory response syndrome. Am J Obstet Gynecol 2006;194(1):153–9.
235. Cinel I, Dellinger RP. Advances in pathogenesis and management of sepsis. Curr Opin Infect Dis 2007;20(4):345–52.
236. Cinel I, Opal SM. Molecular biology of inflammation and sepsis: a primer. Crit Care Med 2009;37(1):291–304.
237. Pfenninger J, Tschaeppeler H, Wagner BP, et al. The paradox of adult respiratory distress syndrome in neonates. Pediatr Pulmonol 1991;10(1):18–24.

238. Engle WA. Surfactant-replacement therapy for respiratory distress in the preterm and term neonate. Pediatrics 2008;121(2):419–32.
239. Ng PC, Lam CW, Fok TF, et al. Refractory hypotension in preterm infants with adrenocortical insufficiency. Arch Dis Child Fetal Neonatal Ed 2001;84(2):F122–4.
240. Das BK, Agarwal P, Agarwal JK, et al. Serum cortisol and thyroid hormone levels in neonates with sepsis. Indian J Pediatr 2002;69(8):663–5.
241. Glavina-Durdov M, Springer O, Capkun V, et al. The grade of acute thymus involution in neonates correlates with the duration of acute illness and with the percentage of lymphocytes in peripheral blood smear. Pathological study. Biol Neonate 2003;83(4):229–34.
242. Itoh K, Aihara H, Takada S, et al. Clinicopathological differences between early-onset and late-onset sepsis and pneumonia in very low birth weight infants. Pediatr Pathol 1990;10(5):757–68.
243. Timens W, Boes A, Rozeboom-Uiterwijk T, et al. Immaturity of the human splenic marginal zone in infancy. Possible contribution to the deficient infant immune response. J Immunol 1989;143(10):3200–6.
244. Toti P, De Felice C, Occhini R, et al. Spleen depletion in neonatal sepsis and chorioamnionitis. Am J Clin Pathol 2004;122(5):765–71.
245. Toti P, De Felice C, Stumpo M, et al. Acute thymic involution in fetuses and neonates with chorioamnionitis. Hum Pathol 2000;31(9):1121–8.
246. van Baarlen J, Schuurman HJ, Huber J. Acute thymus involution in infancy and childhood: a reliable marker for duration of acute illness. Hum Pathol 1988;19(10):1155–60.
247. Hotchkiss RS, Coopersmith CM, Karl IE. Prevention of lymphocyte apoptosis–a potential treatment of sepsis? Clin Infect Dis 2005;41(Suppl 7):S465–9.
248. Kalman L, Lindegren ML, Kobrynski L, et al. Mutations in genes required for T-cell development: IL7R, CD45, IL2RG, JAK3, RAG1, RAG2, ARTEMIS, and ADA and severe combined immunodeficiency: HuGE review. Genet Med 2004;6(1):16–26.
249. Le Tulzo Y, Pangault C, Gacouin A, et al. Early circulating lymphocyte apoptosis in human septic shock is associated with poor outcome. Shock 2002;18(6):487–94.
250. Wynn JL, Scumpia PO, Winfield RD, et al. Defective innate immunity predisposes murine neonates to poor sepsis outcome but is reversed by TLR agonists. Blood 2008;112(5):1750–8.
251. Bauer J, Hentschel R, Linderkamp O. Effect of sepsis syndrome on neonatal oxygen consumption and energy expenditure. Pediatrics 2002;110(6):e69.
252. Romeo C, Eaton S, Spitz L, et al. Nitric oxide inhibits neonatal hepatocyte oxidative metabolism. J Pediatr Surg 2000;35(1):44–8.
253. Eaton S. Impaired energy metabolism during neonatal sepsis: the effects of glutamine. Proc Nutr Soc 2003;62(3):745–51.
254. Dellinger RP, Levy MM, Carlet JM, et al. Surviving Sepsis Campaign: international guidelines for management of severe sepsis and septic shock: 2008. Intensive Care Med 2008;34(1):17–60.
255. Brierley J, Carcillo JA, Choong K, et al. Clinical practice parameters for hemodynamic support of pediatric and neonatal septic shock: 2007 update from the American College of Critical Care Medicine. Crit Care Med 2009;37(2):666–88.
256. Parker MM, Hazelzet JA, Carcillo JA. Pediatric considerations. Crit Care Med 2004;32(Suppl 11):S591–4.
257. Dempsey EM, Al Hazzani F, Barrington KJ. Permissive hypotension in the extremely low birthweight infant with signs of good perfusion. Arch Dis Child Fetal Neonatal Ed 2009;94(4):F241–4.

258. Shiao SY. Effects of fetal hemoglobin on accurate measurements of oxygen saturation in neonates. J Perinat Neonatal Nurs 2005;19(4):348–61.

259. Kluckow M, Seri I, Evans N. Echocardiography and the neonatologist. Pediatr Cardiol 2008;29(6):1043–7.

260. Kluckow M, Seri I, Evans N. Functional echocardiography: an emerging clinical tool for the neonatologist. J Pediatr 2007;150(2):125–30.

261. Evans N, Kluckow M, Simmons M, et al. Which to measure, systemic or organ blood flow? Middle cerebral artery and superior vena cava flow in very preterm infants. Arch Dis Child Fetal Neonatal Ed 2002;87(3):F181–4.

262. Kluckow M, Evans N. Superior vena cava flow in newborn infants: a novel marker of systemic blood flow. Arch Dis Child Fetal Neonatal Ed 2000;82(3):F182–7.

263. Hunt RW, Evans N, Rieger I, et al. Low superior vena cava flow and neurodevelopment at 3 years in very preterm infants. J Pediatr 2004;145(5):588–92.

264. Miletin J, Pichova K, Dempsey EM. Bedside detection of low systemic flow in the very low birth weight infant on day 1 of life. Eur J Pediatr 2009;168(7): 809–13.

265. Fortune PM, Wagstaff M, Petros AJ. Cerebro-splanchnic oxygenation ratio (CSOR) using near infrared spectroscopy may be able to predict splanchnic ischaemia in neonates. Intensive Care Med 2001;27(8):1401–7.

266. Johnson BA, Hoffman GM, Tweddell JS, et al. Near-infrared spectroscopy in neonates before palliation of hypoplastic left heart syndrome. Ann Thorac Surg 2009;87(2):571–7 [discussion: 577–9].

267. Osborn DA, Evans N, Kluckow M, et al. Low superior vena cava flow and effect of inotropes on neurodevelopment to 3 years in preterm infants. Pediatrics 2007; 120(2):372–80.

268. Seri I. Circulatory support of the sick preterm infant. Semin Neonatol 2001;6(1): 85–95.

269. Munro MJ, Walker AM, Barfield CP. Hypotensive extremely low birth weight infants have reduced cerebral blood flow. Pediatrics 2004;114(6):1591–6.

270. Han YY, Carcillo JA, Dragotta MA, et al. Early reversal of pediatric-neonatal septic shock by community physicians is associated with improved outcome. Pediatrics 2003;112(4):793–9.

271. Osborn DA, Evans N. Early volume expansion for prevention of morbidity and mortality in very preterm infants [review]. Cochrane Database Syst Rev 2004; 2:CD002055.

272. Goldberg RN, Chung D, Goldman SL, et al. The association of rapid volume expansion and intraventricular hemorrhage in the preterm infant. J Pediatr 1980;96(6):1060–3.

273. Pellicer A, Valverde E, Elorza MD, et al. Cardiovascular support for low birth weight infants and cerebral hemodynamics: a randomized, blinded, clinical trial. Pediatrics 2005;115(6):1501–12.

274. Osborn D, Evans N, Kluckow M. Randomized trial of dobutamine versus dopamine in preterm infants with low systemic blood flow. J Pediatr 2002;140(2): 183–91.

275. Osborn DA, Paradisis M, Evans N. The effect of inotropes on morbidity and mortality in preterm infants with low systemic or organ blood flow [review]. Cochrane Database Syst Rev 2007;1:CD005090.

276. Barton P, Garcia J, Kouatli A, et al. Hemodynamic effects of i.v. milrinone lactate in pediatric patients with septic shock. A prospective, double-blinded, randomized, placebo-controlled, interventional study. Chest 1996;109(5): 1302–12.

277. Paradisis M, Evans N, Kluckow M, et al. Randomized trial of milrinone versus placebo for prevention of low systemic blood flow in very preterm infants. J Pediatr 2009;154(2):189–95.
278. Leone M, Martin C. Role of terlipressin in the treatment of infants and neonates with catecholamine-resistant septic shock. Best Pract Res Clin Anaesthesiol 2008;22(2):323–33.
279. Meyer S, Gottschling S, Baghai A, et al. Arginine-vasopressin in catecholamine-refractory septic versus non-septic shock in extremely low birth weight infants with acute renal injury. Crit Care 2006;10(3):R71.
280. Annane D, Bellissant E, Bollaert PE, et al. Corticosteroids for severe sepsis and septic shock: a systematic review and meta-analysis. BMJ 2004; 329(7464):480.
281. Annane D, Sebille V, Charpentier C, et al. Effect of treatment with low doses of hydrocortisone and fludrocortisone on mortality in patients with septic shock. JAMA 2002;288(7):862–71.
282. Sprung CL, Annane D, Keh D, et al. Hydrocortisone therapy for patients with septic shock. N Engl J Med 2008;358(2):111–24.
283. Togari H, Sugiyama S, Ogino T, et al. Interactions of endotoxin with cortisol and acute phase proteins in septic shock neonates. Acta Paediatr Scand 1986; 75(1):69–74.
284. Seri I, Tan R, Evans J. Cardiovascular effects of hydrocortisone in preterm infants with pressor-resistant hypotension. Pediatrics 2001;107(5):1070–4.
285. Noori S, Friedlich P, Wong P, et al. Hemodynamic changes after low-dosage hydrocortisone administration in vasopressor-treated preterm and term neonates. Pediatrics 2006;118(4):1456–66.
286. Fernandez EF, Watterberg KL. Relative adrenal insufficiency in the preterm and term infant. J Perinatol 2009;29(Suppl 2):S44–9.
287. Roberts JD Jr, Fineman JR, Morin FC 3rd, et al. Inhaled nitric oxide and persistent pulmonary hypertension of the newborn. The Inhaled Nitric Oxide Study Group. N Engl J Med 1997;336(9):605–10.
288. Farrow KN, Fliman P, Steinhorn RH. The diseases treated with ECMO: focus on PPHN. Semin Perinatol 2005;29(1):8–14.
289. Maclaren G, Butt W. Extracorporeal membrane oxygenation and sepsis. Crit Care Resusc 2007;9(1):76–80.
290. Shankaran S, Laptook AR, Ehrenkranz RA, et al. Whole-body hypothermia for neonates with hypoxic-ischemic encephalopathy. N Engl J Med 2005;353(15): 1574–84.
291. Emery EF, Greenough A, Gamsu HR. Randomised controlled trial of colloid infusions in hypotensive preterm infants. Arch Dis Child 1992;67(10 Spec No): 1185–8.
292. Neu J, Huang Y. Nutrition of premature and critically ill neonates. Nestle Nutr Workshop Ser Clin Perform Programme 2003;8:171–81 [discussion: 181–5].
293. Park W, Paust H, Schroder H. Lipid infusion in premature infants suffering from sepsis. JPEN J Parenter Enteral Nutr 1984;8(3):290–2.
294. Toce SS, Keenan WJ. Lipid intolerance in newborns is associated with hepatic dysfunction but not infection. Arch Pediatr Adolesc Med 1995;149(11):1249–53.
295. Basu R, Muller DP, Eaton S, et al. Lipid peroxidation can be reduced in infants on total parenteral nutrition by promoting fat utilisation. J Pediatr Surg 1999;34(2): 255–9.
296. Pierro A. Metabolism and nutritional support in the surgical neonate. J Pediatr Surg 2002;37(6):811–22.

297. Mathur NB, Singh A, Sharma VK, et al. Evaluation of risk factors for fatal neonatal sepsis. Indian Pediatr 1996;33(10):817–22.
298. Adams-Chapman I, Stoll BJ. Neonatal infection and long-term neurodevelopmental outcome in the preterm infant. Curr Opin Infect Dis 2006;19(3): 290–7.
299. Stoll BJ, Hansen NI, Adams-Chapman I, et al. Neurodevelopmental and growth impairment among extremely low-birth-weight infants with neonatal infection. JAMA 2004;292(19):2357–65.
300. Bassler D, Stoll BJ, Schmidt B, et al. Using a count of neonatal morbidities to predict poor outcome in extremely low birth weight infants: added role of neonatal infection. Pediatrics 2009;123(1):313–8.
301. Shah DK, Doyle LW, Anderson PJ, et al. Adverse neurodevelopment in preterm infants with postnatal sepsis or necrotizing enterocolitis is mediated by white matter abnormalities on magnetic resonance imaging at term. J Pediatr 2008; 153(2):170–5, 175 e171.
302. Hintz SR, Kendrick DE, Stoll BJ, et al. Neurodevelopmental and growth outcomes of extremely low birth weight infants after necrotizing enterocolitis. Pediatrics 2005;115(3):696–703.
303. Manzoni P, Maestri A, Leonessa M, et al. Fungal and bacterial sepsis and threshold ROP in preterm very low birth weight neonates. J Perinatol 2006; 26(1):23–30.
304. Wong HR, Cvijanovich N, Lin R, et al. Identification of pediatric septic shock subclasses based on genome-wide expression profiling. BMC Med 2009;7:34.
305. Wong HR, Cvijanovich N, Allen GL, et al. Genomic expression profiling across the pediatric systemic inflammatory response syndrome, sepsis, and septic shock spectrum. Crit Care Med 2009;37(5):1558–66.
306. Wong HR, Odoms K, Sakthivel B. Divergence of canonical danger signals: the genome-level expression patterns of human mononuclear cells subjected to heat shock or lipopolysaccharide. BMC Immunol 2008;9:24.
307. Cvijanovich N, Shanley TP, Lin R, et al. Validating the genomic signature of pediatric septic shock. Physiol Genomics 2008;34(1):127–34.
308. Shanley TP, Cvijanovich N, Lin R, et al. Genome-level longitudinal expression of signaling pathways and gene networks in pediatric septic shock. Mol Med 2007; 13(9–10):495–508.
309. Tang BM, McLean AS, Dawes IW, et al. Gene-expression profiling of Gram-positive and Gram-negative sepsis in critically ill patients. Crit Care Med 2008;36(4): 1125–8.
310. Tang BM, McLean AS, Dawes IW, et al. The use of gene-expression profiling to identify candidate genes in human sepsis. Am J Respir Crit Care Med 2007; 176(7):676–84.
311. Tang BM, McLean AS, Dawes IW, et al. Gene-expression profiling of peripheral blood mononuclear cells in sepsis. Crit Care Med 2009;37(3):882–8.
312. Karvunidis T, Mares J, Thongboonkerd V, et al. Recent progress of proteomics in critical illness. Shock 2009;31(6):545–52.
313. Buhimschi CS, Bhandari V, Hamar BD, et al. Proteomic profiling of the amniotic fluid to detect inflammation, infection, and neonatal sepsis. PLoS Med 2007;4(1):e18.
314. Feezor RJ, Cheng A, Paddock HN, et al. Functional genomics and gene expression profiling in sepsis: beyond class prediction. Clin Infect Dis 2005; 41(Suppl 7):S427–35.
315. Levy O, Sisson RB, Kenyon J, et al. Enhancement of neonatal innate defense: effects of adding an N-terminal recombinant fragment of bactericidal/

permeability-increasing protein on growth and tumor necrosis factor-inducing activity of Gram-negative bacteria tested in neonatal cord blood ex vivo. Infect Immun 2000;68(9):5120–5.

316. Reinhart K, Gluck T, Ligtenberg J, et al. CD14 receptor occupancy in severe sepsis: results of a phase I clinical trial with a recombinant chimeric CD14 monoclonal antibody (IC14). Crit Care Med 2004;32(5):1100–8.

317. Lauterbach R, Pawlik D, Kowalczyk D, et al. Effect of the immunomodulating agent, pentoxifylline, in the treatment of sepsis in prematurely delivered infants: a placebo-controlled, double-blind trial. Crit Care Med 1999;27(4):807–14.

318. Tracey KJ. Physiology and immunology of the cholinergic antiinflammatory pathway. J Clin Invest 2007;117(2):289–96.

319. Pleiner J, Schaller G, Mittermayer F, et al. Simvastatin prevents vascular hyporeactivity during inflammation. Circulation 2004;110(21):3349–54.

320. Ikegami M, Carter K, Bishop K, et al. Intratracheal recombinant surfactant protein d prevents endotoxin shock in the newborn preterm lamb. Am J Respir Crit Care Med 2006;173(12):1342–7.

321. Mohan P, Abrams SA. Oral lactoferrin for the treatment of sepsis and necrotizing enterocolitis in neonates [review]. Cochrane Database Syst Rev 2009;1: CD007138.

322. Venkatesh M, Abrams S. Can lactoferrin prevent neonatal sepsis and necrotizing enterocolitis? Expert Rev Anti Infect Ther 2009;7(5):515–25.

323. Suri M, Harrison L, Van de Ven C, et al. Immunotherapy in the prophylaxis and treatment of neonatal sepsis. Curr Opin Pediatr 2003;15(2):155–60.

Adjunctive Immunologic Interventions in Neonatal Sepsis

William Tarnow-Mordi, MBChB, MRCP(UK), DCH, FRCPCH[a],*,
David Isaacs, MBChB, MD, FRCP, FRACP[b], Sourabh Dutta, MD, PhD[c]

KEYWORDS

- Colony-stimulating factors • Intravenous immunoglobulin
- Neonatal sepsis • Randomized controlled trials

It is widely accepted that randomized controlled trials (RCTs) are essential to minimize bias when testing therapies. Trials must also minimize random error, however, to avoid being misled by the play of chance. This requires surprisingly large numbers. To detect reliably a moderate risk difference of 5% in mortality or in disability-free survival (eg, from 35% to 30%), an adequately powered two-arm trial needs around 4000 patients, whereas a risk difference of 10% (eg, from 30% to 20%) requires over 800. Most trials are too small to provide reliable evidence about any but the largest treatment effects. As a result, most adjunctive immunologic interventions, and most neonatal therapies, remain incompletely evaluated.[1,2]

Despite a profusion of promising hypotheses arising from basic science, lack of adequately powered trials remains a major barrier to progress in translational research. Meta-analysis is one strategy to overcome this problem, but it cannot provide reliable evidence when available trials are of poor quality, or are unrepresentative because of publication bias or other forms of selection.

Table 1 shows the immunologic interventions to be considered in this article, categorized by the reliability of the evidence of their impact on sepsis, inflammatory disorders, mortality, or disability.

[a] Westmead International Network for Neonatal Education and Research (WINNER) Institute, Centre for Newborn Care, Westmead Hospital, University of Sydney, Hawkesbury Road, New South Wales 2145, Australia
[b] Department of Immunology and Infectious Diseases, University of Sydney, Children's Hospital at Westmead, Hawkesbury Road, New South Wales 2145, Australia
[c] Newborn Unit, Department of Pediatrics, Sector 12, Postgraduate Institute of Medical Education and Research, Chandigarh 160012, India
* Corresponding author.
E-mail address: williamtm@med.usyd.edu.au

Clin Perinatol 37 (2010) 481–499
doi:10.1016/j.clp.2009.12.002
0095-5108/10/$ – see front matter © 2010 Elsevier Inc. All rights reserved.

perinatology.theclinics.com

Table 1
Interventions, postulated immunologic mechanisms, and evidence of effects on sepsis, inflammatory disease, disability, and morbidity in newborn infants

Intervention	Postulated Immunologic Mechanisms	Level of Evidence	No. of Infants	Outcomes and Conclusions
Granulocyte transfusion	Enhance neutrophil numbers and function	Systematic review of three therapeutic RCTs[3]	44	No difference shown in mortality or sepsis: more RCTs needed
G-CSF or GM-CSF	Enhance neutrophil (G-CSF) or neutrophil and macrophage (GM-CSF) numbers	Systematic review of seven therapeutic RCTs[4]	257	No difference shown in mortality or sepsis: more RCTs needed
		Subgroup analysis of three therapeutic RCTs[4]	97	? GM-CSF improves survival in sepsis with neutropenia[6]: more RCTs needed
	Enhance neutrophil function	Systematic reviews of four prophylactic RCTs[5]	639	No difference shown in mortality or sepsis: more RCTs needed
Activated protein C	Fibrinolytic, anti-inflammatory	No RCTs in newborns		Not recommended
Exchange transfusion	Remove toxins and harmful circulating cytokines, enhance immunoglobulins	Two therapeutic RCTs[7,8]	70	? Exchange transfusion improves survival in gram-negative sepsis: more RCTs needed
Pentoxifylline	Xanthine derivative, phosphodiesterase inhibitor, increase adenylyl cyclase and cAMP, decrease TNF-α, anti-inflammatory	Two therapeutic RCTs[9]	140	? Pentoxifylline improves survival in proved sepsis: more RCTs needed
Reduce oxidative stress: Selenium Melatonin	Component of glutathione peroxidase, antioxidant Free radical scavenger	Systematic review of three prophylactic RCTs[10] No RCTs in newborns	583	? Selenium reduces sepsis: more RCTs needed RCTs needed
Glutamine	Anabolic for dividing immune and gut cells	Systematic review of seven prophylactic RCTs[11]	2365	No difference shown in mortality or sepsis or disability free survival: More RCTs not a high priority

Intervention	Mechanism	Evidence	N	Comments
Lactoferrin	Antimicrobial by iron sequestration or direct effect on microbial cell membranes. Anti-inflammatory by suppressing TNF-α and other cytokines by leukocytes and respiratory and gut epithelial cells	Three-arm prophylactic RCT of lactoferrin versus lactoferrin + L rhamnosus GG versus placebo[12]	472	Lactoferrin and Lactoferrin + L rhamnosus reduce late-onset sepsis RCTs needed to evaluate effects on disability-free survival
Probiotics	Enhance local and systemic immunity, anti-inflammatory cytokines and gut impermeability to bacteria and toxins; suppress pathogenic organisms associated with NEC	Systematic reviews of prophylactic RCTs[13-15]	2167	Probiotics reduce all-cause mortality and NEC. Large equivalence and cost-effectiveness RCTs of multiple probiotic regimens are needed. Continuing to include placebo or no-treatment groups is ethically problematic
Prebiotics	Promote growth of bifidobacteria and other probiotics in colon	Systematic review of four RCTs[16]	126	Increased bifidobacteria in stools. No difference shown in mortality, NEC, Sepsis. No data on disability free survival
	Reduce growth of Potentially allergeneic pathogens in gut	Systematic review of seven RCTs[17]	432	Insufficient evidence: further RCTs needed
Broad-spectrum peripartum antibiotics	Reduce probiotic colonization in gut; down-regulate major histocompatibility class Ib and II genes and genes coding for Paneth cell antimicrobial products (defensins, matrilysin, and phospholipase A_2) and for metalloproteinase	Prophylactic RCTs of antenatal antibiotics[18,19]	4221	Broad-spectrum antenatal antibiotics increase NEC, functional impairment and cerebral palsy at 7 years
		Cohort study in extremely low birth weight infants[20]	5693	Prolonged postnatal antibiotic therapy after sterile cultures is associated with increased risk of death and NEC RCTs needed to evaluate effect of early curtailment of antibiotics after sterile cultures on disability-free survival

(continued on next page)

Table 1
(continued)

Intervention	Postulated Immunologic Mechanisms	Level of Evidence	No. of Infants	Outcomes and Conclusions
Breast milk	Contains secretory IgA, cellular defenses, antimicrobial proteins and peptides, such as lysozyme and lactoferrin, which restrict growth of gut pathogens; immunoregulatory cytokines, such as TGF-β; prebiotic oligosaccharides, which enhance growth of gut probiotics and prevent attachment of pathogenic bacteria to mucosal receptors; IL-7, which enhances lymphocyte production by thymus; soluble receptors, which bind TNF-α and IL-1β	Prophylactic RCT of expressed breast milk versus formula in low birth weight infants[21]	62	Breast milk reduced sepsis
		Prophylactic cluster RCT of breastfeeding promotion: all infants[22]	17,046	Breastfeeding reduced gastroenteritis and atopic eczema in first 12 months after birth
		Cohort study in less developed country: all infants[23]	10,947	Initiation of breast feeding within 1 hour of birth versus later initiation is associated with 22% reduction in mortality RCTs of early initiation with colostrum needed in preterm infants
		Individual patient data meta-analysis of six cohort studies in less developed countries: all infants[24]	17,982	Breast milk is associated with lower risk of death from gastroenteritis and infectious respiratory disease
		Cohort study in preterm infants[25]	926	Breast milk is associated with lower risk of NEC and death
		Cohort study in VLBW infants[26]	212	Breast milk is associated with lower risk of infection

			N	
IVIG (polyclonal): IgG	Multiple proinflammatory actions: binds to cell surface receptors, enhances opsonic activity, complement, cytotoxicity, and neutrophil function	Systematic review of therapeutic RCTs in clinically suspected infection: all infants[27]	318	No difference shown in mortality or disability free survival in suspected infection, but marginally significant reduction in mortality in subsequently proved infection (N = 262). INIS trial (N = 3493) awaited[32]
	IVIG also has multiple immunomodulatory actions; down-regulation of the cytokine cascade, IL-1 system and complement-mediated inflammation, blockade of Fc-receptors on phagocytic cells, modulation of Fc receptor expression, cytoprotective effect on TNF-α–induced cell death in fibroblasts and regulation of B cell differentiation, immunoglobulin production and CD8 mediated suppressor or cytotoxic T cell function	Systematic review of therapeutic RCTs for sepsis and septic shock: all infants[28]	241	Meta-analysis does not support a reduction in mortality
		Systematic review of prophylactic RCTs in preterm infants[29]	4986	Meta-analysis shows 3% reduction in sepsis but no effect on mortality No further similar RCTs needed
IgM enriched	Pentameric IgM confers superior toxin neutralization and bacterial agglutination	Two therapeutic RCTs[30,31]	104	No difference shown in mortality or disability survival: Further RCTs needed
IVIG (monoclonal)	Hyperimmune titers of Ab directed against a single microbial antigen	Systematic review of prophylactic RCTs of antistaphylococcal IgG in VLBW infants[33]	2694	No difference shown in mortality, sepsis, or other adverse outcomes Further RCTs needed

Abbreviations: G-CSF, granulocyte colony-stimulating factor; GM-CSF, granulocyte-macrophage colony-stimulating factor; IL, interleukin; IVIG, intravenous immunoglobulin; NEC, necrotizing enterocolitis; RCT, randomized controlled trials; TGF, transforming growth factor; TNF, tumor necrosis factor; VLBW, very low birth weight.

GRANULOCYTE TRANSFUSIONS

Neonates, particularly preterm neonates, have defective humoral and phagocytic immunity, predisposing to increased incidence of bacterial and fungal infection. Neonatal neutrophil granulocytes exhibit both quantitative and qualitative abnormalities. Immaturity of granulopoiesis in preterm neonates results in a low neutrophil cell mass, a reduced capacity for increasing progenitor cell proliferation, and frequent occurrence of neutropenia in response to sepsis. Neutropenia is common in growth-restricted babies and predisposes to sepsis, but can also develop following sepsis.[34] Neutropenic neonates with sepsis have a higher mortality rate than nonneutropenic neonates with sepsis.[34] Neonatal neutrophils also have reduced function.[3]

In neutropenic neonates with sepsis transfusions of granulocytes could potentially reduce mortality and morbidity, but there is insufficient evidence on safety and efficacy to justify routine use. Granulocytes, predominantly neutrophils, are prepared in a concentrated form for transfusion to reduce the volume of the transfusion. Granulocyte concentrates are prepared either by leukophoresis or by centrifugation of whole blood (buffy coats). Buffy coats are easier to prepare but contain a lower dose of granulocytes and are less effective in reducing mortality in infected, neutropenic adults than leukopheresis granulocyte concentrates.[3] Early, nonrandomized studies suggested a possible reduction in mortality associated with the use of granulocyte transfusions in newborns with sepsis.[35] It can take several hours, however, to prepare granulocyte concentrates. In addition, there are potential severe complications of leukocyte transfusions in neonates, notably fluid overload, transmission of blood-borne infection, graft-versus-host disease caused by mature lymphocytes in the transfusion, pulmonary complications secondary to leukocyte aggregation and sequestration, and sensitization to donor erythrocyte and leukocyte antigens.[3]

A Cochrane systematic review of the role of granulocyte transfusions as an adjunct to antibiotics in the treatment of neutropenic newborns with sepsis identified four small, eligible trials.[3] Forty-four infants with sepsis and neutropenia were randomized in three trials to granulocyte transfusions, or placebo with no transfusion. In another trial, 35 infants with sepsis and neutropenia were randomized to granulocyte transfusion or intravenous immunoglobulin (IVIG).[36]

When granulocyte transfusion was compared with placebo or no transfusion, there was no significant difference in all-cause mortality (typical relative risk [RR] 0.89; [95% confidence interval (CI), 0.43 to 1.86]; typical risk difference [RD] −0.05; [95% CI, −0.31 to−0.21]). When granulocyte transfusion was compared with IVIG, there was a reduction in all-cause mortality of borderline statistical significance (RR 0.06 [95% CI, 0.00 to 1.04]; RD −0.34 [95% CI, −0.60 to −0.09]; number needed to treat [NNT] 2.7 [95% CI, 1.6 to 9.1]). The authors recommend adequately powered multicenter RCTs in neutropenic newborns with sepsis. Pulmonary complications were reported in four babies in two trials that used buffy coat transfusions. None of the trials reported neurologic outcome.

COLONY-STIMULATING FACTORS

Although neutrophil transfusions are expensive and potentially hazardous, the rationale for improving neutrophil numbers and function in sepsis still exists. The discovery and synthesis of hemopoietic colony-stimulating factors (CSFs) created new opportunities for sepsis prevention and treatment. Granulocyte-macrophage–colony-stimulating factor (GM-CSF) and granulocyte colony-stimulating factor (G-CSF) are naturally occurring cytokines that stimulate the production and antibacterial function of neutrophils and monocytes. They are routinely used to accelerate neutrophil recovery in adults and children receiving chemotherapy, in whom they cause only minor adverse events, such as low-grade fever.

In neonates, CSFs could potentially be used therapeutically to treat established or suspected sepsis, with or without neutropenia, or prophylactically to prevent sepsis. A Cochrane systematic review of G-CSF or GM-CSF in neonates[4] found seven treatment studies including 257 infants with suspected systemic bacterial infection and three prophylaxis studies with 359 neonates.

The treatment studies did not show that G-CSF or GM-CSF, added to antibiotic therapy in preterm infants with suspected systemic infection, reduced all-cause mortality 14 days from the start of therapy (typical RR 0.71 [95% CI, 0.38 to 1.33]; typical RD −0.05 [95% CI, −0.14 to −0.04]). The seven treatment studies were all small, however, with only 60 infants in the largest study. A subgroup analysis of 97 infants from three treatment studies who, in addition to systemic infection, had clinically significant neutropenia (<1.7 × 10^9/L) at trial entry did show a significant reduction in mortality by day 14 (RR 0.34 [95% CI, 0.12 to 0.92]; RD −0.18 [95% CI, −0.33 to −0.03]; NNT 6 [95% CI, 3 to 33]).

Studies of G-CSF or GM-CSF given prophylactically did not show a significant reduction in mortality in neonates receiving GM-CSF (RR 0.59 [95% CI, 0.24 to 1.44]; RD −0.03 [95% CI, −0.08 to −0.02]).[4] Inadequately stringent definitions of systemic infection meant that the primary outcome of sepsis was uncertain and not comparable. Only one study recruited a subgroup of infants less than 32 weeks gestation who were neutropenic or at high risk of developing neutropenia.[6] The incidence of systemic infection in this subgroup was reduced from 53% to 31%, but the numbers were small (N = 31) and the difference not statistically significant (RR 0.59 [95% CI, 0.25 to 1.39]; RD −0.22 [95% CI, −0.56 to −0.12]).[6]

Since the Cochrane Review,[4] a larger, multicenter trial has randomized 280 neonates less than 31 weeks gestation and small for gestational age (<10th percentile) within 72 hours of birth to receive GM-CSF for 5 days or standard care. Although neutrophil counts rose more rapidly in the GM-CSF babies, there was no significant difference in sepsis-free survival for all infants (93 of 139 treated infants, 105 of 141 control infants; difference −8%, 95% CI,−18 to −3). A meta-analysis of this trial and previous published prophylactic trials did not show evidence of survival benefit.[5]

There are limited data suggesting that CSF treatment may reduce mortality when systemic infection is accompanied by severe neutropenia. The data do not suggest that CSF can prevent sepsis or reduce mortality in babies with or at risk of neutropenia. The evidence is too weak to support the prophylactic use of G-CSF or GM-CSF, and CSFs are not recommended to treat established infection without further evidence from adequately powered trials.

ACTIVATED PROTEIN C

Endotoxins or other microbiologic products produced by infecting organisms activate host immunologic defense systems including complement, proinflammatory, anti-inflammatory, procoagulation, anticoagulation, fibrinolytic, and immunologic cascades. Although the host proinflammatory response is an essential response against invading organisms, an inadequate or excessive host response may lead to apoptosis, organ failure, and death. Microvascular thrombus formation and the host anticoagulation process they induce can cause disseminated intravascular coagulation and contribute to organ dysfunction. An endothelial cell glycoprotein, thrombomodulin, combines with thrombin and converts protein C to its activated form. Activated protein C (APC) promotes fibrinolysis and has anti-inflammatory action by blocking production of tumor necrosis factor (TNF). APC has a short half-life and, in sepsis, conversion to the activated form is reduced and the circulating pool of protein C is rapidly depleted. This can lead to an increase in inflammation, intravascular coagulation, and multiorgan failure.

In a RCT of adults with severe sepsis, recombinant human APC or drotrecogin alfa reduced 28-day all-cause mortality by 6.1%, at the cost of an increase in serious bleeding complications in the treatment group (3.5%) compared with the placebo group (2%).[37] The NNT to prevent one death, extrapolated from this trial, was 16. The number needed to harm[38] (for serious bleeding) was 66. A subsequent Cochrane systematic review, however, found that APC did not reduce mortality in 4434 adults (pooled RR 0.92; 95% CI, 0.72 to 1.18) but did increase bleeding.[39] In a RCT of 477 children with severe sepsis, APC did not reduce mortality (RR 0.98; 95% CI, 0.66 to 1.46) but bleeding was not increased.[40]

The mortality for neonatal sepsis is higher than for older children, and trials in newborn infants might be able to show an effect using smaller numbers of participants if APC had a positive but marginal benefit. Neonates with or without sepsis are at increased risk for major bleeding, however, and APC might well cause more harm than good. At present there are no RCTs of APC in neonates[41] and the authors advise against the use of APC in neonatal sepsis because there is no evidence of benefit and the potential for harm from bleeding.

EXCHANGE TRANSFUSION

The rationale for the use of exchange transfusion using fresh, whole, adult blood to treat sepsis is to remove toxic bacterial products, such as endotoxins and harmful, circulating cytokines, to improve perfusion and tissue oxygenation, replace clotting factors, and enhance humoral and cellular inflammatory responses. Neutropenia, if present, may also be corrected. Exchange transfusion has predominantly been used to treat overwhelming sepsis. Most reports are anecdotal or of poor quality. Some anecdotes sound persuasive, such as a report of 10 babies with severe sepsis and sclerema unresponsive to antibiotics, who were each treated with up to four exchange transfusions. Seven babies were reported to have improved immediately and eventually survived.[42] A quasirandomized controlled trial of exchange transfusion in neutropenic neonates reported a mortality of 35% (7 of 20) in the transfusion group and 70% (7 of 10) in the controls ($P = .07$).[7] A RCT from the same institution randomly assigned consecutive culture-positive neonates with sepsis and sclerema to exchange transfusion or no exchange transfusion. Ten of 20 babies in the study group died and 19 of 20 controls died ($P = .003$). Gram-negative organisms accounted for 85% in the study group and 90% in controls. IgG, IgA, and IgM levels rose significantly after exchange transfusion, but complement (C3) levels did not change.[8]

In a study from Turkey, 88 infants with sepsis and gestational ages ranging from 32 to less than 37 weeks were enrolled consecutively. Seven (21%) of 33 babies treated with exchange transfusion died, compared with 9 (27%) of 33 who received IVIG and 9 (41%) of 22 controls ($P > .05$).[43] Exchange transfusion may be beneficial as a last resort in babies with severe sepsis, particularly in babies who are failing appropriate antibiotic and full supportive therapy, but the evidence is weak.

PENTOXIFYLLINE

Pentoxifylline is a xanthine derivative. It is a phosphodiesterase inhibitor that suppresses TNF-α production by activating adenyl cyclase and increasing cellular cyclic AMP concentration. TNF-α activates polymorphonuclear leukocytes and increases its own production, so excess TNF-α can amplify the inflammatory response. Pentoxifylline improves endothelial cell function and reduces excessive coagulation in sepsis. In adult humans with sepsis, pentoxifylline improves renal blood flow and can prevent transition from a hyperdynamic to a hypodynamic cardiovascular response. It also improves inflammatory lung injury after chronic endotoxemia.[44] In adults and neonates, pentoxifylline decreases serum levels of TNF-α, interleukin (IL)-1, and IL-10 but not IL-6 or IL-8. Pentoxifylline reduced the incidence and severity of necrotizing enterocolitis (NEC) in a rat model.[45]

A Cochrane systematic review of pentoxifylline as an adjunct to antibiotics for treatment of suspected or confirmed sepsis or NEC in neonates identified Two RCTs that enrolled a total of 140 preterm (<36 weeks gestation) neonates with suspected late-onset (>7 days) sepsis.[9] Outcomes were reported for only 107 randomized patients with confirmed sepsis. A reduction was noted in all-cause mortality during hospital stay following pentoxifylline treatment (typical RR 0.14 [95% CI, 0.03 to 0.76]; typical RD −0.16 [95% CI, −0.27 to −0.04]; NNT 6 [95% CI, 4 to 25]). No adverse effects caused by pentoxifylline or other outcomes of interest were reported. These results are promising, but need to be confirmed in larger studies.

REDUCTION OF OXIDATIVE STRESS: SELENIUM

Newborns, especially if born preterm, are at risk of oxidative stress. Newborn infants have lower levels of plasma antioxidants, such as vitamin E, betacarotene, and sulphydryl groups, than adults; lower levels of plasma metal binding proteins including ceruloplasmin and transferrin; and reduced activity of erythrocyte superoxide dismutase. Strategies to reduce oxidative stress might be helpful in such conditions as asphyxia, respiratory distress syndrome, and sepsis, where oxidative stress is thought to be an important contributor to morbidity and mortality.

Selenium is an essential trace element and component of a number of proteins including glutathione peroxidase, which has a role in protecting against oxidative damage. Selenium deficiency is associated with impairment of both cell-mediated immunity and B-cell function.[46] In experimental animals, selenium deficiency has been associated with increased susceptibility to oxidative lung injury. Sick preterm neonates are exposed to many sources of oxygen radicals, from high concentrations of inspired oxygen, frequent alteration of blood flow to major organs, and inflammation with accumulation of neutrophils and macrophages. Low blood selenium concentrations in preterm infants have been suggested as a potential risk factor for sepsis, chronic neonatal lung disease, and retinopathy of prematurity.

A Cochrane systematic review identified three RCTs that compared clinical outcomes in preterm or very low birth weight infants given parenteral or enteral selenium supplementation with placebo or nothing from shortly after birth.[10] Two trials were conducted in populations that had low selenium concentrations. Meta-analysis of the pooled data (N = 583) showed that selenium supplementation was associated with a significant reduction in the number of infants with sepsis (summary RR 0.73 [0.57 to 0.93]; RD −0.10 [−0.17 to −0.02]; NNT 10 [5.9 to 50]). Supplementation with selenium was not associated with improved survival or with reduction in neonatal chronic lung disease or retinopathy of prematurity. The role of selenium supplementation is unclear, although it might be considered in areas where soil selenium levels are extremely low.

REDUCTION OF OXIDATIVE STRESS: MELATONIN

Melatonin reduces oxidative stress from toxic free radicals in animals and there are theoretical reasons that it might be helpful in sepsis.[47] Melatonin has been used in one nonrandomized clinical trial in which 10 neonates with sepsis given oral melatonin had lower serum levels of free radicals and all survived, compared with survival of 7 of 10 control infants with sepsis.[48] RCTs are warranted.

GLUTAMINE

Endogenous biosynthesis of glutamine may be insufficient for tissue needs in states of metabolic stress. Trials in critically ill adults suggest that glutamine supplementation improves clinical outcomes. It has been postulated that glutamine supplementation may benefit preterm infants, particularly very low birth weight infants. A Cochrane systematic review found seven good quality trials of glutamine supplementation, three enteral and four parenteral, involving 2365 very low birth weight neonates.[11] Glutamine supplementation had no statistically significant effect on mortality: RR 0.98 (95% CI, 0.80 to 1.20); RD 0.00 (95% CI, −0.03 to −0.02). In addition, glutamine supplementation had no statistically significant effect on other neonatal morbidities including invasive infection, NEC, or neurodevelopment at 18 months. The available data from good quality RCTs do not support glutamine supplementation to prevent sepsis in preterm infants.

LACTOFERRIN

Lactoferrin is a glycoprotein found mainly in human colostrum and to a lesser extent in human milk, tears, saliva, seminal fluid, and neutrophils. It forms part of the innate immune response to infection and has broad-spectrum antimicrobial activity against bacteria, fungi, viruses, and protozoa. Antimicrobial activity may be caused by either sequestration of iron or a direct effect on microbial cell membranes. Acid proteolysis of lactoferrin (eg, in the stomach or in neutrophil phagolysosomes) yields peptides called "lactoferricins" with enhanced antimicrobial activity. Lactoferrin inhibits the growth of *Streptococcus epidermidis* and *Candida albicans* in vitro, and lactoferrin and lactoferricins are highly effective against antibiotic-resistant *Klebsiella* species and *Staphylococcus aureus* in vitro. Lactoferrin is effective in animal models of systemic and intestinal infection. A Cochrane systematic review found no eligible studies of lactoferrin in treatment of sepsis neonates.[49] In a recent three-arm RCT in 472 very low birth weight infants, however, which compared prophylaxis with bovine lactoferrin alone, with bovine lactoferrin in combination with a probiotic (*Lactobacillus rhamnosus* GG) versus placebo, lactoferrin, alone and in combination with *L rhamnosus* GG, substantially reduced late-onset sepsis.[12] A large multicenter RCT to confirm these findings, and to assess the effects of lactoferrin on disability-free survival in preterm infants, is being planned.

PROBIOTICS AND PREBIOTICS

Probiotic bacteria are defined as live microbial supplements that colonize the gut and provide health benefits to the host.[50] The establishment of a normal microbiota in the neonatal period is crucial to the development of the intestinal mucosal immune system.[51] In babies born after normal birth at term, the gut is colonized with probiotic organisms from the mother, such as lactobacilli and bifidobacteria, which upregulate local and systemic immunity, increase anti-inflammatory cytokines, decrease the permeability of the gut to bacteria and toxins, and suppress pathogens associated with NEC. Preterm neonates often have aberrant intestinal colonization. In a systematic review of six studies on bacterial intestinal colonization of preterm infants, Westerbeek and colleagues[52] found that there are low numbers of bifidobacteria and lactobacilli in the feces of preterm infants, whereas potentially pathogenic bacteria, such as *Escherichia coli*, *Bacteroides*, enterococci, and streptococci, are found in large numbers. Pathogenic bacteria, such as clostridia, staphylococci, pseudomonas, and klebsiella, are found in variable numbers. Pathogenic intestinal bacteria are more likely to translocate to the bloodstream and regional lymph nodes.[53] Probiotics have been shown to increase phagocytic capacity[53–56]; increase natural killer cell activity[57,58]; stimulate IgA production[59–61]; increase cell-mediated immunity[62]; and promote the production of a variety of cytokines (IL-6, IL-8, IL-1β, TNF-α, IL-15) in the intestine.[57,63–66] Probiotics also inhibit the transmigration of bacteria and competitively inhibit pathogenic bacteria.[67,68] Many of these effects are strain-specific.

A systematic review of seven RCTs of probiotics versus control in 1393 newborn infants showed no difference in the incidence of sepsis, but substantial reductions in all-cause mortality and in NEC.[13] A subsequent Cochrane meta-analysis evaluated nine eligible trials in which 1425 newborn infants were randomized to receive probiotics or control supplements.[14] Data for culture-proved nosocomial sepsis were available for 1284 infants. Overall, there was no evidence of significant reduction of sepsis by probiotics (typical RR 0.93 [95% CI, 0.73 to 1.19]). None of the individual studies included in the Cochrane meta-analysis demonstrated a significant reduction of sepsis, although the study by Lin and colleagues[69] did show a trend (RR 0.63 [95% CI, 0.39 to 1.04]). A more recent study conducted by Lin and colleagues[70] showed a trend toward an increased incidence of culture-proved sepsis (RR 1.67 [95% CI, 1.04 to 2.67]), whereas a smaller trial showed a significant decline in the incidence of sepsis (RR 0.48 [95% CI, 0.27 to 0.88]).[71] An updated systematic review that included the two eligible trials published after the Cochrane review found no evidence of reduction of sepsis (typical RR 0.97 [95% CI, 0.80 to 1.19]).[15,72]

It is difficult to pinpoint any specific reasons for the difference in the studies by Lin and colleagues[69] and Samanta and colleagues,[71] and the rest of the studies included in the meta-analysis. Whether the difference in reduction of sepsis is attributable to the strain of probiotics used, the baseline sepsis rate, the concurrent use of human milk, or random error is speculative. Current probiotic products are safe and effective in reducing all-cause mortality and NEC by over half (P <0.00001), with no increase in sepsis.[13–15,68,69,70] This makes further RCTs with a placebo group ethically problematic.[70] Probiotics are different from conventional drugs; there are many types and optimum production, transport, dosage, and contra-indications are unclear. There are also theoretical concerns that probiotics could enhance transfer of antibiotic resistance genes. However, large RCTs comparing multiple probiotic regimens and Phase IV surveillance will address these issues more reliably than two-arm placebo RCTs.[70] A commentary from the European Society of Paediatric Gastroenterology, Hepatology and Nutrition Committee on Nutrition did not recommend probiotics for preterm infants,[71] but was submitted for publication before the most recent evidence became available.[13–15,68–70]

Human milk contains nondigestible prebiotic components which promote the growth of non-pathogenic, probiotic flora including bifidobacteria and lactobacilli in the colon. Prebiotics (commonly oligosaccharides) added to infant feeds might prevent death, NEC, death and allergy but current evidence is inconclusive.[71,72] A large RCT of prebiotic supplements versus probiotics on mortality, NEC, growth, allergy, and long term outcome is needed in preterm and term newborns fed with formula and/or breast milk. Large RCTs of prebiotic plus probiotic (synbiotics) versus probiotics or prebiotics will be informative.

BROAD-SPECTRUM ANTIBIOTICS

The first organisms ingested into the gut induce gene expression in the epithelium to gain an advantage in colonization over competing organisms that arrive later.[74] For example, probiotics given perinatally have been shown to persist in some infants for months or years,[75] whereas probiotics administered after 6 months persisted only transiently.[76] Two mechanisms postulated to explain this are that the initial colonizing organisms induce epithelial cells to synthesize a protective biofilm within the luminal glycocalyx, and induce Paneth cells to synthesize antibacterial proteins, such as defensins, matrilysin, and phospholipase A_2, which act against competing organisms.[74,77,78] The administration of broad-spectrum antibiotics to neonatal rats eradicates normal populations of commensal bacteria in the intestine and downregulates genes expressing major histocompatibility II molecules.[78] This parallels findings in germ-free neonatal mice,[79] in which expression of major histocompatibility molecules is also downregulated, supporting the concept that bacterial colonization with commensal bacteria is important for normal maturation of immune function in the gut. In newborn infants, broad-spectrum antibiotic treatment in the perinatal period may deplete commensal populations in the gut; alter the normal maturation of intestinal immune and barrier function; and promote persistent colonization by gram-negative pathogens, predisposing to infection and inflammatory disease.[74]

In a large RCT, antenatal treatment of women at risk of preterm birth with up to ten days of broad-spectrum antibiotics increased the risks of NEC in infants after preterm rupture of membranes[18] and of cerebral palsy in infants after preterm labor with intact membranes.[19] In a risk-adjusted cohort study of 5693 extremely low birth weight infants, prolonged antibiotic therapy after sterile initial cultures was associated with increased risks of NEC and death.[20] This underlines the need to curtail antibiotic therapy when cultures are negative.

BREAST MILK

Lack of breast milk may be the commonest immunodeficiency of infancy.[80] In a RCT in 62 low birth weight infants, expressed human milk reduced the incidence of infection compared with formula.[21] Early human milk is rich in a variety of immune, nonimmune, and anti-inflammatory components that may accelerate intestinal maturation, resistance to infection, and epithelial recovery from infection.[80]

Breast milk provides secretory IgA antibodies against the microbial flora of the mother and her environment. These antibodies bind microbes on the infant's mucosal surfaces, preventing proinflammatory activation. The milk protein lactoferrin can destroy microbes and modulate inflammatory responses. The nonabsorbed milk oligosaccharides (also known as "prebiotics") block attachment of microbes to the infant's mucosal surfaces, preventing infection, and provide nutrients that promote the growth of commensal organisms in the gut. The breast milk cytokine IL-7 may explain why the thymus is larger and why development of intestinal T$\gamma\delta$ lymphocytes is enhanced in breastfed versus non-breastfed infants.[80] Total protein and immunoglobulin levels in breast milk decrease markedly over the first days of life: concentrations are highest on day 1, halve by day 2, and slowly decrease thereafter.[23] This may explain why in a less developed country initiation of breastfeeding within an hour of birth was associated with a 22% reduction in mortality compared with later initiation of breastfeeding.[23] A large RCT of the effect of earlier introduction of colostrum in preterm infants on disability-free survival would be valuable.

These and other mechanisms may explain the strong inverse associations between breast milk and (1) gastroenteritis, septicemia, meningitis, and NEC in low birth weight or preterm infants[21,25,26]; (2) mortality from gastroenteritis and respiratory illness in all infants in less developed countries[23,25,81]; and (3) gastroenteritis and atopic disease[20] in all infants.

IVIG

Newborn infants have immunoglobulin and complement deficiencies, particularly those born before 32 weeks gestation, when very little maternal IgG has crossed the placenta to the fetus. The rationale for prophylaxis or treatment of neonatal infections with polyclonal IVIG is that IgG, by its proinflammatory actions, can bind to cell surface receptors, provide opsonic activity, activate complement, promote antibody-dependent cytotoxicity, and improve neutrophil chemoluminescence.[27] IVIG also has a broad array of other immunomodulatory effects. It modulates the cytokine cascade, downregulates the IL-1 system, blocks Fc-receptors on phagocytic cells, and modulates Fc receptor expression. It has a cytoprotective effect on TNF-α–induced cell death in fibroblasts and can regulate B-cell differentiation, immunoglobulin production, and CD8-mediated suppressor or cytotoxic T-cell function. IVIG has been shown to reduce infiltration of neutrophils in inflamed tissues and reduce C3 activation and complement-mediated inflammation.[82] High-dose polyclonal IVIG is effective in the treatment of several inflammatory disorders of the nervous system in adults.[83,84] Neurodevelopmental impairment and disability-free survival are important measures of outcome in RCTs of IVIG in newborn infants.

THERAPEUTIC RCTS USING POLYCLONAL IVIG

In a systematic review of RCTs of treatment of suspected or proved clinical sepsis in newborns of all gestations, Ohlsson and Lacy[27] found six studies (N = 318) that reported mortality from any cause. They showed a reduction in mortality of borderline statistical significance (typical RR 0.63 [95% CI, 0.40 to 1.00]; typical RD −0.09 [95% CI, 0.00 to −0.17]; $P = .05$). There was no statistically significant heterogeneity between studies for this outcome ($I^2 = 0\%$). A total of 262 newborns with subsequently proved infection were enrolled in seven RCTs to evaluate the effectiveness of IVIG versus placebo or no treatment to prevent mortality. Treatment with IVIG resulted in a statistically significant reduction in mortality in cases of subsequently proved infection (typical RR 0.55 [95% CI, 0.31 to 0.98]; $P = .04$). This marginal benefit, however, is of limited value. Furthermore, IVIG is an expensive product.

In another systematic review, Alejandria and colleagues[28] found no difference in mortality in a subgroup analysis of five therapeutic RCTs of polyclonal IVIG in 241 newborn infants. Neither systematic review included measures of neurodevelopmental impairment as outcomes. Polyclonal IVIG containing pentameric IgM has been postulated to confer superior toxin neutralization and bacterial agglutination and to reduce mortality in gram-negative septic shock in all age groups.[85] Two RCTs in newborn infants, however, did not show a difference in mortality.[30,31]

Publication bias and other forms of selection bias are a major concern when interpreting meta-analyses of RCTs. In a systematic review of 14 RCTs in critically ill adults with severe sepsis and septic shock, IVIG was associated with a substantial and highly significant reduction in the odds of mortality (odds ratio 0.66; 95% CI, 0.53 to 0.83; $P<.0005$).[86] There was significant heterogeneity, however, between trials ($I^2 = 53.8$). The funnel plot was strikingly asymmetric, suggesting that the apparent benefit of IVIG was explained by a preponderance of smaller trials. When the meta-analysis was restricted to larger, high-quality RCTs, the treatment benefit was lost (odds ratio 0.96; 95% CI, 0.71 to 1.3; $P = .78$). This raises the possibility that the smaller trials may not have been truly representative of all trials performed, or may have overestimated the true treatment effect.

Further information will be available from the International Neonatal Immunotherapy Study, a placebo-controlled RCT of polyclonal IVIG that has recruited 3493 newborn infants with suspected or proved infection. The primary outcome is survival or major disability at 2 years corrected for gestation.[32]

PROPHYLACTIC RCTS OF POLYCLONAL IVIG

A systematic review of 16 RCTs of prophylactic polyclonal IVIG in 4986 preterm or very low birth weight infants demonstrated a 4% risk difference in one or more episodes of any serious infection (RR 0.82 [95% CI, 0.74 to 0.92]; $P = .0005$), but no reductions in mortality, NEC, intraventricular haemorrhage, or length of hospital stay.[29] Prophylactic IVIG was not associated with any short-term serious side effects. There was significant heterogeneity between studies ($I^2 = 50\%$). The reduction in serious infection, with no difference in other adverse outcomes, was of marginal clinical significance.

ANTISTAPHYLOCOCCAL IVIG TO PREVENT STAPHYLOCOCCAL INFECTION IN VERY LOW BIRTH WEIGHT INFANTS

Staphylococci, especially coagulase-negative staphylococci, are responsible for over 75% of late-onset infections in very low birth weight infants. These infections increase length of hospital stay, the cost of medical care, and mortality. Recently, IVIG preparations containing various type-specific antibodies targeted at different antigenic markers of staphylococcus have been developed. These include INH-A21 (or Veronate) (antibody against "microbial surface components recognizing adhesive matrix molecules") and Altastaph (antibody against capsular polysaccharide antigen type 5 and 8). A systematic review[33,87,88] of three RCTs of antistaphylococcal IVIG showed no difference in sepsis, mortality, or other adverse outcomes in two RCTs of HNA1 (Veronate) versus placebo (N = 2488) (RR 1.07 [95% CI, 0.94 to 1.22]) and in a RCT of Altastaph versus placebo (N = 206) (RR 0.86 [95% CI, 0.32 to 2.28]). Further RCTs of antistaphylococcal IVIG are in progress or await publication.

SUMMARY

Few immunologic interventions to treat or prevent neonatal sepsis have been reliably evaluated in RCTs, because of inadequate sample sizes. Promising or possible therapeutic interventions in severe or gram-negative sepsis include exchange transfusions, pentoxifylline, and IgM-enriched IVIG. Promising or possible prophylactic interventions include lactoferrin, with or without a probiotic; selenium; early curtailment of antibiotics after sterile cultures; and earlier initiation of breast milk (colostrum) in high-risk preterm infants. Current probiotic products are safe and effective in substantially reducing all-cause mortality and NEC, with no increase in sepsis. International collaboration is essential in achieving adequate samples to reliably assess reductions in disability-free survival.

REFERENCES

1. Tarnow-Mordi WO, Healy MJ. Distinguishing between "no evidence of effect" and "evidence of no effect" in randomised controlled trials and other comparisons. Arch Dis Child 1999;80(3):210–1.
2. Brok J, Thorlund K, Wetterslev J, et al. Apparently conclusive meta-analyses may be inconclusive: trial sequential analysis adjustment of random error risk due to

repetitive testing of accumulating data in apparently conclusive neonatal meta-analyses. Int J Epidemiol 2009;38(1):287–98.

3. Mohan P, Brocklehurst P. Granulocyte transfusions for neonates with confirmed or suspected sepsis and neutropaenia. Cochrane Database Syst Rev 2003;4: CD003956.DOI:10.1002/14651858.

4. Carr R, Modi N, Doré CJ. G-CSF and GM-CSF for treating or preventing neonatal infections. Cochrane Database Syst Rev 2003;3:CD003066.DOI:10.1002/14651858.

5. Carr R, Brocklehurst P, Doré CJ, et al. Granulocyte-macrophage colony stimulating factor administered as prophylaxis for reduction of sepsis in extremely preterm, small for gestational age neonates (the PROGRAMS trial): a single-blind, multicentre, randomised controlled trial. Lancet 2009;373:226–33.

6. Carr R, Modi N, Doré CJ, et al. A randomised controlled trial of prophylactic GM-CSF in human newborns less than 32 weeks gestation. Pediatrics 1999;103:796–802.

7. Vain NE, Mazlumian JR, Swarner OW, et al. Role of exchange transfusion in the treatment of severe septicemia. Pediatrics 1980;66:693–7.

8. Sadana S, Mathur NB, Thakur A. Exchange transfusion in septic neonates with sclerema: effect on immunoglobulin and complement levels. Indian Pediatr 1997;34:20–5.

9. Haque KN, Mohan P. Pentoxifylline for treatment of sepsis and necrotizing enterocolitis in neonates. Cochrane Database Syst Rev 2003;2:CD004205.DOI: 10.1002/14651858.

10. Darlow BA, Austin N. Selenium supplementation to prevent short-term morbidity in preterm neonates. Cochrane Database Syst Rev 2003;4:CD003312.DOI: 10.1002/14651858.

11. Tubman RTRJ, Thompson S, McGuire W. Glutamine supplementation to prevent morbidity and mortality in preterm infants. Cochrane Database Syst Rev 2008;1: CD001457. DOI:10.1002/14651858.

12. Manzoni P, Rinaldi M, Cattani S, et al. Italian Task Force for the Study and Prevention of Neonatal Fungal Infections, Italian Society of Neonatology. Bovine lactoferrin supplementation for prevention of late-onset sepsis in very low-birth-weight neonates: a randomized trial. JAMA 2009;302(13):1421–8.

13. Deshpande G, Rao S, Patole S. Probiotics for prevention of necrotising enterocolitis in preterm neonates with very low birthweight: a systematic review of randomised controlled trials. Lancet 2007;369(9573):1614.

14. Alfaleh K, Bassler D. Probiotics for prevention of necrotizing enterocolitis in preterm infants. Cochrane Database Syst Rev 2008;1:CD005496.

15. Deshpande G, Rao S, Patole S. Updated systematic review and meta analysis of probiotics supplementation in preterm very low birth weight neonates- do we need more trials? Pediatrics, in press

16. Srinivasjois R, Rao S, Patole S. Prebiotic supplementation of formula in preterm neonates: a systematic review and meta-analysis of randomised controlled trials. Clin Nutr 2009;28:237–42.

17. Osborn DA, Sinn JKH, Patole S. Prebiotics in infants for prevention of allergic disease and food hypersensitivity. Cochrane Database Syst Rev 2007;4: CD006474. DOI:10.1002/14651858.CD006474.pub2.

18. Kenyon SL, Taylor DJ, Tarnow-Mordi W, et al. Broad-spectrum antibiotics for preterm, prelabour rupture of fetal membranes: the ORACLE I randomised trial. ORACLE Collaborative Group. Lancet 2001;357(9261):979–88.

19. Kenyon S, Pike K, Jones DR, et al. Childhood outcomes after prescription of antibiotics to pregnant women with spontaneous preterm labour: 7-year follow-up of the ORACLE II trial. Lancet 2008;372(9646):1319–27.

20. Cotten CM, Taylor S, Stoll B, et al. NICHD Neonatal Research Network. Prolonged duration of initial empirical antibiotic treatment is associated with increased rates of necrotizing enterocolitis and death for extremely low birth weight infants. Pediatrics 2009;123(1):58–66.

21. Narayanan I, Prakash K, Gujral VV. The value of human milk in the prevention of infection in the high-risk low-birth-weight infant. J Pediatr 1981;99(3):496–8.

22. Kramer MS, Chalmers B, Hodnett ED, et al. PROBIT Study Group (Promotion of Breastfeeding Intervention Trial). Promotion of Breastfeeding Intervention Trial (PROBIT): a randomized trial in the Republic of Belarus. JAMA 2001;285(4): 413–20.

23. Edmond KM, Zandoh C, Quigley MA, et al. Delayed breastfeeding initiation increases risk of neonatal mortality. Pediatrics 2006;117(3):e380–6.

24. WHO Collaborative Study Team on the Role of Breastfeeding on the Prevention of Infant Mortality. Effect of breastfeeding on infant and child mortality due to infectious diseases in less developed countries: a pooled analysis. Lancet 2000;355: 451–5.

25. Lucas A, Cole TJ. Breast milk and neonatal necrotising enterocolitis. Lancet 1990; 336(8730):1519–23.

26. Hylander MA, Strobino DM, Dhanireddy R. Human milk feedings and infection among very low birth weight infants. Pediatrics 1998;102(3):E38.

27. Ohlsson A, Lacy JB. Intravenous immunoglobulin for suspected or subsequently proven infection in neonates. Cochrane Database Syst Rev. 2004;1:CD001239.

28. Alejandria MM, Lansang MA, Dans LF, et al. Intravenous immunoglobulin for treating sepsis and septic shock. Cochrane Database Syst Rev. 2002;1: CD001090.

29. Ohlsson A, Lacy J. Intravenous immunoglobulin for preventing infection in preterm and/or low birth weight infants. Cochrane Database Syst Rev 2004;1: CD000361. DOI:10.1002/14651858.

30. Haque KN, Zaidi MH, Bahakim H. IgM-enriched intravenous immunoglobulin therapy in neonatal sepsis. Am J Dis Child 1988;142:1293–6.

31. Erdem G, Yurdakok M, Gulsevin T, et al. The use of IgM-enriched intravenous immunoglobulin for the treatment of neonatal sepsis in preterm infants. Turk J Pediatr 1993;35:277–81.

32. INIS Study Collaborative Group. International Neonatal Immunotherapy Study: non-specific intravenous immunoglobulin therapy for suspected or proven neonatal sepsis: an international, placebo controlled, multicentre randomised trial. BMC Pregnancy Childbirth 2008;8:52.

33. Shah PS, Kaufman DA. Antistaphylococcal immunoglobulins to prevent staphylococcal infection in very low birth weight infants. Cochrane Database Syst Rev 2009;2:CD006449. DOI:10.1002/14651858.

34. Rodwell RL, Taylor KM, Tudehope DI, et al. Hematologic scoring system in early diagnosis of sepsis in neutropenic newborns. Pediatr Infect Dis J 1993;12:372–6.

35. Cairo MS, Rucker R, Bennetts GA, et al. Improved survival of newborns receiving leukocyte transfusions for sepsis. Pediatrics 1984;74:887–92.

36. Cairo MS, Worcester CC, Rucker RW, et al. Randomized trial of granulocyte transfusions versus intravenous immune globulin therapy for neonatal neutropenia and sepsis. J Pediatr 1992;120:281–5.

37. Bernard GR, Vincent JL, Laterre PF, et al. Recombinant human protein C Worldwide Evaluation in Severe Sepsis (PROWESS) study group. Efficacy and safety of recombinant human activated protein C for severe sepsis. N Engl J Med 2001; 344:699–709.

38. Bernard GR, Margolis BD, Shanies HM, et al. Extended evaluation of recombinant human activated protein C United States Trial (ENHANCE US): a single-arm, phase 3B, multicenter study of drotrecogin alfa (activated) in severe sepsis. Chest 2004;125:2206–16.
39. Martí-Carvajal AJ, Salanti G, Cardona-Zorrilla AF. Human recombinant activated protein C for severe sepsis. Cochrane Database Syst Rev 2008;1:CD004388. DOI:10.1002/14651858.
40. Nadel S, Goldstein B, Williams MD, et al. Drotrecogin alfa (activated) in children with severe sepsis: a multicentre phase III randomised controlled trial. Lancet 2007;369:836–43.
41. Kylat RI, Ohlsson A. Recombinant human activated protein C for severe sepsis in neonates. Cochrane Database Syst Rev 2006;2:CD005385. DOI:10.1002/14651858.
42. Mathur NB, Subramanian BK, Sharma VK, et al. Exchange transfusion in neutropenic septicemic neonates: effect on granulocyte functions. Acta Paediatr 1993; 82:939–43.
43. Gunes T, Koklu E, Buyukkayhan D, et al. Exchange transfusion or intravenous immunoglobulin therapy as an adjunct to antibiotics for neonatal sepsis in developing countries: a pilot study. Ann Trop Paediatr 2006;26:39–42.
44. Michetti C, Coimbra R, Hoyt DB, et al. Pentoxifylline reduces acute lung injury in chronic endotoxemia. J Surg Res 2003;115:92–9.
45. Travadi J, Patole S, Charles A, et al. Pentoxifylline reduces the incidence and severity of necrotizing enterocolitis in a neonatal rat model. Pediatr Res 2006;60:185–9.
46. Rayman MP. The importance of selenium to human health. Lancet 2000;356: 233–41.
47. Gitto E, Pellegrino S, Gitto P, et al. Oxidative stress of the newborn in the pre- and postnatal period and the clinical utility of melatonin. J Pineal Res 2009; 46:128–39.
48. Gitto E, Karbownik M, Reiter RJ, et al. Effects of melatonin treatment in septic newborns. Pediatr Res 2001;50:756–60.
49. Mohan P, Abrams SA. Oral lactoferrin for the treatment of sepsis and necrotizing enterocolitis in neonates. Cochrane Database Syst Rev 2009;1:CD007138. DOI: 10.1002/14651858.
50. Fuller R. Probiotics in man and animals. J Appl Bacteriol 1989;66:365–78.
51. Delcenserie V, Martel D, Lamoureux M, et al. Immunomodulatory effects of probiotics in the intestinal tract. Curr Issues Mol Biol 2008;10:37–54.
52. Westerbeek EA, van den BA, Lafeber HN, et al. The intestinal bacterial colonisation in preterm infants: a review of the literature. Clin Nutr 2006;25:361–8.
53. Lichtman SM. Bacterial translocation in humans. J Pediatr Gastroenterol Nutr 2001;33:1–10.
54. Arunachalam K, Gill HS, Chandra RK. Enhancement of natural immune function by dietary consumption of Bifidobacterium lactis (HN019). Eur J Clin Nutr 2000;54:263–7.
55. Donnet-Hughes A, Rochat F, Serrant P, et al. Modulation of nonspecific mechanisms of defense by lactic acid bacteria: effective dose. J Dairy Sci 1999;82: 863–9.
56. Schiffrin EJ, Brassart D, Servin AL, et al. Immune modulation of blood leukocytes in humans by lactic acid bacteria: criteria for strain selection. Am J Clin Nutr 1997;66:515S–20S.
57. Ogawa T, Asai Y, Tamai R, et al. Natural killer cell activities of symbiotic *Lactobacillus casei ssp.* casei in conjunction with Dextran. Clin Exp Immunol 2006;143: 103–9.

58. Sheih YH, Chiang BL, Wang LH, et al. Systemic immunity-enhancing effects in healthy subjects following dietary consumption of the lactic acid bacterium *Lactobacillus rhamnosus* HN001. J Am Coll Nutr 2001;20:149–56.

59. Fukushima Y, Kawata Y, Hara H, et al. Effect of a probiotic formula on intestinal immunoglobulin A production in healthy children. Int J Food Microbiol 1998;42: 39–44.

60. Park JH, Um JI, Lee BJ, et al. Encapsulated *Bifidobacterium bifidum* potentiates intestinal IgA production. Cell Immunol 2002;219:22–7.

61. Mohan R, Koebnick C, Schildt J, et al. Effects of *Bifidobacterium lactis* Bb12 supplementation on body weight, fecal pH, acetate, lactate, calprotectin, and IgA in preterm infants. Pediatr Res 2008;64:418–22.

62. de Waard R, Claassen E, Bokken GC, et al. Enhanced immunological memory responses to *Listeria monocytogenes* in rodents, as measured by delayed-type hypersensitivity (DTH), adoptive transfer of DTH, and protective immunity, following *Lactobacillus casei* Shirota ingestion. Clin Diagn Lab Immunol 2003; 10:59–65.

63. Haller D, Bode C, Hammes WP, et al. Non-pathogenic bacteria elicit a differential cytokine response by intestinal epithelial cell/leucocyte co-cultures. Gut 2000;47: 79–87.

64. Lammers KM, Helwig U, Swennen E, et al. Effect of probiotic strains on interleukin 8 production by HT29/19A cells. Am J Gastroenterol 2002;97:1182–6.

65. Ruiz PA, Hoffmann M, Szcesny S, et al. Innate mechanisms for *Bifidobacterium lactis* to activate transient pro-inflammatory host responses in intestinal epithelial cells after the colonization of germ-free rats. Immunology 2005;115:441–50.

66. Zhang L, Li N, Caicedo R, et al. Alive and dead *Lactobacillus rhamnosus* GG decrease tumor necrosis factor-alpha-induced interleukin-8 production in Caco-2 cells. J Nutr 2005;135:1752–6.

67. Mattar AF, Drongowski RA, Coran AG, et al. Effect of probiotics on enterocyte bacterial translocation in vitro. Pediatr Surg Int 2001;17:265–8.

68. Reid G, Howard J, Gan BS. Can bacterial interference prevent infection? Trends Microbiol 2001;9:424–8.

69. Lin HC, Su BH, Chen AC, et al. Oral probiotics reduce the incidence and severity of necrotizing enterocolitis in very low birth weight infants. Pediatrics 2005;115:1–4.

70. Lin HC, Hsu CH, Chen HL, et al. Oral probiotics prevent necrotizing enterocolitis in very low birth weight preterm infants: a multicenter, randomized, controlled trial. Pediatrics 2008;122:693–700.

71. Samanta M, Sarkar M, Ghosh P, et al. Prophylactic probiotics for prevention of necrotizing enterocolitis in very low birth weight newborns. J Trop Pediatr 2009; 55:128–31.

72. Tarnow-Mordi WO, Wilkinson D, Trivedi A, et al. Probiotics reduce all-cause mortality and necrotizing enterocolitis: it is time to change practice. Pediatrics, in press.

73. Agostoni C, Buonocore G, Carnielli VP, et al. ESPGHAN Committee on Nutrition. Enteral nutrient supply for preterm infants: commentary from the European Society of Paediatric Gastroenterology, Hepatology and Nutrition Committee on Nutrition. J Pediatr Gastroenterol Nutr 2010;50(1):85–91.

74. Bedford Russell AR, Murch SH. Could peripartum antibiotics have delayed health consequences for the infant? BJOG 2006;113(7):758–65.

75. Kalliomäki M, Salminen S, Poussa T, et al. Probiotics and prevention of atopic disease: 4-year follow-up of a randomised placebo-controlled trial. Lancet 2003;361(9372):1869–71.

76. Heilig HG, Zoetendal EG, Vaughan EE, et al. Molecular diversity of *Lactobacillus spp.* and other lactic acid bacteria in the human intestine as determined by specific amplification of 16S ribosomal DNA. Appl Environ Microbiol 2002; 68(1):114–23.

77. Sonnenburg JL, Angenent LT, Gordon JI. Getting a grip on things: how do communities of bacterial symbionts become established in our intestine? Nat Immunol 2004;5(6):569–73.

78. Schumann A, Nutten S, Donnicola D, et al. Neonatal antibiotic treatment alters gastrointestinal tract developmental gene expression and intestinal barrier transcriptome. Physiol Genomics 2005;23(2):235–45.

79. Matsumoto S, Setoyama H, Umesaki Y. Differential induction of major histocompatibility complex molecules on mouse intestine by bacterial colonization. Gastroenterology 1992;103:1777–82.

80. Hanson LA. Session 1: feeding and infant development breast-feeding and immune function. Proc Nutr Soc 2007;66(3):384–96.

81. Darmstadt GL, Bhutta ZA, Cousens S, et al. Evidence-based, cost-effective interventions: how many newborn babies can we save? Lancet 2005;365:977–88.

82. Mohan PV, Tarnow-Mordi W, Stenson B, et al. Can polyclonal intravenous immunoglobulin limit cytokine mediated cerebral damage and chronic lung disease in preterm infants? Arch Dis Child Fetal Neonatal Ed 2004;89(1):F5–8.

83. Eftimov F, Winer JB, Vermeulen M, et al. Intravenous immunoglobulin for chronic inflammatory demyelinating polyradiculoneuropathy. Cochrane Database Syst Rev 2009;1:CD001797.

84. Elovaara I, Apostolski S, van Doorn P, et al. EFNS guidelines for the use of intravenous immunoglobulin in treatment of neurological diseases: EFNS task force on the use of intravenous immunoglobulin in treatment of neurological diseases. Eur J Neurol 2008;15(9):893–908.

85. Norrby-Teglund A, Haque KN, Hammarström L. Intravenous polyclonal IgM-enriched immunoglobulin therapy in sepsis: a review of clinical efficacy in relation to microbiological aetiology and severity of sepsis. J Intern Med 2006;260(6): 509–16.

86. Laupland KB, Kirkpatrick AW, Delaney A. Polyclonal intravenous immunoglobulin for the treatment of severe sepsis and septic shock in critically ill adults: a systematic review and meta-analysis. Crit Care Med 2007;35(12):2686–92.

87. De Angelis CD, Drazen JM, Frizelle FA, et al. Clinical trial registration: a statement from the International Committee of Medical Journal Editors. N Engl J Med 2004; 352:1250–1.

88. Baigent C, Keech A, Kearney PM, et al. Efficacy and safety of cholesterol-lowering treatment: prospective meta-analysis of data from 90,056 participants in 14 randomised trials of statins. Lancet 2005;366(9493):1267–78.

International Perspective on Early-Onset Neonatal Sepsis

Hammad A. Ganatra, MBBS[a], Barbara J. Stoll, MD[b],
Anita K.M. Zaidi, MBBS, SM[a],*

KEYWORDS

- Neonate • Sepsis • Infection • Early-onset
- Developing countries

Global neonatal mortality continues to be unacceptably high, with 4 million neonatal deaths each year.[1] Of these, 99% occur in the developing world, with South Asia and sub-Saharan Africa having the highest burden.[2] Of the several contributors to neonatal mortality, infections form the single largest cause of death, responsible for an estimated 35% of all neonatal deaths.[3] The early neonatal period, which extends from birth to the seventh day of life, is the most dangerous period for a neonate, with increased risk of morbidity and mortality from perinatal causes, including birth asphyxia, prematurity, and infection. Three-fourths of the 4 million neonatal deaths occur during this period,[2] underscoring the importance of interventions, including measures to prevent and manage infections in the early neonatal period, as a means to reducing neonatal mortality worldwide.

DEFINITION OF EARLY-ONSET NEONATAL SEPSIS

The term, *neonatal sepsis*, has been traditionally defined as bacteremia accompanied by hemodynamic compromise and systemic signs of infection.[4] The literature on neonatal sepsis is confused by the inclusion of the entity clinical sepsis, meaning, in developed countries, significant symptoms or laboratory abnormalities, suggesting sepsis with a negative blood culture. In resource-poor countries, blood cultures and adjunct laboratory tests are often not possible and the diagnosis of neonatal sepsis is often based solely on clinical signs. The signs of sepsis in the neonate are often

[a] Department of Pediatrics and Child Health, Aga Khan University, Stadium Road, PO Box 3500, Karachi 74800, Pakistan
[b] Department of Pediatrics, Emory University School of Medicine, 2040 Ridgewood Drive, Atlanta, GA 30322, USA
* Corresponding author.
E-mail address: anita.zaidi@aku.edu

Clin Perinatol 37 (2010) 501–523
doi:10.1016/j.clp.2010.02.004
0095-5108/10/$ – see front matter © 2010 Elsevier Inc. All rights reserved.
perinatology.theclinics.com

nonspecific and include lethargy or irritability, poor feeding, vomiting, jaundice, respiratory distress, apnea, fever, or hypothermia.[4–6] These symptoms overlap with those of perinatal asphyxia and with normal findings in preterm infants, further complicating the diagnosis. Furthermore, neonatal pneumonia and meningitis may be included within the term, neonatal sepsis, particularly in the developing world where microbiology laboratories are not available. In addition, the clinical syndromes overlap and pneumonia and meningitis are variably accompanied by bacteremia.

Neonatal sepsis is generally divided into early-onset neonatal sepsis (EONS) and late-onset neonatal sepsis (LONS). The cutoff for these definitions is variable throughout the literature. EONS is typically defined as sepsis occurring within the first 3 or 7 days after birth. Seven days is typically used for GBS sepsis; 3 days is more commonly used in epidemiologic studies. Depending on the parameters defining EONS, LONS occurs as early as 4 or 8 days after birth and as late as 28 days after birth. Again, there are variations in the timing of onset used to define LONS, particularly in epidemiologic surveys of neonatal intensive care units, because very low-birth-weight preterm infants often develop sepsis beyond the traditionally defined neonatal period of 28 days from birth. The designation of EONS or LONS is important because it implies particular routes of infection and organisms and thus can help to guide therapy. EONS is associated with maternal risk factors and acquisition of pathogens from the birth canal whereas LONS is associated with infection with environmental pathogens acquired in the home or hospital settings.[4] The distinction between EONS and LONS routes of infection and pathogens does not necessarily hold true in the developing world, where unsanitary birth practices and newborn care at home or in hospitals expose newborns to the risk of acquiring environmental pathogens at or soon after birth.[7]

This review identifies the burden and risk factors of EONS with a focus on developing countries and discusses evidence-based preventive and treatment strategies. Developing countries are defined by the World Bank as those with low or middle levels of gross national income up to $11,905 per capita as of this writing.[8] Also included in this review is a discussion of the global burden of tetanus, omphalitis, and pneumonia in the early neonatal period. Other pathogens causing infections in the newborn, such as viral infections, nosocomial infections, tuberculosis, and congenital syphilis, are beyond the scope of this review.

GLOBAL BURDEN OF EONS

Determining the true burden of EONS in the developing world is not an easy task. Most births and deaths in developing countries take place at home and are unrecorded.[9] Assessment of the burden of disease is hampered by limited community-based surveillance and inadequate laboratory resources to identify EONS. Most of the available information comes from Demographic and Health Surveys, which are believed to underreport early neonatal deaths.[10] Accurate diagnosis of EONS and EONS-related deaths is further complicated by the uncertainties involved in distinguishing the clinical syndrome of sepsis from those of birth asphyxia and prematurity in the early neonatal period.

To determine the global burden of EONS, the authors conducted searches of PubMed and the World Health Organization (WHO) regional databases published between 1990 and 2008 to identify studies reporting EONS rates or case fatality attributed to EONS. The authors' searches identified 108 studies that reported the incidence of neonatal sepsis across the world.[11–118] Few of these studies differentiated early-onset from late-onset sepsis. Only 4 studies from developing countries

serves to guide empiric therapy while awaiting culture and antimicrobial susceptibility results. The longest running database on neonatal sepsis in the developed world has been maintained by the Yale-New Haven Hospital, which has published findings for a 75-year period, from 1928 to 2003.[16] Their findings showed that *Streptococcus pneumoniae* and group A streptococci comprised almost half the cases from 1933 to 1943. The incidence of infections due to *S pneumoniae* or group A streptococci have decreased steadily during the past 15 years and have been replaced by GBS and *Escherichia coli*. The intrapartum use of antibiotics to reduce vertical transmission of GBS, recommended since the 1990s, has contributed to a decline in the percentage of EONS secondary to GBS in recent years.[132] Organisms such as coagulase-negative staphylococci are usually nosocomially acquired and not considered in this review.[133]

Etiologic information on causes of EONS in developing countries is limited. A recent review found 44 studies that reported the causes of EONS in developing countries.[134] Only 4 of these focused on community-acquired infections (the rest were facility-based studies) and, therefore, were not representative of home environments with high neonatal mortality rates. Information on causes of EONS in home-delivered babies was minimal. The limited data available in the review showed that 25% of all episodes of EONS were caused by *Klebsiella*, 15% were caused by *E coli*, 18% were caused by *Staphylococcus aureus*, 7% were caused by GBS, and 12% were caused collectively by *Acinetobacter* and *Pseudomonas* (**Table 1**). The overall ratio of gram-negative organisms to gram-positive organisms was 2:1 in the global data set. In African countries, the ratio of gram-positive organisms to gram-negative organisms was equal, due to a larger proportion of infections caused by *S aureus* and GBS as compared with other regions of the world. *Pseudomonas* and *Acinetobacter* were more common in East Asia, Pacific, and South Asian countries, and *S aureus* was uncommon in East Asia and Latin America as compared with other regions.

Although GBS is one of the predominant organisms causing EONS in developed countries, it was uncommon in developing countries.[134] In developing countries, South Asia had the lowest rates of GBS. The reason for this difference in distribution of GBS between developed and developing countries is not clearly understood. Stoll and Schuchat[135] reviewed 34 studies published between 1980 and 1996 that evaluated GBS colonization rates in women in developing countries. Studies using adequate culture methods found differences in the prevalence of colonization in different regions (Middle East/North Africa, 22%; Asia/Pacific, 19%; sub-Saharan Africa, 19%; Americas, 14%; and India/Pakistan, 12%). Other factors, such as strain virulence, maternally derived antibody levels, or cultural practices, are also thought to contribute to observed differences in GBS rates in different populations.[9] It is also possible that in developing countries, GBS is a very early-onset illness causing death within a few hours of birth, and the lack of information on very early-onset deaths misses the vast majority of GBS cases.

BURDEN OF NEONATAL TETANUS

Neonatal tetanus is predominantly a disease of poorer developing countries where lack of maternal tetanus immunization, unhygienic birth practices, and poor neonatal care continue to contribute to high rates of disease. Tetanus in developing countries usually affects newborns in the early neonatal period before they ever come into contact with a health care worker.[9] Therefore, it is often underreported and the true burden remains unknown. Historically, tetanus was a major cause of neonatal mortality worldwide, with a case fatality rate of 85% if untreated. With the introduction of maternal vaccination with tetanus toxoid in the developed world, neonatal tetanus

Table 1				
Causes of sepsis in neonates up to 7 days of age in developing countries				
	≤3 Days of Life		**≤7 Days of Life**	
Organism Isolated	**N**	**%**	**N**	**%**
Total	834	100	3209	100
Staphylococcus aureus	144	17.3	560	17.5
Streptococcus pyogenes	3	0.4	33	1
GBS	109	13.1	207	6.5
Group D streptococci/Enterococcus	44	5.3	80	2.5
Group G streptococci			1	0.03
Viridans streptococci	3	0.4	5	0.2
Streptococcus pneumoniae	9	1.1	49	1.5
Other Streptococcus species/unspecified	19	2.3	32	1.0
Listeria monocytogenes	4	0.5	5	0.2
Other gram positives			69	2.2
All gram positives	335	40.2	1041	32.4
Klebsiella species	220	26.4	813	25.3
E coli	105	12.6	490	15.3
Pseudomonas species	49	5.9	224	7.0
Enterobacter species	30	3.6	141	4.4
Serratia species	4	0.5	10	0.3
Proteus species	5	0.6	27	0.8
Salmonella species	6	0.7	37	1.2
Citrobacter species	3	0.4	43	1.3
Haemophilus influenzae	1	0.1	5	0.2
Nisseria meningitidis			1	0.03
Acinetobacter species	18	2.2	153	4.8
Other gram negatives	37	4.4	167	5.2
All gram negatives	478	57.4	2111	65.8
Other	21	2.5	57	1.8

Data from Zaidi AK, Thaver D, Ali SA, et al. Pediatr Infect Dis J 2009;28:S10–8.

was eliminated more than 50 years ago.[136] Although improvements also took place in the developing world, neonatal tetanus continues to be a significant problem with some communities reporting rates as high as 22 to 82 per 1000 live births during the late 1990s.[136] Many neonatal nurseries in developing countries still have tetanus wards. According to the WHO, the number of neonatal deaths secondary to tetanus was estimated at 180,000 in the year 2002, and 48 countries have yet to meet the target of decreasing the incidence of neonatal tetanus to less than 1 per 1000 live births.[137]

BURDEN OF OMPHALITIS

The necrotic tissue of the umbilical stump is an excellent medium for bacterial growth and undergoes early colonization from the maternal genital tract and the environment.[131] Omphalitis or umbilical stump infections may remain localized to the stump or they may spread to the peritoneum and eventually cause bacteremia due to the close proximity of the umbilical vessels.[131] In developed countries, where hygienic birth practices and clean cord care in the neonatal period are standard practices, omphalitis is uncommon. Unsanitary practices, however, such as use of unsterile instruments to cut or tie the cord and application of cow dung or other materials continue to predispose newborns in developing countries to omphalitis.

Studies from developing countries in the 1990s reported incidence rates of omphalitis of 2 to 77 per 1000 live births,[138–141] with 1 center reporting an incidence of 15.6 per 1000 admissions and a case fatality rate of 15%.[142] The burden of disease is thought much higher in community settings in areas where most births occur at home. Limited incidence data from community settings show high incidence rates ranging from 55 to 197 per 1000 live births.[143,144]

Knowledge of etiologic agents of omphalitis from community settings is also scarce. *S aureus* and polymicrobial flora, including gram-negative rods, seem to be commonly encountered.

BURDEN OF EARLY-ONSET PNEUMONIA

Due to syndromic overlap, it is difficult to differentiate early-onset neonatal pneumonia from neonatal sepsis even in developed countries. The signs of pneumonia in the early neonatal period are nonspecific; neonates present with grunting, tachypnea, retractions, and hypoxemia,[145] but these are also features of sepsis. Furthermore, pneumonia may be accompanied by bacteremia. In premature infants, respiratory distress syndrome and pneumonia are also difficult to differentiate clinically.

The incidence of blood culture-confirmed neonatal pneumonia (bacteremic pneumonia) has been reported in 4 studies and ranged from 0.4 to 12.6 per 1000 live births in developing countries,[11,81] and 1.4 to 4.8 per 1000 live births in developed countries.[62,146] Studies evaluating case fatality rates have reported rates of 14% to 31%.[81,147,148] None of these reports separated early-onset from late-onset pneumonia. Therefore, reliable estimates for the burden of early-onset neonatal pneumonia cannot be derived from the published literature.

DIAGNOSIS OF EONS

The presentation of neonatal sepsis can be subtle and nonspecific, leading to underdiagnosis and overdiagnosis. Signs of neonatal sepsis may include lethargy, poor feeding, irritability, temperature instability, fever or hypothermia, apnea, tachypnea, and chest retractions. A high index of suspicion needs to be maintained to detect all cases and to begin antibiotic therapy as soon as possible. That results, however, in unnecessary evaluations and overuse of antibiotics. The blood culture remains the gold standard of diagnosis and is required to document the organism causing bacteremia. Blood cultures lack sensitivity, however, and are often reported as negative even in the presence of strong clinical evidence of sepsis.[122] The administration of intrapartum antibiotics may lead to a decreased bacterial load and thus avoid detection of EONS through blood cultures. In addition, the volume of blood that can be drawn from neonates is often insufficient to establish diagnosis through cultures.[149] In developing countries, laboratory facilities are often lacking at district and community hospitals, and blood cultures are often not feasible. In an effort to improve detection of serious illness, including EONS, in low-resource settings, a large multicenter study was recently conducted to assess the usefulness of simple clinical signs that could be used by minimally trained health care providers to identify newborns in need of referral care.[6] The study identified 7 easily identifiable clinical signs that had a high sensitivity and specificity for detecting serious illness, including sepsis in the early neonatal period (**Box 1**). Training and scale up of an algorithm using these clinical signs could lead to earlier identification and improved management of EONS in resource-limited settings.

STRATEGIES TO PREVENT EONS IN DEVELOPING COUNTRIES

Several interventions have been demonstrated to prevent neonatal sepsis and are standard of care in developed countries. Administration of intrapartum antibiotics to women with chorioamnionitis reduces the incidence of EONS and selective use of intrapartum antibiotics in women colonized with GBS reduces EONS with this pathogen. Also, in developed countries, many newborns with risk factors for EONS, including infants who are asymptomatic, undergo testing and treatment to rule out sepsis, resulting in many more evaluations than infants with true EONS. These interventions are costly and not feasible in many developing countries where most births occur at home. To prevent EONS in these settings, cost-effective interventions must be introduced at the community level, with prevention strategies applied during the antenatal, intrapartum, and early neonatal period. Several such interventions with documented benefits are listed in **Box 2** and discussed later in further detail. It is estimated that implementation of these interventions with coverage of 99% can prevent 41% to 72% of neonatal deaths globally.[150] The knowledge and implementation of these interventions, however, is lacking in the poorest countries, where they are most needed.[150]

Antenatal Care

Preventive measures for EONS start before a baby is born and are closely related to overall maternal well-being. Antenatal care is a neglected component of maternal and child health in developing countries and almost 40% of women do not receive the minimum of 4 antenatal care visits recommended by the WHO.[151] Maternal tetanus toxoid immunization is an important component of antenatal care in any developing country and its role in preventing neonatal tetanus is well established. Some estimates suggest an 88% to 100% decrease in neonatal tetanus with antenatal use of tetanus toxoid.[150] Screening and treatment of maternal STDs, especially

---

Box 1
Clinical signs with high sensitivity and specificity for severe illness, including sepsis, when used by minimally trained health workers in infants under 2 months of age at primary level health facilities

History of difficulty in feeding

History of convulsions

Movement only when stimulated

Respiratory rate $\geq$60 breaths per minute

Severe chest indrawing

Axillary temperature $\geq$37.5°C

Axillary temperature <35.5°C

Data from The Young Infants Clinical Signs Study Group. Clinical signs that predict severe illness in children under age 2 months: a multicentre study. Lancet 2008;371:135–42; with permission.

Box 2
Interventions available to prevent EONS and its associated mortality

Antenatal Care

Adequate antenatal care with at least 4 antenatal care visits to a skilled health professional

Maternal tetanus toxoid vaccination

Screening and treatment of sexually transmitted diseases (STDs) and other infections along with treatment of asymptomatic bacteriuria and urinary tract infection

Educating mothers about importance of clean birth practices

Improved nutrition

Intrapartum Care

Delivery by a skilled birth attendant

Clean birth practices

Appropriate management and referral of complications

Clean cord cutting with sterile instruments

Risk-based administration of intrapartum antibiotics

Postnatal Care

Encouragement of early and exclusive breastfeeding

Hygienic skin and cord care

Use of chlorhexidine to decrease skin colonization

Kangaroo mother care, especially for low-birth-weight babies

Training of community health worker cadres to take health care to the home

Health System Approaches

Promotion of female literacy and education

Creating health awareness about appropriate care seeking

Prioritization of limited resources to improve maternal-newborn care delivery

---

syphilis and HIV, are also known to decrease the burden of neonatal infectious disease[9,150] as are detection and treatment of asymptomatic bacteriuria.[150] STDs and maternal urinary tract infections increase the maternal risk of puerperal sepsis with the associated risk of EONS.[9] Antenatal care also serves to educate mothers regarding nutrition, birth preparedness, and danger signs during pregnancy and the early neonatal period.[9] At the same time, expectant mothers can be counseled on the importance of clean delivery and the healthful benefits of early and exclusive breastfeeding.

Improved maternal nutrition during pregnancy is an important component of antenatal care, with possible beneficial effects leading to improved birth outcomes, which may decrease the risk of neonatal sepsis. Recent reviews have synthesized the evidence for effects of micronutrient and caloric supplementation during pregnancy.[152–154] Although a direct link between nutritional supplementation during pregnancy and decreased risk of EONS remains unproved, evidence suggests that improved maternal caloric intake reduces intrauterine growth restriction and preterm births,[154] both of which are important risk factors for EONS. Additionally, meta-analyses of several trials indicate that micronutrient supplementation reduces small-for-gestational-age births,[152] and zinc supplementation lowers the rate of preterm births.[153] Other studies have found no benefit of multiple micronutrient supplementation on improving pregnancy outcomes, however.[155]

Intrapartum Care

Most pathogens causing EONS are acquired during labor and delivery, and appropriate intrapartum care has the most potential to significantly reduce the number of infants with EONS. In developing countries, where only 35% of births are attended by a skilled health worker, there is a dire need for provision of skilled birth attendants at the community level who are trained in the prevention, identification, management, and referral of neonates with sepsis. Birth attendants need to be educated about safe and aseptic delivery practices, including hand hygiene, avoiding unnecessary vaginal examinations, and aseptic cutting of the umbilical cord.[9] Birth attendants also need to be provided with clean delivery kits (containing plastic sheets, soap, gloves, sterile razor for cord cutting, and cord clamps), possibly through social marketing strategies,[156] to ensure a clean delivery for the mother and baby.

Administration of antibiotics to women with preterm prolonged rupture of membranes is another intervention that may decrease incidence of neonatal infections by up to a third.[150] Risk-based intrapartum prophylactic antibiotics have contributed significantly to the reduction of EONS in developed countries, in particular infections attributable to GBS.[157] These antibiotics have not been tested in developing country settings. Risk-based intrapartum prophylactic antibiotics would be challenging to implement in home births because of the requirement of close monitoring of duration of ruptured members, maternal temperature, and other factors. The value of using vaginal chlorhexidine during labor is unclear. Although it has not been proved useful in the developed world,[158,159] studies from developing countries suggest that it might prevent EONS and EONS-specific mortality.[160,161] Given the low cost of chlorhexidine, it may be a promising and cost-effective intervention for prevention of neonatal sepsis in developing countries.

Postnatal Care

The benefits of breast milk in preventing neonatal infections and infection-related neonatal mortality are well established.[9] Fresh human milk contains lysozyme, secretory IgA, and lactoferrin, which inhibit the growth of E coli and other gram-negative pathogens responsible for EONS.[125] Yet only about a third of neonates in developing countries are exclusively breastfed.[162] Encouragement of early and exclusive breastfeeding in developing country settings is perhaps the most important postnatal intervention to prevent EONS. Breastfeeding in the context of maternal HIV is a more complex issue beyond the scope of this article. Readers are referred to the WHO and UNAIDS Web sites for the most up-to-date recommendations.

Hygienic newborn care also needs to be encouraged to prevent infections in the early neonatal period. This includes sanitary disposal of waste, provision of clean water in homes, and hand washing by care providers.[131] Appropriate cord and skin care is also essential and recent trials have shown the benefit of cord and skin cleansing with chlorhexidine.[163] Similarly, massage of newborns with topical sunflower oil, which is traditionally practiced in some communities, has been shown to produce significant reductions in hospital-acquired neonatal infections among preterm infants in randomized controlled trials in developing countries.[164,165]

Kangaroo care by mothers is another intervention that can decrease EONS.[150] Kangaroo care involves skin-to-skin contact between mother and infant in a strict vertical position between a mother's breasts and frequent and exclusive breastfeeding.[166] Although it remains to be assessed in community settings, a recent meta-analysis of randomized controlled trials of kangaroo care has shown significant reduction in infection rates in low-birth-weight babies in hospital settings.[167] Some of the proven physiologic benefits of kangaroo care include increase in body temperature and weight of the child and reduced stress level of the infant.[168] These factors combined with the increased rate of exclusive breastfeeding might be responsible for the lower rates of infections in neonates receiving kangaroo care.

Health System Approaches

To bring about sustainable improvements in child survival, major changes are needed to reform the health care infrastructure providing maternal-newborn care in most developing countries. Although resource constraints pose major impediments, especially in sub-Saharan Africa, poverty alone is not an excuse for the high neonatal mortality rates observed. Prioritization of developmental resources to promote female literacy, and provision of high quality primary care, antenatal care, and skilled delivery can make a big difference. This model has been successfully adopted by Sri Lanka, one of the poorer Asian countries, which now has a neonatal mortality rate of only 8 per 1000 live births and an infant mortality rate of 11 per 1000 live births,[169] figures comparable with industrialized countries despite per capita gross national income of only $1780.[170]

Although the infrastructure for improved health systems providing care to women and children will take some time to develop, several short-term solutions do exist and can be scaled up immediately in many developing countries where access to health facilities is limited. The concept of family-community care has been proposed, whereby community health workers visit mothers at home to provide the simple interventions (discussed previously) and educate and promote established healthful practices, such as breastfeeding, cord and skin care, and immunization.[156] These community workers should also be trained to detect maternal and neonatal danger signs and provide basic treatment and referral. Training of traditional birth attendants to provide early neonatal care in addition to maternal care has been proposed. A successful demonstration of this approach has been shown by Bang and colleagues[46] in rural India.

TREATMENT STRATEGIES FOR EONS IN DEVELOPING COUNTRIES

In developed countries, the standard of care for management of EONS is inpatient administration of parenteral antibiotics (generally a penicillin combined with an aminoglycoside) and supportive care, often in an intensive care unit setting.[171] Ampicillin and gentamicin provide good empiric coverage for common neonatal pathogens, such as GBS and E coli.[171] Hospitalization allows for provision of supportive care, such as intravenous fluids; oxygen therapy, when needed; and a controlled thermal environment. WHO recommends this same standard of care for newborns in developing countries.[172] More advanced therapies, such as mechanical ventilation, surfactant therapy for respiratory distress of the premature neonate, inhaled nitric oxide for pulmonary hypertension, pressor therapy for shock, and extracorporeal membrane oxygenation, are life-saving interventions available in neonatal intensive care units in developed nations but are not feasible in most developing country settings.

Unfortunately, most newborns with severe illness in developing countries never reach a health care facility. Therefore, treatment strategies in developing countries need to be tailored to deliver care at the community level (home or primary care facility) with close interaction between the community health workers, mothers, and other family members and linkages with the formal health system. WHO and United Nations Children's Fund (UNICEF) have developed the Neonatal Integrated Management of Childhood Illnesses (nIMCI) program, which trains community health workers to identify severely ill infants and provide treatment and referral.[6,173,174] Essential features of the nIMCI program are listed in **Box 3**.

A recent review on the management of neonatal sepsis in primary care settings highlighted the dearth of data on community-based management options.[175] It suggested, however, the use of parenteral antibiotics integrated into home- or community-based packages as an effective option. The lack of etiologic data for EONS from community settings makes it difficult to design empiric antibiotic regimens. Among the various parenteral antibiotic options possible, there is considerable experience with the use of penicillins, cephalosporins, and aminoglycosides in health-facility settings of developed and developing countries. At the community level, the preferred parenteral antibiotic combination is procaine penicillin G given by intramuscular injection once daily and gentamicin at intervals of greater than or equal to 24

Box 3
Essential components of the WHO/UNICEF nIMCI training program for primary healthcare workers in low resource settings

Assessment of child

Examining the child and assessing for danger signs

Checking for feeding problems and low birth weight

Checking vaccination status

Classification of illness

Color-coded triage system used to classify illness according to the need for

- Urgent referral,
- Specific medical treatment and advice, or
- Simple advice and home-based care

Identification of specific therapy

- Algorithm-based identification of specific therapy based on classification of illness
- Essential treatment (eg, intramuscular antibiotic injections) given before transfer for serious urgent conditions
- First dose of oral antibiotic therapy given in clinic for children requiring therapy at home
- Vaccinations provided according to immunization status

Counseling

Counseling mother about exclusive breastfeeding and any feeding problems with child

Counseling mother about her own health

Counseling mother on techniques to keep low-weight infants warm at home

Teaching caretaker to recognize danger signs and importance of seeking timely care

Teaching caretaker to give oral drugs and general care for child

Asking caretaker to return for follow-up at appropriate time

Follow-up care

Reassess child for any new problems

hours.[176] This is an attractive combination due to its efficacy, safety, and extended interval dosing and can be administered through intramuscular route at home or in primary care facilities.[176] A community-based study in rural Sylhet, Bangladesh, studied the impact of a perinatal care package, which included the administration of intramuscular procaine penicillin and gentamicin at home for neonates with presumed infection who could not be referred to hospitals.[177] The trial showed a 34% reduction in overall neonatal mortality. Whether or not 7 to 10 days of parenteral penicillin and gentamicin can be shortened by switching to oral amoxicillin is being investigated in ongoing trials in Bangladesh and Pakistan.

For many families in the developing world living in remote communities, even injectable antibiotic therapy is not easily accessible, and alternate management strategies may save many newborn lives. Administration of oral antibiotics is the preferred alternative in such neonates and is superior to no therapy.[178] Although no studies have compared the efficacy of oral with parenteral antibiotics (and none is possible for ethical reasons), the existing evidence corroborates the recommendation to provide parenteral antibiotics whenever feasible.[178] A recent review discussed oral agents available for managing neonatal sepsis in developing countries.[178] Oral cotrimoxazole for neonatal sepsis in the community has been studied most extensively. A meta-analysis assessing the impact of oral cotrimoxazole for pneumonia in newborns reported significant benefits.[170] Total mortality was found to decrease by 27% and pneumonia-specific mortality was reduced by 42%.[179] Concerns have been raised over the rapid development of resistance; thus, utility of this oral antibiotic is likely to be limited. Oral amoxicillin has also been extensively used in neonates and has an excellent safety record. High-dose oral amoxicillin (80–90 mg/kg/day) reaches therapeutic serum levels[180,181] and may be a good option, especially because it is also the drug of choice for severe pneumonia. Amoxicillin-clavulanate is also approved for use in neonates and would provide antistaphylococcal coverage; however, the possible association of neonatal necrotizing enterocolitis with maternal use during childbirth is concerning and has resulted in limited use in the neonatal period.[178] Second-generation cephalosporins, such as oral cefuroxime, may also be considered, because their antibacterial spectrum includes common gram-positive and gram-negative organisms causing neonatal sepsis. Second-generation cephalosporins have an excellent safety profile but are more expensive. Ciprofloxacin is increasingly accepted as safe in neonates and warrants further investigation for treatment of infections in newborns where injectable therapy is not feasible.[178]

Neonatal pathogens in developing countries are increasingly antibiotic resistant and reports of multidrug-resistant pathogens in neonatal nurseries are common.[7] A recent review identified studies documenting resistance among pathogens causing EONS or community-acquired neonatal sepsis in developing countries (*Klebsiella* species, *E coli*, and *S aureus*).[182] Few reports describing antimicrobial resistance spectra in community-acquired infections were found, and there were almost no data on pathogens causing EONS in home-delivered babies. The limited data from the community on microbes causing neonatal sepsis showed resistance to gentamicin was low among *E coli* (13%) but was notably high among *Klebsiella* (60%). Significant resistance to ampicillin has been observed among *E coli* with recent data showing more than 70% resistance.[182] Resistance to third-generation cephalosporins was also high among *Klebsiella* (66%), and 1 in 5 *E coli* isolates were also resistant. All 3 pathogens showed high levels of resistance to cotrimoxazole, an oral antibiotic used as the first-line drug in childhood pneumonia control programs in most developing countries. Methicillin resistance among *S aureus* was observed rarely in community settings but is widespread in EONS in hospital-born babies.[7]

More information on antimicrobial resistance patterns of pathogens causing EONS in the community in different regions of the world is needed to devise appropriate empiric treatment regimens.

SUMMARY

Infections are a major cause of neonatal death in developing countries. High-quality information on the burden of EONS and sepsis-related deaths is limited in most of these settings. Simple preventive and treatment strategies have the potential to save many newborns from a sepsis-related death. Scaling up of these cost-effective interventions by implementation in public health programs at the national level will reduce child mortality rates of countries lagging behind the United Nations Millennium Development Goals targets of reduction in child mortality.

Simple, cost-effective diagnostic tests for neonatal sepsis, which can be applied to resource-limited settings, are also needed. Improved diagnosis of sepsis, as well as identification of etiologic agents responsible for disease, would help in the timely management of newborns with EONS. Better information on the burden of specific pathogens will also allow exploration of maternal vaccination approaches.

Although rapid initiation of antibiotic therapy and referral to a hospital facility is optimal, treatment of EONS at the community level may save many lives.

REFERENCES

1. Zupan J, Aahman E. Perinatal mortality for the year 2000: estimates developed by WHO. Geneva: World Health Organization; 2005.
2. Lawn JE, Cousens S, Zupan J. 4 Million neonatal deaths: when? Where? Why? Lancet 2005;365(9462):891–900.
3. Lawn JE, Wilczynska-Ketende K, Cousens SN. Estimating the causes of 4 million neonatal deaths in the year 2000. Int J Epidemiol 2006;35(3):706–18.
4. Klein JO. Bacterial sepsis and meningitis. In: Remington JS, Klein JO, editors. Infectious diseases of the fetus and newborn infant. Philadelphia: WB Saunders; 2006. p. 247–95.
5. Edwards MS, Baker CJ. Bacterial infections in the neonate. In: Long SS, Pickering LK, Prober CG, editors. Principles and practice of pediatric infectious disease. New York: Churchill Livingstone; 2003. p. 536–42.
6. Young Infants Clinical Signs Study Group. Clinical signs that predict severe illness in children under age 2 months: a multicentre study. Lancet 2008; 371(9607):135–42.
7. Zaidi AK, Huskins WC, Thaver D, et al. Hospital-acquired neonatal infections in developing countries. Lancet 2005;365(9465):1175–88.
8. The World Bank. DEPweb: beyond economic growth, glossary. Available at: http://www.worldbank.org/depweb/english/beyond/global/glossary.html. Accessed December 30, 2009.
9. Stoll BJ. Neonatal infections: a global perspective. In: Remington JS, Klein JO, editors. Infectious diseases of the fetus and newborn infant. Philadelphia: WB Saunders; 2006. p. 27–57.
10. Lawn JE, Osrin D, Adler A, et al. Four million neonatal deaths: counting and attribution of cause of death. Paediatr Perinat Epidemiol 2008;22(5):410–6.
11. Aurangzeb B, Hameed A. Neonatal sepsis in hospital-born babies: bacterial isolates and antibiotic susceptibility patterns. J Coll Physicians Surg Pak 2003;13(11):629–32.

12. Karthikeyan G, Premkumar K. Neonatal sepsis: staphylococcus aureus as the predominant pathogen. Indian J Pediatr 2001;68(8):715–7.
13. Kuruvilla KA, Pillai S, Jesudason M, et al. Bacterial profile of sepsis in a neonatal unit in south India. Indian Pediatr 1998;35(9):851–8.
14. Chacko B, Sohi I. Early onset neonatal sepsis. Indian J Pediatr 2005;72(1):23–6.
15. Baltimore RS, Huie SM, Meek JI, et al. Early-onset neonatal sepsis in the era of group B streptococcal prevention. Pediatrics 2001;108(5):1094–8.
16. Bizzarro MJ, Raskind C, Baltimore RS, et al. Seventy-five years of neonatal sepsis at Yale: 1928–2003. Pediatrics 2005;116(3):595–602.
17. Borderon E, Desroches A, Tescher M, et al. Value of examination of the gastric aspirate for the diagnosis of neonatal infection. Biol Neonate 1994;65(6):353–66.
18. Bromiker R, Arad I, Peleg O, et al. Neonatal bacteremia: patterns of antibiotic resistance. Infect Control Hosp Epidemiol 2001;22(12):767–70.
19. Chen KT, Tuomala RE, Cohen AP, et al. No increase in rates of early-onset neonatal sepsis by non-group B Streptococcus or ampicillin-resistant organisms. Am J Obstet Gynecol 2001;185(4):854–8.
20. Cordero L, Rau R, Taylor D, et al. Enteric gram-negative bacilli bloodstream infections: 17 years' experience in a neonatal intensive care unit. Am J Infect Control 2004;32(4):189–95.
21. Davies HD, Raj S, Adair C, et al. Population-based active surveillance for neonatal group B streptococcal infections in Alberta, Canada: implications for vaccine formulation. Pediatr Infect Dis J 2001;20(9):879–84.
22. Galanakis E, Krallis N, Levidiotou S, et al. Neonatal bacteraemia: a population-based study. Scand J Infect Dis 2002;34(8):598–601.
23. Haque KN, Khan MA, Kerry S, et al. Pattern of culture-proven neonatal sepsis in a district general hospital in the United Kingdom. Infect Control Hosp Epidemiol 2004;25(9):759–64.
24. Hervas JA, Ballesteros F, Alomar A, et al. Increase of enterobacter in neonatal sepsis: a twenty-two-year study. Pediatr Infect Dis J 2001;20(2):134–40.
25. Hyde TB, Hilger TM, Reingold A, et al. Trends in incidence and antimicrobial resistance of early-onset sepsis: population-based surveillance in San Francisco and Atlanta. Pediatrics 2002;110(4):690–5.
26. Isaacs D, Barfield C, Clothier T, et al. Late-onset infections of infants in neonatal units. J Paediatr Child Health 1996;32(2):158–61.
27. Isaacs D, Barfield CP, Grimwood K, et al. Systemic bacterial and fungal infections in infants in Australian neonatal units. Australian Study Group for Neonatal Infections. Med J Aust 1995;162(4):198–201.
28. Isaacs D, Royle JA. Intrapartum antibiotics and early onset neonatal sepsis caused by group B Streptococcus and by other organisms in Australia. Australasian Study Group for Neonatal Infections. Pediatr Infect Dis J 1999;18(6):524–8.
29. Labenne M, Michaut F, Gouyon B, et al. A population-based observational study of restrictive guidelines for antibiotic therapy in early-onset neonatal infections. Pediatr Infect Dis J 2007;26(7):593–9.
30. Laugel V, Kuhn P, Beladdale J, et al. Effects of antenatal antibiotics on the incidence and bacteriological profile of early-onset neonatal sepsis. A retrospective study over five years. Biol Neonate 2003;84(1):24–30.
31. Mercer BM, Carr TL, Beazley DD, et al. Antibiotic use in pregnancy and drug-resistant infant sepsis. Am J Obstet Gynecol 1999;181(4):816–21.
32. Moreno MT, Vargas S, Poveda R, et al. Neonatal sepsis and meningitis in a developing Latin American country. Pediatr Infect Dis J 1994;13(6):516–20.

33. Schuchat A, Zywicki SS, Dinsmoor MJ, et al. Risk factors and opportunities for prevention of early-onset neonatal sepsis: a multicenter case-control study. Pediatrics 2000;105(1 Pt 1):21–6.
34. Stoll BJ, Gordon T, Korones SB, et al. Early-onset sepsis in very low birth weight neonates: a report from the National Institute of Child Health and Human Development Neonatal Research Network. J Pediatr 1996;129(1):72–80.
35. Stoll BJ, Hansen N, Fanaroff AA, et al. Changes in pathogens causing early-onset sepsis in very-low-birth-weight infants. N Engl J Med 2002;347(4):240–7.
36. Stoll BJ, Hansen NI, Higgins RD, et al. Very low birth weight preterm infants with early onset neonatal sepsis: the predominance of gram-negative infections continues in the National Institute of Child Health and Human Development Neonatal Research Network, 2002–2003. Pediatr Infect Dis J 2005; 24(7):635–9.
37. Neonatal morbidity and mortality: report of the National Neonatal-Perinatal Database. Indian Pediatr 1997;34(11):1039–42.
38. Aavitsland P, Hoiby EA, Lystad A. Systemic group B streptococcal disease in neonates and young infants in Norway 1985–94. Acta Paediatr 1996;85(1):104–5.
39. Adejuyigbe EA, Adeodu OO, ko-Nai KA, et al. Septicaemia in high risk neonates at a teaching hospital in Ile-Ife, Nigeria. East Afr Med J 2001;78(10):540–3.
40. Ali Z. Neonatal bacterial septicaemia at the Mount Hope Women's Hospital, Trinidad. Ann Trop Paediatr 2004;24(1):41–4.
41. Al-Zwaini EJ. Neonatal septicaemia in the neonatal care unit, Al-Anbar governorate, Iraq. East Mediterr Health J 2002;8(4–5):509–14.
42. Anyebuno M, Newman M. Common causes of neonatal bacteraemia in Accra, Ghana. East Afr Med J 1995;72(12):805–8.
43. Ascher DP, Becker JA, Yoder BA, et al. Failure of intrapartum antibiotics to prevent culture-proved neonatal group B streptococcal sepsiss. J Perinatol 1993;13(3):212–6.
44. Bang AT, Bang RA, Baitule S, et al. Burden of morbidities and the unmet need for health care in rural neonates–a prospective observational study in Gadchiroli, India. Indian Pediatr 2001;38(9):952–65.
45. Bang AT, Bang RA, Baitule SB, et al. Effect of home-based neonatal care and management of sepsis on neonatal mortality: field trial in rural India. Lancet 1999;354(9194):1955–61.
46. Bang AT, Bang RA, Stoll BJ, et al. Is home-based diagnosis and treatment of neonatal sepsis feasible and effective? Seven years of intervention in the Gadchiroli field trial (1996 to 2003). J Perinatol 2005;25(Suppl 1):S62–71.
47. Bell Y, Barton M, Thame M, et al. Neonatal sepsis in Jamaican neonates. Ann Trop Paediatr 2005;25(4):293–6.
48. Berardi A, Lugli L, Baronciani D, et al. Group B streptococcal infections in a northern region of Italy. Pediatrics 2007;120(3):e487–93.
49. Berkley JA, Lowe BS, Mwangi I, et al. Bacteremia among children admitted to a rural hospital in Kenya. N Engl J Med 2005;352(1):39–47.
50. Boo NY, Chor CY. Six year trend of neonatal septicaemia in a large Malaysian maternity hospital. J Paediatr Child Health 1994;30(1):23–7.
51. Bromberger P, Lawrence JM, Braun D, et al. The influence of intrapartum antibiotics on the clinical spectrum of early-onset group B streptococcal infection in term infants. Pediatrics 2000;106(2 Pt 1):244–50.
52. Carbonell-Estrany X, Lawrence JM, Braun D, et al. Probable early-onset group B streptococcal neonatal sepsis: a serious clinical condition related to intrauterine infection. Arch Dis Child Fetal Neonatal Ed 2008;93(2):F85–9.

53. Chen KT, Puopolo KM, Eichenwald EC, et al. No increase in rates of early-onset neonatal sepsis by antibiotic-resistant group B Streptococcus in the era of intrapartum antibiotic prophylaxis. Am J Obstet Gynecol 2005;192(4):1167–71.

54. Dahl MS, Tessin I, Trollfors B. Invasive group B streptococcal infections in Sweden: incidence, predisposing factors and prognosis. Int J Infect Dis 2003; 7(2):113–9.

55. Daley AJ, Isaacs D. Ten-year study on the effect of intrapartum antibiotic prophylaxis on early onset group B streptococcal and escherichia coli neonatal sepsis in Australasia. Pediatr Infect Dis J 2004;23(7):630–4.

56. Daoud AS, al-Sheyyab M, bu-Ekteish F, et al. Neonatal meningitis in northern Jordan. J Trop Pediatr 1996;42(5):267–70.

57. Das PK, Basu K, Chakraborty P, et al. Clinical and bacteriological profile of neonatal infections in metropolitan city based medical college nursery. J Indian Med Assoc 1999;97(1):3–5.

58. Das PK, Basu K, Chakraborty S, et al. Early neonatal morbidity and mortality in a city based medical college nursery. Indian J Public Health 1998;42(1):9–14.

59. Dobson SR, Isaacs D, Wilkinson AR, et al. Reduced use of surface cultures for suspected neonatal sepsis and surveillance. Arch Dis Child 1992;67(Spec No 1): 44–7.

60. Edwards RK, Jamie WE, Sterner D, et al. Intrapartum antibiotic prophylaxis and early-onset neonatal sepsis patterns. Infect Dis Obstet Gynecol 2003;11(4): 221–6.

61. English M, Mohammed S, Ross A, et al. A randomised, controlled trial of once daily and multi-dose daily gentamicin in young Kenyan infants. Arch Dis Child 2004;89(7):665–9.

62. Escobar GJ, Li DK, Armstrong MA, et al. Neonatal sepsis workups in infants >/= 2000 grams at birth: a population-based study. Pediatrics 2000;106(2 Pt 1): 256–63.

63. Etuk SJ, Etuk IS, Ekott MI, et al. Perinatal outcome in pregnancies booked for antenatal care but delivered outside health facilities in Calabar, Nigeria. Acta Trop 2000;75(1):29–33.

64. Fluegge K, Siedler A, Heinrich B, et al. Incidence and clinical presentation of invasive neonatal group B streptococcal infections in Germany. Pediatrics 2006;117(6):e1139–45.

65. Garcia-Prats JA, Cooper TR, Schneider VF, et al. Rapid detection of microorganisms in blood cultures of newborn infants utilizing an automated blood culture system. Pediatrics 2000;105(3 Pt 1):523–7.

66. Gebremariam A. Neonatal meningitis in Addis Ababa: a 10-year review. Ann Trop Paediatr 1998;18(4):279–83.

67. Ghiorghis B. Neonatal sepsis in Addis Ababa, Ethiopia: a review of 151 bacteremic neonates. Ethiop Med J 1997;35(3):169–76.

68. Gransden WR, Eykyn SJ, Phillips I. Septicaemia in the newborn and elderly. J Antimicrob Chemother 1994;34(Suppl A):101–19.

69. Greenberg D, Shinwell ES, Yagupsky P, et al. A prospective study of neonatal sepsis and meningitis in southern Israel. Pediatr Infect Dis J 1997;16(8): 768–73.

70. Grimwood K, Darlow BA, Gosling IA, et al. Early-onset neonatal group B streptococcal infections in New Zealand 1998–1999. J Paediatr Child Health 2002; 38(3):272–7.

71. Gupta P, Murali MV, Faridi MM, et al. Clinical profile of klebsiella septicemia in neonates. Indian J Pediatr 1993;60(4):565–72.

72. Hakansson S, Kallen K. Impact and risk factors for early-onset group B strepto-coccal morbidity: analysis of a national, population-based cohort in Sweden 1997–2001. BJOG 2006;113(12):1452–8.

73. Herbst A, Kallen K. Time between membrane rupture and delivery and septi-cemia in term neonates. Obstet Gynecol 2007;110(3):612–8.

74. Hervas JA, Alomar A, Salva F, et al. Neonatal sepsis and meningitis in Mallorca, Spain, 1977–1991. Clin Infect Dis 1993;16(5):719–24.

75. Holt DE, Halket S, de LJ, et al. Neonatal meningitis in England and Wales: 10 years on. Arch Dis Child Fetal Neonatal Ed 2001;84(2):F85–9.

76. Isaacs D, Fraser S, Hogg G, et al. Staphylococcus aureus infections in Austral-asian neonatal nurseries. Arch Dis Child Fetal Neonatal Ed 2004;89(4):F331–5.

77. Jenkins J, Alderdice F, McCall E. Making information available for quality improvement and service planning in neonatal care. Ir Med J 2003;96(6):171–4.

78. Johnson CE, Whitwell JK, Pethe K, et al. Term newborns who are at risk for sepsis: are lumbar punctures necessary? Pediatrics 1997;99(4):E10.

79. Kallman J, Kihlstrom E, Sjoberg L, et al. Increase of staphylococci in neonatal septicaemia: a fourteen-year study. Acta Paediatr 1997;86(5):533–8.

80. Karunasekera KA, Jayawardena DR, Chandra NP. The use of commercially prepared 10% dextrose reduces the incidence of neonatal septicaemia. Ceylon Med J 1997;42(4):207–8.

81. Kaushik SL, Parmar VR, Grover N, et al. Neonatal sepsis in hospital born babies. J Commun Dis 1998;30(3):147–52.

82. Levine EM, Strom CM, Ghai V, et al. Intrapartum management relating to the risk of perinatal transmission of group B streptococcus. Infect Dis Obstet Gynecol 1998;6(1):25–9.

83. Lim NL, Wong YH, Boo NY, et al. Bacteraemic infections in a neonatal intensive care unit—a nine-month survey. Med J Malaysia 1995;50(1):59–63.

84. Lopez Sastre JB, Coto Cotallo GD, Fernandez CB. Neonatal sepsis of vertical transmission: an epidemiological study from the "Grupo de Hospitales Castrillo". J Perinat Med 2000;28(4):309–15.

85. Lopez Sastre JB, Fernandez CB, Coto Cotallo GD, et al. Trends in the epidemi-ology of neonatal sepsis of vertical transmission in the era of group B strepto-coccal prevention. Acta Paediatr 2005;94(4):451–7.

86. Mansour E, Eissa AN, Nofal LM, et al. Morbidity and mortality of low-birth-weight infants in Egypt. East Mediterr Health J 2005;11(4):723–31.

87. Martius JA, Roos T, Gora B, et al. Risk factors associated with early-onset sepsis in premature infants. Eur J Obstet Gynecol Reprod Biol 1999;85(2):151–8.

88. Maxwell FC, Bourchier D. Neonatal septicaemia: a changing picture? N Z Med J 1991;104(922):446–7.

89. May M, Daley AJ, Donath S, et al. Early onset neonatal meningitis in Australia and New Zealand, 1992–2002. Arch Dis Child Fetal Neonatal Ed 2005;90(4): F324–7.

90. Mayor-Lynn K, Gonzalez-Quintero VH, O'Sullivan MJ, et al. Comparison of early-onset neonatal sepsis caused by Escherichia coli and group B streptococcus. Am J Obstet Gynecol 2005;192(5):1437–9.

91. McDonald M, Moloney A, Clarke TA, et al. Blood cultures and antibiotic use in a neonatal intensive care unit. Ir J Med Sci 1992;161(1):3–4.

92. McIntire DD, Bloom SL, Casey BM, et al. Birth weight in relation to morbidity and mortality among newborn infants. N Engl J Med 1999;340(16):1234–8.

93. McIntire DD, Leveno KJ. Neonatal mortality and morbidity rates in late preterm births compared with births at term. Obstet Gynecol 2008;111(1):35–41.

94. Modi N, Kirubakaran C. Reasons for admission, causes of death and costs of admission to a tertiary referral neonatal unit in India. J Trop Pediatr 1995; 41(2):99–102.
95. Mokuolu AO, Jiya N, Adesiyun OO. Neonatal septicaemia in Ilorin: bacterial pathogens and antibiotic sensitivity pattern. Afr J Med Med Sci 2002;31(2):127–30.
96. Morken NH, Kallen K, Jacobsson B. Outcomes of preterm children according to type of delivery onset: a nationwide population-based study. Paediatr Perinat Epidemiol 2007;21(5):458–64.
97. Moses LM, Heath PT, Wilkinson AR, et al. Early onset group B streptococcal neonatal infection in Oxford 1985–96. Arch Dis Child Fetal Neonatal Ed 1998; 79(2):F148–9.
98. Neto MT. Group B streptococcal disease in Portuguese infants younger than 90 days. Arch Dis Child Fetal Neonatal Ed 2008;93(2):F90–3.
99. Oddie S, Embleton ND. Risk factors for early onset neonatal group B streptococcal sepsis: case-control study. BMJ 2002;325(7359):308.
100. Park CH, Seo JH, Lim JY, et al. Changing trend of neonatal infection: experience at a newly established regional medical center in Korea. Pediatr Int 2007;49(1): 24–30.
101. Patel DM, Rhodes PG, LeBlanc MH, et al. Role of postnatal penicillin prophylaxis in prevention of neonatal group B streptococcus infection. Acta Paediatr 1999; 88(8):874–9.
102. Persson E, Trollfors B, Brandberg LL, et al. Septicaemia and meningitis in neonates and during early infancy in the Goteborg area of Sweden. Acta Paediatr 2002;91(10):1087–92.
103. Piper JM, Georgiou S, Xenakis EM, et al. Group B streptococcus infection rate unchanged by gestational diabetes. Obstet Gynecol 1999;93(2):292–6.
104. Robillard PY, Nabeth P, Hulsey TC, et al. Neonatal bacterial septicemia in a tropical area. Four-year experience in Guadeloupe (French West Indies). Acta Paediatr 1993;82(8):687–9.
105. Robillard PY, Perez JM, Hulsey TC, et al. Evaluation of neonatal sepsis screening in a tropical area. Part I: major risk factors for bacterial carriage at birth in Guadeloupe. West Indian Med J 2000;49(4):312–5.
106. Ronnestad A, Abrahamsen TG, Medbo S, et al. Late-onset septicemia in a Norwegian national cohort of extremely premature infants receiving very early full human milk feeding. Pediatrics 2005;115(3):e269–76.
107. Salem SY, Sheiner E, Zmora E, et al. Risk factors for early neonatal sepsis. Arch Gynecol Obstet 2006;274(4):198–202.
108. Sanghvi KP, Tudehope DI. Neonatal bacterial sepsis in a neonatal intensive care unit: a 5 year analysis. J Paediatr Child Health 1996;32(4):333–8.
109. Tallur SS, Kasturi AV, Nadgir SD, et al. Clinico-bacteriological study of neonatal septicemia in Hubli. Indian J Pediatr 2000;67(3):169–74.
110. Tan KW, Tay L, Lin R, et al. Group B Streptococcal septicaemia/meningitis in neonates in a Singapore teaching hospital. Aust N Z J Obstet Gynaecol 1998; 38(4):418–23.
111. Trijbels-Smeulders M, de Jonge GA, Pasker-de Jong PC, et al. Epidemiology of neonatal group B streptococcal disease in the Netherlands before and after introduction of guidelines for prevention. Arch Dis Child Fetal Neonatal Ed 2007;92(4):F271–6.
112. Trotman H, Bell Y. Neonatal group B streptococcal infection at the University Hospital of the West Indies, Jamaica: a 10-year experience. Ann Trop Paediatr 2006;26(1):53–7.

113. Velaphi S, Siegel JD, Wendel GD Jr, et al. Early-onset group B streptococcal infection after a combined maternal and neonatal group B streptococcal chemo-prophylaxis strategy. Pediatrics 2003;111(3):541–7.

114. Vergani P, Patane L, Colombo C, et al. Impact of different prevention strategies on neonatal group B streptococcal disease. Am J Perinatol 2002;19(6):341–8.

115. Watson RS, Carcillo JA, Linde-Zwirble WT, et al. The epidemiology of severe sepsis in children in the United States. Am J Respir Crit Care Med 2003; 167(5):695–701.

116. Wolf H, Schaap AH, Smit BJ, et al. Liberal diagnosis and treatment of intra-uterine infection reduces early-onset neonatal group B streptococcal infection but not sepsis by other pathogens. Infect Dis Obstet Gynecol 2000;8(3–4): 143–50.

117. Yancey MK, Duff P, Kubilis P, et al. Risk factors for neonatal sepsis. Obstet Gynecol 1996;87(2):188–94.

118. Zaleznik DF, Rench MA, Hillier S, et al. Invasive disease due to group B strep-tococcus in pregnant women and neonates from diverse population groups. Clin Infect Dis 2000;30(2):276–81.

119. Darmstadt GL, Saha SK, Choi Y, et al. Population-based incidence and etiology of community-acquired neonatal bacteremia in Mirzapur, Bangladesh: an obser-vational study. J Infect Dis 2009;200(6):906–15.

120. Seale AC, Mwaniki M, Newton CR, et al. Maternal and early onset neonatal bac-terial sepsis: burden and strategies for prevention in sub-Saharan Africa. Lancet Infect Dis 2009;9(7):428–38.

121. Gray KJ, Bennett SL, French N, et al. Invasive group B streptococcal infection in infants, Malawi. Emerg Infect Dis 2007;13(2):223–9.

122. Thaver D, Zaidi AK. Burden of neonatal infections in developing countries: a review of evidence from community-based studies. Pediatr Infect Dis J 2009;28(Suppl 1):S3–9.

123. Marodi L. Innate cellular immune responses in newborns. Clin Immunol 2006; 118(2–3):137–44.

124. Kenzel S, Henneke P. The innate immune system and its relevance to neonatal sepsis. Curr Opin Infect Dis 2006;19(3):264–70.

125. Levy O. Innate immunity of the newborn: basic mechanisms and clinical corre-lates. Nat Rev Immunol 2007;7(5):379–90.

126. Bauer K, Zemlin M, Hummel M, et al. Diversification of Ig heavy chain genes in human preterm neonates prematurely exposed to environmental antigens. J Immunol 2002;169(3):1349–56.

127. Darmstadt G, Saha S, Ahmed A, et al. The skin as a potential portal of entry for invasive infections in neonates. Perinatology 2003;5:205–12.

128. Darmstadt GL, Dinulos JG. Neonatal skin care. Pediatr Clin North Am 2000; 47(4):757–82.

129. World Health Organization, Department of Reproductive Health and Research. Factsheet proportion of births attended by a skilled health worker. Geneva: World Health Organization; 2008.

130. Thaver D, Zaidi AK. Neonatal infections in South Asia. In: Bhutta Z, editor. Peri-natal and newborn care in South Asia: priorities for action. Oxford (UK): Oxford University Press; 2007. p. 241–67.

131. Stoll BJ. The global impact of neonatal infection. Clin Perinatol 1997;24(1):1–21.

132. Schrag S, Gorwitz R, Fultz-Butts K, et al. Prevention of perinatal group B strep-tococcal disease. Revised guidelines from CDC. MMWR Recomm Rep 2002; 51(RR-11):1–22.

133. Brodie SB, Sands KE, Gray JE, et al. Occurrence of nosocomial bloodstream infections in six neonatal intensive care units. Pediatr Infect Dis J 2000;19(1): 56–65.
134. Zaidi AK, Thaver D, Ali SA, et al. Pathogens associated with sepsis in newborns and young infants in developing countries. Pediatr Infect Dis J 2009;28(Suppl 1):S10–8.
135. Stoll BJ, Schuchat A. Maternal carriage of group B streptococci in developing countries. Pediatr Infect Dis J 1998;17(6):499–503.
136. Roper MH, Vandelaer JH, Gasse FL. Maternal and neonatal tetanus. Lancet 2007;370(9603):1947–59.
137. Tetanus vaccine. Wkly Epidemiol Rec 2006;81(20):198–208.
138. Airede AI. Pathogens in neonatalomphalitis. J Trop Pediatr 1992;38(3):129–31.
139. Garner P, Lai D, Baea M, et al. Avoiding neonatal death: an intervention study of umbilical cord care. J Trop Pediatr 1994;40(1):24–8.
140. Guvenc H, Guvenc M, Yenioglu H, et al. Neonatal omphalitis is still common in eastern Turkey. Scand J Infect Dis 1991;23(5):613–6.
141. Sawardekar KP. Changing spectrum of neonatal omphalitis. Pediatr Infect Dis J 2004;23(1):22–6.
142. Faridi MM, Rattan A, Ahmad SH. Omphalitis neonatorum. J Indian Med Assoc 1993;91(11):283–5.
143. Bang AT, Reddy HM, Baitule SB, et al. The incidence of morbidities in a cohort of neonates in rural Gadchiroli, India: seasonal and temporal variation and a hypothesis about prevention. J Perinatol 2005;25(Suppl 1):S18–28.
144. Mullany LC, Darmstadt GL, Katz J, et al. Risk factors for umbilical cord infection among newborns of southern Nepal. Am J Epidemiol 2007;165(2): 203–11.
145. Wardlaw T, Johansson E, Hodge M. Pneumonia: the forgotten killer of children. New York: United Nations Children's Fund/UNICEF/WHO. 2006.
146. Sinha A, Yokoe D, Platt R. Epidemiology of neonatal infections: experience during and after hospitalization. Pediatr Infect Dis J 2003;22(3):244–51.
147. Bang AT, Bang RA, Morankar VP, et al. Pneumonia in neonates: can it be managed in the community? Arch Dis Child 1993;68(Spec No 5):550–6.
148. Parkash J, Das N. Pattern of admissions to neonatal unit. J Coll Physicians Surg Pak 2005;15(6):341–4.
149. Neal PR, Kleiman MB, Reynolds JK, et al. Volume of blood submitted for culture from neonates. J Clin Microbiol 1986;24(3):353–6.
150. Darmstadt GL, Bhutta ZA, Cousens S, et al. Evidence-based, cost-effective interventions: how many newborn babies can we save? Lancet 2005; 365(9463):977–88.
151. AbouZahr C, Wardlaw T. Antenatal care in developing countries: promises, achievements and missed opportunities-an analysis of trends, levels and differentials, 1990–2001. Geneva: World Health Organization; 2003.
152. Haider BA, Bhutta ZA. Multiple-micronutrient supplementation for women during pregnancy. Cochrane Database Syst Rev 2006;4:CD004905.
153. Mahomed K, Bhutta Z, Middleton P. Zinc supplementation for improving pregnancy and infant outcome. Cochrane Database Syst Rev 2007;2:CD000230.
154. Rasmussen KM, Habicht JP. Maternal supplementation differentially affects the mother and newborn. J Nutr 2010;140(2):402–6.
155. Christian P, Darmstadt GL, Wu L, et al. The effect of maternal micronutrient supplementation on early neonatal morbidity in rural Nepal: a randomised, controlled, community trial. Arch Dis Child 2008;93(8):660–4.

156. Knippenberg R, Lawn JE, Darmstadt GL, et al. Systematic scaling up of neonatal care in countries. Lancet 2005;365(9464):1087–98.
157. Ohlsson A, Shah VS. Intrapartum antibiotics for known maternal Group B streptococcal colonization. Cochrane Database Syst Rev 2009;3:CD007467.
158. Lumbiganon P, Thinkhamrop J, Thinkhamrop B, et al. Vaginal chlorhexidine during labour for preventing maternal and neonatal infections (excluding Group B streptococcal and HIV). Cochrane Database Syst Rev 2004;4:CD004070.
159. Stade B, Shah V, Ohlsson A. Vaginal chlorhexidine during labour to prevent early-onset neonatal group B streptococcal infection. Cochrane Database Syst Rev 2004;3:CD003520.
160. McClure EM, Goldenberg RL, Brandes N, et al. The use of chlorhexidine to reduce maternal and neonatal mortality and morbidity in low-resource settings. Int J Gynaecol Obstet 2007;97(2):89–94.
161. Taha TE, Biggar RJ, Broadhead RL, et al. Effect of cleansing the birth canal with antiseptic solution on maternal and newborn morbidity and mortality in Malawi: clinical trial. BMJ 1997;315(7102):216–9 [discussion: 220].
162. UNICEF. Nutrition indicators—exclusive breastfeeding. Available at: http://www.unicef.org/progressforchildren/2006n4/index_breastfeeding.html. 2006. Accessed September 26, 2009.
163. Mullany LC, Darmstadt GL, Khatry SK, et al. Topical applications of chlorhexidine to the umbilical cord for prevention of omphalitis and neonatal mortality in southern Nepal: a community-based, cluster-randomised trial. Lancet 2006; 367(9514):910–8.
164. Darmstadt GL, Badrawi N, Law PA, et al. Topically applied sunflower seed oil prevents invasive bacterial infections in preterm infants in Egypt: a randomized, controlled clinical trial. Pediatr Infect Dis J 2004;23(8):719–25.
165. Darmstadt GL, Mao-Qiang M, Chi E, et al. Impact of topical oils on the skin barrier: possible implications for neonatal health in developing countries. Acta Paediatr 2002;91(5):546–54.
166. Charpak N, Ruiz JG, Zupan J, et al. Kangaroo mother care: 25 years after. Acta Paediatr 2005;94(5):514–22.
167. Conde-Agudelo A, Diaz-Rossello JL, Belizan JM. Kangaroo mother care to reduce morbidity and mortality in low birthweight infants. Cochrane Database Syst Rev 2003;2:CD002771.
168. Maulik PK, Darmstadt GL. Community-based interventions to optimize early childhood development in low resource settings. J Perinatol 2009;29(8):531–42.
169. WHO Statistical Information System - WHOSIS. Available at: http://www.who.int/statistics. Accessed September 26, 2009.
170. World Bank - Key development data and statistics. Available at: http://web.worldbank.org/WBSITE/EXTERNAL/DATASTATISTICS/0,,contentMDK:20535285~menuPK:1390200~pagePK:64133150~piPK:64133175~theSitePK:239419,00.html. Accessed September 26, 2009.
171. Saez-Llorens X, McCracken GH. Clinical pharmacology of antimicrobial agents. In: Remington JS, Klein JO, editors. Infectious diseases of the fetus and newborn infant. Philadelphia: WB Saunders; 2006. p. 1223–67.
172. World Health Organization. Management of the child with a serious infection or severe malnutrition: Guidelines for care at the first-referral level in developing countries. Geneva: World Health Organization; 2000.
173. WHO. Integrated Management of Childhood Illness (IMCI). Available at: http://www.who.int/child_adolescent_health/topics/prevention_care/child/imci/en/index.html. Accessed September 26, 2009.

174. WHO. Integrated management of childhood illnesses chart booklet 2008. Available at: http://whqlibdoc.who.int/publications/2008/9789241597289_eng.pdf. Accessed December 30, 2009.
175. Bhutta ZA, Zaidi AK, Thaver D, et al. Management of newborn infections in primary care settings: a review of the evidence and implications for policy? Pediatr Infect Dis J 2009;28(Suppl 1):S22–30.
176. Darmstadt GL, Batra M, Zaidi AK. Parenteral antibiotics for the treatment of serious neonatal bacterial infections in developing country settings. Pediatr Infect Dis J 2009;28(Suppl 1):S37–42.
177. Baqui AH, El-Arifeen S, Darmstadt GL, et al. Effect of community-based newborn-care intervention package implemented through two service-delivery strategies in Sylhet district, Bangladesh: a cluster-randomised controlled trial. Lancet 2008;371(9628):1936–44.
178. Darmstadt GL, Batra M, Zaidi AK. Oral antibiotics in the management of serious neonatal bacterial infections in developing country communities. Pediatr Infect Dis J 2009;28(Suppl 1):S31–6.
179. Sazawal S, Black RE. Effect of pneumonia case management on mortality in neonates, infants, and preschool children: a meta-analysis of community-based trials. Lancet Infect Dis 2003;3(9):547–56.
180. Cohen MD, Raeburn JA, Devine J, et al. Pharmacology of some oral penicillins in the newborn infant. Arch Dis Child 1975;50(3):230–4.
181. Gras-Le Guen C, Boscher C, Godon N, et al. Therapeutic amoxicillin levels achieved with oral administration in term neonates. Eur J Clin Pharmacol 2007;63(7):657–62.
182. Thaver D, Ali SA, Zaidi AK. Antimicrobial resistance among neonatal pathogens in developing countries. Pediatr Infect Dis J 2009;28(Suppl 1):S19–21.

Index

Note: Page numbers of article titles are in **boldface** type.

A

Abscess, in chorioamnionitis, 346
Acetaminophen, for chorioamnionitis, 348
Acute phase reactants, 318, 427–431, 452
Adaptive immunity, versus innate immunity, 308
Adhesion molecules, in sepsis, 448–449
Advanced glycation end product receptors, in chorioamnionitis, 366–368
Airway
    antimicrobial proteins and peptides in, 320–321
    management of, in septic shock, 456–457
Amniotic fluid testing, for chorioamnionitis, 344–345
Amyloid, immune function of, 318
Antibiotics
    for chorioamnionitis, 347–349
    for group B streptococcal infection prevention, 378–385
    for sepsis, 483, 492, 511–513
    for *Ureaplasma* infections, 401–402
    resistance to, in intrapartum antibiotic prophylaxis, 383
Antigen-presenting cells, 313–314
Antimicrobial proteins and peptides, 319–321
Azithromycin
    for chorioamnionitis, 348
    for *Ureaplasma* infections, 401–402

B

Bacteremia, molecular diagnosis of, **411–419**
Bacterial vaginosis, chorioamnionitis in, 345–346
Bactericidal permeability increasing protein (BPI), immune function of, 319, 322
Bacteriuria, in chorioamnionitis, 340
Bifidobacteria, for sepsis, 483, 490–491
Biomarkers, for sepsis, 321–322, 360–368
Blood counts, 425–427
Blood culture, **411–419,** 422–423
BPI protein, immune function of, 319, 322
Brain injury, in *Ureaplasma* infections, 399–400
Breast milk, for sepsis, 484, 492–493
Breathing, management of, in septic shock, 456–457
Bronchopulmonary dysplasia, in *Ureaplasma* infections, 396–398, 402

Clin Perinatol 37 (2010) 525–534
doi:10.1016/S0095-5108(10)00060-6
0095-5108/10/$ – see front matter © 2010 Elsevier Inc. All rights reserved.

perinatology.theclinics.com

Moving?

Make sure your subscription moves with you!

To notify us of your new address, find your **Clinics Account Number** (located on your mailing label above your name), and contact customer service at:

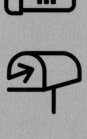

Email: journalscustomerservice-usa@elsevier.com

800-654-2452 (subscribers in the U.S. & Canada)
314-447-8871 (subscribers outside of the U.S. & Canada)

Fax number: 314-447-8029

Elsevier Health Sciences Division
Subscription Customer Service
3251 Riverport Lane
Maryland Heights, MO 63043

*To ensure uninterrupted delivery of your subscription, please notify us at least 4 weeks in advance of move.